DERMATOLOGICAL SIGNS of INTERNAL DISEASE

Jeffrey P. Callen, M.D.
Department of Dermatology
University of Louisville
Louisville, Kentucky

Joseph Jorizzo, M.D.
Department of Dermatology
Bowman Gray School of Medicine
of Wake Forest University
Winston-Salem, North Carolina

Kenneth E. Greer, M.D.
University of Virginia Hospital
Department of Dermatology
Charlottesville, Virginia

Neal Penneys, M.D.
University of Miami School of Medicine
Department of Dermatology
Miami, Florida

Warren Piette, M.D.
University of Iowa Hospital
Department of Dermatology
Iowa City, Iowa

John J. Zone, M.D.
Division of Dermatology
Salt Lake City, Utah

1988
W. B. SAUNDERS COMPANY
Harcourt Brace Jovanovich, Inc.

Philadelphia ○ London ○ Toronto
Montreal ○ Sydney ○ Tokyo

W. B. SAUNDERS COMPANY
Harcourt Brace Jovanovich, Inc.

The Curtis Center
Independence Square West
Philadelphia, PA 19106

Library of Congress Cataloging-in-Publication Data

Dermatological signs of internal disease/Jeffrey P.
Callen . . . [et al].
    p.   cm.

    Includes index.
    ISBN 0-7216-1860-X

    1. Cutaneous manifestations of general diseases.
I. Callen, Jeffrey P., 1947–
[DNLM: 1. Skin Manifestations.   WR 143 D435]

RL100.D47 1988   616.07′5—dc19
DNLM/DLC   88-11495
for Library of Congress   CIP

Editor: William Lamsback
Developmental Editor: Kathleen McCullough
Designer: Karen Giacomucci
Production Manager: Bill Preston
Manuscript Editor: Tom Stringer
Illustration Coordinator: Peg Shaw
Indexer: Linda Caravelli

Dermatological Signs of Internal Disease   ISBN 0–7216–1860–X

Last digit is the print number: 9   8   7   6   5   4   3   2   1

Preface

Dermatological Signs of Internal Disease is a teaching text, which explores the relationship of the skin and systemic diseases. As dermatologists with a common interest in the interface between internal medicine and dermatology, we have attempted to present a practical, succinct, and affordable textbook. This text is not intended to be all inclusive in either its approach to skin disease or its approach to internal medicine. It is intended to be a guide for rapid study of those cutaneous changes most commonly associated with systemic manifestations, principally for the primary care physician (family practitioner, internist, or pediatrician), or the physician in training, or the dermatologist. We have divided the text in a traditional system-oriented approach. You will notice that on several occasions subjects are covered in more than one section. This is intentional, since such coverage is necessary for the message of each section. This text differs from previous texts written on this topic in our brevity, our emphasis on practical teaching points, and our selection of suggested readings, as opposed to extensive reference lists. We have emphasized aspects of clinical and therapeutic information that are applicable to the clinical practice setting over an extensive discussion of pathogenesis. The text is extensively illustrated and includes color plates that are not overutilized so that the price of the text is kept to a minimum. Thus, we have filled a gap in the literature. It is our sincere hope that you will be able to use the information presented to improve your ability to recognize the important cutaneous signs of systemic disease and the important systemic manifestations seen in patients with cutaneous disease, and that this will ultimately lead to better care for your patients.

JEFFREY P. CALLEN, M.D.
JOSEPH L. JORIZZO, M.D.
EDITORS

Acknowledgements

Dr. Callen wishes to acknowledge Ms. Sandra Lingle, who typed many drafts and has assisted with many administrative complexities involved in the production of this text. He wishes to acknowledge the following physicians: L. G. Owen, M.D.; M. W. McCall, M.D.; E. M. Ahrens, M.D.; S. J. Hodge, M.D.; and J. F. Fowler, M.D., for allowing him the time to write by caring for his patients during his absence. Dr. Callen would like to dedicate the book to Susan, Amy, and David.

Dr. Jorizzo wishes to acknowledge Ms. Lynn Boyles, for preparing his manuscripts, and Barry Leshin, M.D., and Michael Zanolli, M.D., for their friendship and support. Dr. Jorizzo would like to dedicate the book to Susan and John. He would also like to acknowledge the support of his mother, late father, and Johanna and Paul.

Contents

Color plates

(A) Annular subacute cutaneous lupus erythematosus. This erythematous, annular lesion lacks scarring or atrophy, yet represents a histologically specific pattern of lupus erythematosus.

(B) Subacute cutaneous lupus erythematosus, papulosquamous variant. This patient developed an exquisitely photosensitive eruption with minimal sun exposure.

(C) Erythematous papular lesion of polymorphous light eruption representing a clinical picture similar to that seen in subacute cutaneous lupus erythematosus.

(D) Dermatomyositis. This female has a history of uterine carcinoma and has developed inflammatory myopathy in conjunction with very typical heliotrope eruption around the eyelids and typical lesions elsewhere on her body.

(E) Photosensitivity dermatitis found in dermatomyositis. Note the sparing of the interdigital webs and the prominences in the lesions occurring over the joints.

(F) Poikilodermatous eruption in the photosensitive distribution is present in this woman with malignancy and dermatomyositis.

(G) Typical palpable purpuric lesions seen in a patient with a hypersensitivity angiitis (cutaneous leukocytoclastic vasculitis).

(H) Erythema elevatum diutinum. These violaceous nodular lesions on the extensor surfaces and over bone prominences represent a localized leukocytoclastic vasculitis. (Courtesy of Dr. Neil A. Fenske, Tampa, FL.)

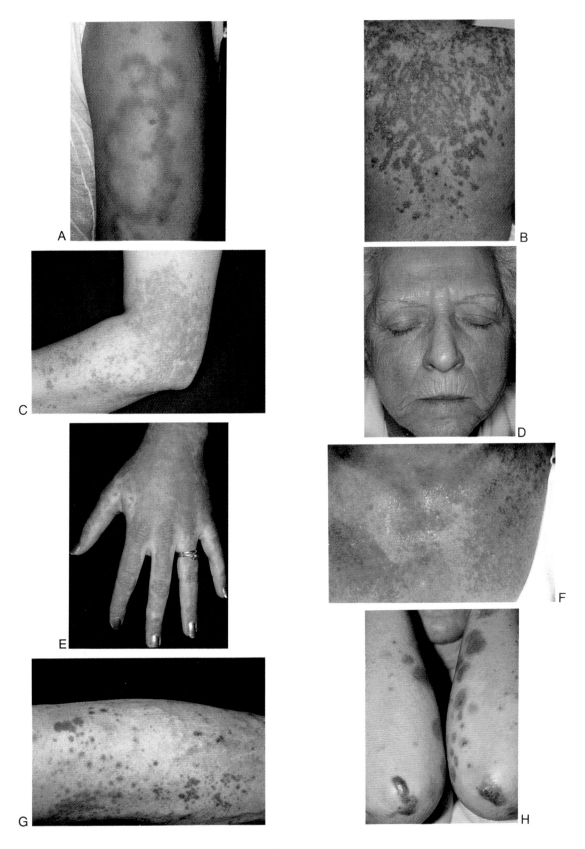

Plate I

Plate II

(A) Kawasaki's syndrome.

(B) Multiple yellowish nodular lesions are seen, which are representative of tophi.

(C) Palmar erythema in a patient with an acute graft versus host syndrome following bone marrow transplant. (Courtesy of Dr. Richard Sturm, Atlanta, GA.)

(D) Same patient as in *C*, demonstrating mucosal surface lesions. (Courtesy of Dr. Richard Sturm, Atlanta, GA.)

(E) Erythema multiforme with typical target lesions.

(F) Stevens-Johnson syndrome—conjunctivitis.

(G) Toxic epidermal necrolysis as a result of phenytoin (Dilantin) therapy. This individual demonstrates loss of multiple sheets of skin with denuded areas below the loss.

(H) Large areas of purpura with necrosis in a patient with diffuse intravascular coagulopathy and gram-negative sepsis. (Courtesy of Dr. Neil A. Fenske, Tampa, FL.)

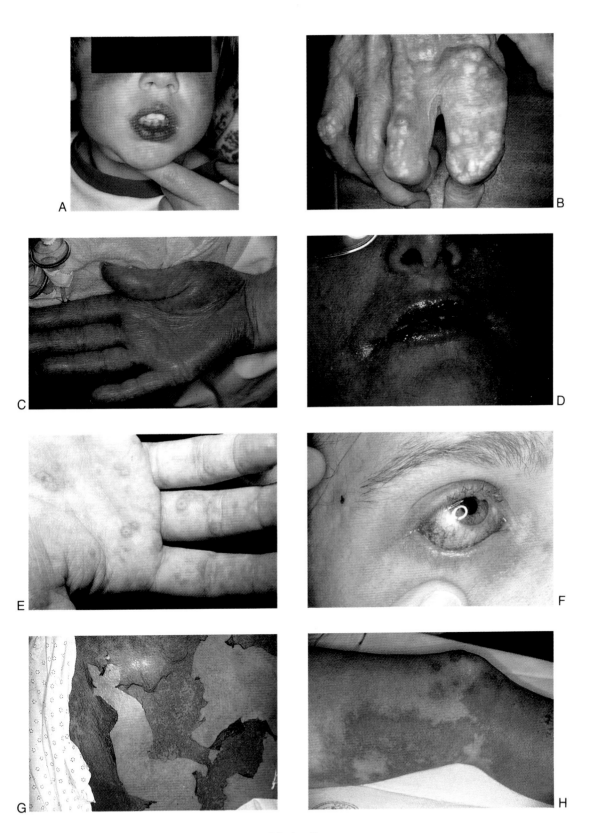

Plate II

Plate III

(A) Acanthosis nigricans and multiple seborrheic keratoses and skin tags in an individual with adenocarcinoma of the stomach. (Courtesy of Dr. Neil A. Fenske, Tampa, FL.)

(B) Acrokeratosis paraneoplastica. This patient demonstrates violaceous plaques in the acral areas. He also had a squamous cell carcinoma of the larynx. (Courtesy of Dr. Charles Camisa, Columbus, OH.)

(C) Paget's disease of the breast. An erythematous plaque surrounds the nipple in this female with ductal adenocarcinoma of the breast.

(D) Metastatic carcinoma with a cellulitic appearance on the anterior chest wall as a result of carcinoma of the lung.

(E) Multiple erythematous to violaceous nodules are present in this man with lymphoblastic lymphoma.

(F) Multiple small violaceous papules and small nodules are present in this man with a blast cell crisis.

(G) Letterer-Siwe disease. Erythematous, slightly scaly plaques are present in the scalp of this child.

(H) Multiple xanthogranulomas representative of non-X histiocytosis in an 18-year-old man with no evidence of internal disease.

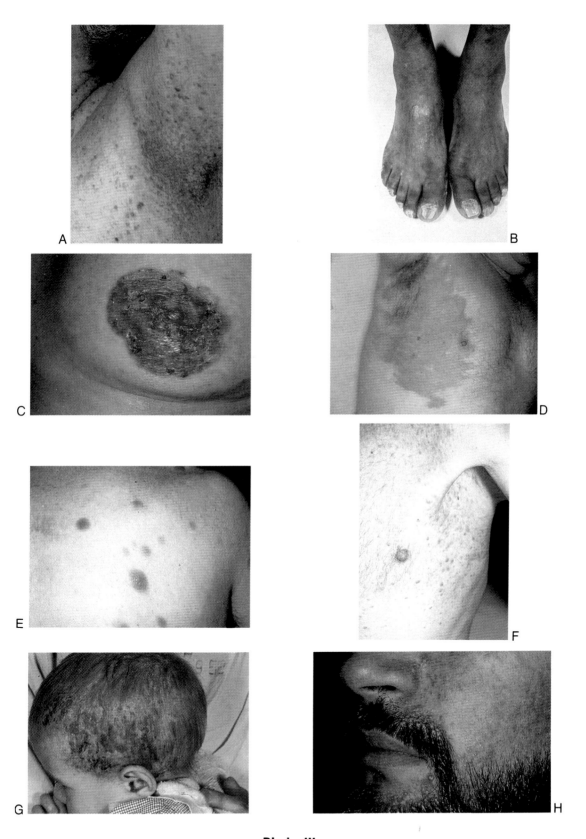

Plate III

Plate IV

(A) Multiple irregular erythematous plaques are present in a man with mycosis fungoides.

(B) An irregular margin with multiple colors of black, blue, slight red, and white are seen in this superficial spreading melanoma.

(C) Multiple variations and colors are seen in this elderly man with lentigo maligna melanoma.

(D) Acrolentiginous melanoma. (Courtesy of Dr. Neil A. Fenske, Tampa, FL.)

(E) Multiple irregular pigmented lesions are seen in a patient with a familial dysplastic nevus syndrome.

(F) Necrobiosis lipoidica dibeticorum.

(G) Multiple eruptive xanthomas in poorly controlled diabetic.

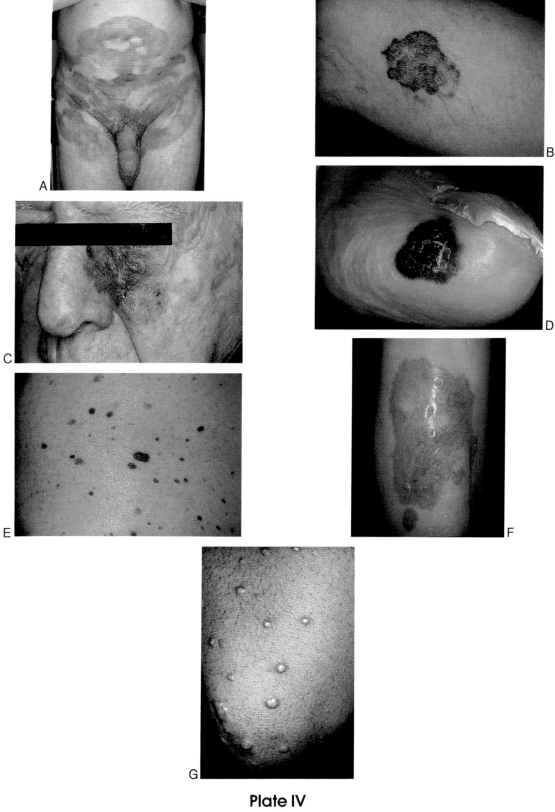

Plate IV

Plate V

(A) Plain xanthomas (xanthelasmas of the eyelids).

(B) Pseudoxanthoma elasticum.

(C) Hereditary hemorrhagic telangiectasia. Multiple, small, telangiectatic mats are present on the lips and tongue of this individual.

(D) Acrodermatitis enteropathica.

(E) Multiple, plain xanthomas in primary biliary cirrhosis.

(F) Verrucous plaque on the chin in a patient with North American blastomycosis.

(G) Erythematous, cellulitic-appearing rash on the malar skin as well as on the nose in a man with coccidioidomycosis.

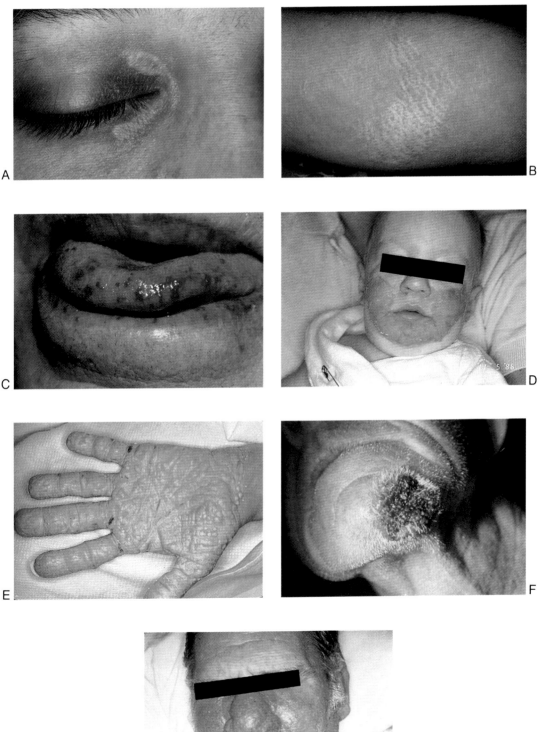

Plate V

Plate VI

(A) Crusted and vesiculated skin in a patient with staphylococcal scalded skin syndrome.
(B) Erythematous lesions representative of toxic shock syndrome.
(C) Hypopigmented anesthetic skin in an East Indian physician with tuberculoid leprosy.
(D) Multiple annular lesions are present in this female with sarcoidosis.
(E) Violaceous, scarring lesions representative of lupus pernio are present in this patient with sarcoidosis of the upper respiratory tract.
(F) Erythematous eruption of the earlobe representative of relapsing polychondritis.

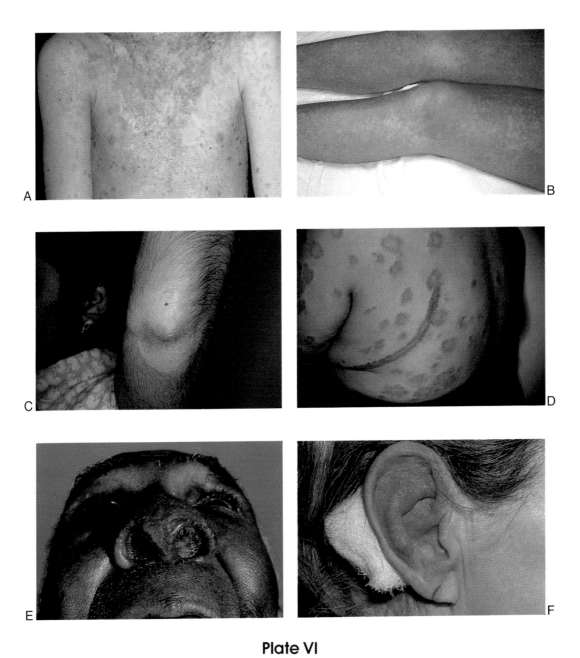

Plate VI

Plate VII

(A) The nodular lesion shown represents metastatic calcification in a patient with chronic renal failure on hemodialysis.

(B) Fabry's disease.

(C) Fabry's disease (same patient as in *B*).

(D) A hypopigmented spot on the thigh in the shape of an ash leaf is present in this patient with tuberous sclerosis.

(E) A unilateral port-wine stain is present in this man with Sturge-Weber syndrome.

(F) Hypopigmented swirls of skin in a patient with incontinentia pigmenti achromians.

(G) The patient shown has epidermal nevus syndrome with multiple anomalies, hemangiomas, and epidermal nevi, as represented by the fine, slightly pigmented skin.

(H) Multiple bruises in a patient with Gardner-Diamond syndrome. (Courtesy of Dr. Neil A. Fenske, Tampa, FL.)

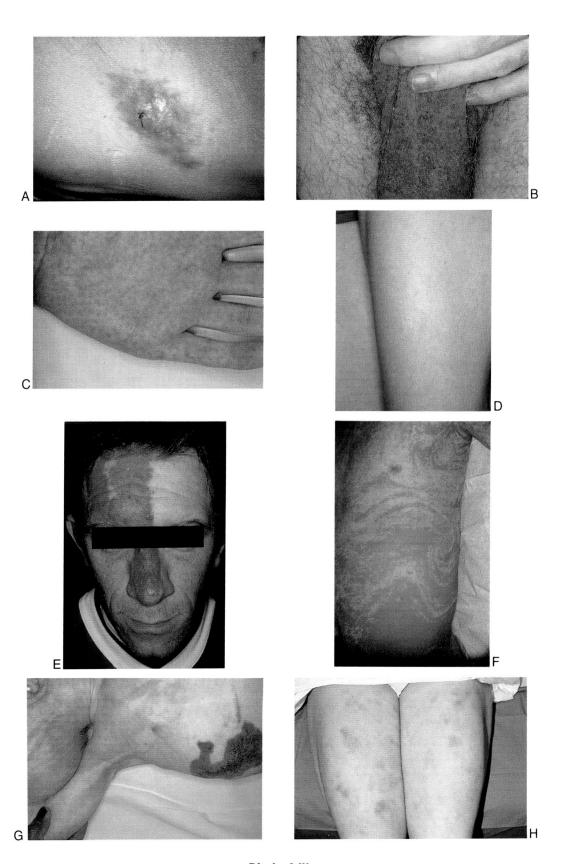

Plate VII

Plate VIII

Violaceous plaque of a fixed drug reaction as a result of therapy with thioridazine hydro-chloride (Mellaril).

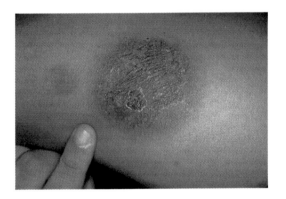

Plate VIII

CUTANEOUS
RHEUMATOLOGY

I

Lupus Erythematosus

JEFFREY P. CALLEN

Lupus erythematosus (LE) is a multisystem disorder whose spectrum runs from a relatively benign, self-limited cutaneous eruption to a severe, often fatal, systemic disease. Prior to Hargrave's recognition of the LE cell, lupus erythematosus was diagnosed by a constellation of clinical findings. Ultimately, the American Rheumatism Association (ARA) developed a set of criteria that could be used for the classification of systemic lupus erythematosus (SLE). The criteria were revised in 1982 (Table 1–1). When a patient has 4 or more of the criteria either concurrently or serially during any period of observation, the patient can be classified as having SLE. Occasionally patients with overlapping features of the various collagen-vascular diseases (mixed or undifferentiated connective tissue disease—MCTD/UCTD) will also fulfill 4 of these criteria. However, patients with rheumatoid arthritis, various infections, and/or neoplastic disease rarely fulfill the criteria, and are excluded from consideration. Thus, the ARA criteria for LE are useful because they are relatively sensitive and specific.

In the 1940s and 1950s, dermatologists first recognized that most of their patients with chronic, scarring, discoid LE (DLE) lesions had few, if any, systemic findings, whereas those with photosensitivity and/or malar erythema frequently had systemic disease. They also recognized a middle group in whom the skin lesions were more transient, those with systemic disease but in whom the prognosis was not as poor as that of patients with SLE. These patients were categorized as having subacute LE or disseminated discoid LE or subacute disseminated LE. This was the beginning of what we now

recognize as the subset theory of LE. The classification of cutaneous subsets was stressed by Gilliam and his coworkers. Gilliam proposed that patients be classified by the type of skin disease present: chronic cutaneous (discoid) LE, subacute cutaneous LE (SCLE), or acute cutaneous LE (ACLE). Although some refinements have occurred, the basic classification remains valuable. However, one must still keep in mind that each patient need not behave according to the generalization from the subset. Thus, some individuals in the generally benign subset can have severe systemic disease.

CHRONIC CUTANEOUS LUPUS ERYTHEMATOSUS

Chronic cutaneous LE can be manifested by several clinical variations. The most common subset is the patient with DLE lesions. These patients may be classified as having *localized DLE*, when lesions are only on the head and neck, or *widespread DLE*, when lesions are on other body surfaces as well as on the head and neck. Other, less common forms of chronic cutaneous LE include hypertrophic or verrucous (wart-like) lesions, lesions on the palms and/or soles, oral discoid LE, and lupus panniculitis (lupus profundus). In addition, there exists a group of patients in whom the discoid LE lesion is only one manifestation of SLE (DLE-SLE subset).

The discoid LE lesion is characterized by erythema; telangiectasia; adherent scale, varying from fine to thick; follicular plugging; dyspigmentation; and atrophy and scarring (Fig. 1–1). The lesions are usually

Table 1–1. CRITERIA FOR THE DIAGNOSIS OF SYSTEMIC LE (SLE)

If 4 or more of the following criteria are present serially or simultaneously during any period of observation, the patient is said to have SLE.

1. Malar rash
2. Discoid LE lesions
3. Photosensitivity: by history or observation
4. Oral ulcers: usually painless, observed by physician
5. Arthritis: non-erosive, involving 2 or more joints
6. Serositis: pleuritis or pericarditis
7. Renal disorder: proteinuria (> 500 mg/day) or cellular casts
8. CNS disorder: seizures or psychosis (absence of known cause)
9. Hematologic disorder: hemolytic anemia, leukopenia ($< 4000/mm^3$); lymphopenia ($< 1500/mm^3$); or thrombocytopenia ($< 100,000/mm^3$)
10. Immunologic disorder: +LE prep, abnormal titer of anti-nDNA and anti-Sm, false positive VDRL
11. Antinuclear antibody

sharply demarcated, and can be round, thus giving rise to the term discoid (or disc-like). The presence of scarring and/or atrophy is what separates these lesions from those of subacute cutaneous LE. Often DLE lesions are distinct, allowing the physician to feel certain about the diagnosis. The differential diagnosis most often includes papulosquamous diseases, such as psoriasis, lichen planus, secondary syphilis, superficial fungal infection, polymorphous light eruption, and sarcoidosis. Histopathologic examination is usually very helpful in confirming a diagnosis, and only rarely is immunofluorescence microscopy necessary.

Patients with localized DLE have their lesions located solely on the head and/or neck. In studies of DLE patients, this subset represents only one half of those seen, whether the population is derived from a referral center or from a private practice setting. These patients differ from those with widespread DLE in a number of ways. Those with localized disease rarely are among the subset of DLE-SLE. They have fewer manifestations suggestive of systemic disease, and they less frequently demonstrate a positive antinuclear antibody (ANA) or leukopenia. Lastly, on follow-up examination those patients with localized DLE have a better chance of having inactive disease (>50%) at 5 years than those with widespread DLE (<10%). Also, it appears that the rare patient with DLE who progressively develops more of these criteria is generally in the widespread DLE subset. Thus, it seems that it is prognostically worthwhile to separate the localized versus the widespread DLE patients into different subsets.

Hypertrophic or verrucous DLE (HLE) is a unique subset in which an unusual lesion occurs. The thick, adherent scale is replaced by massive hyperkeratosis, and lesions that look like warts or squamous cell carcinomas

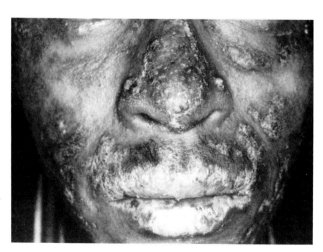

Figure 1–1. Discoid lupus erythematosus. This young black male demonstrates multiple features of discoid lupus erythematosus, including follicular plugging, scarring, atrophy of lesions, and involvement of the mucosal surfaces.

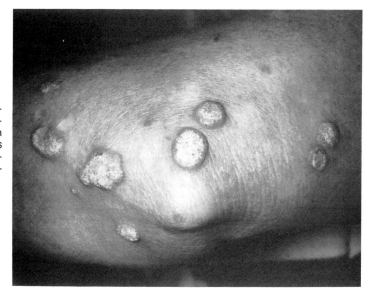

Figure 1–2. Hypertrophic (verrucous) lupus erythematosus. These wart-like lesions were present in a patient with typical discoid lupus erythematosus elsewhere. They simulate warts, keratoacanthoma, or squamous cell carcinoma.

develop (Fig. 1–2). These lesions occur in the setting of other, more typical DLE lesions, and although histologically less distinctive than the DLE lesion, they can be separated from warts or squamous cell carcinoma. In an occasional patient with HLE, immunofluorescence microscopy of lesional skin is useful for diagnosis. These patients tend to have chronic disease, to have little in the way of systemic symptoms or laboratory findings, and to be extremely difficult to treat with conventional therapy.

Lesions of DLE can occur on the palms and/or soles (Fig. 1–3). The incidence of this occurence is small, and there is no specific clinical or serologic correlation. These patients can have chronic non-systemic disease, or the lesions can be present in the patient with SLE. These palmar or plantar lesions are difficult to treat.

Oral discoid LE is histopathologically and clinically similar to cutaneous DLE. These lesions are different from the oral and nasal ulcerations that occur in SLE. Those occurring in the SLE patient are associated with active systemic disease and are histopathologically non-specific. Lesions that look like those of DLE in the oral mucosa have similar associations to those seen with localized or widespread DLE.

Lupus panniculitis (profundus) (LEP) is a lobular panniculitis that occurs in a rare DLE patient (Fig. 1–4). Fewer than 100 cases have been reported in the world literature,

and in our practice, lupus panniculitis has been seen only once in over 300 cutaneous LE patients. Whether LEP is histopathologically distinct is controversial; thus, in our opinion, the patient must have documented

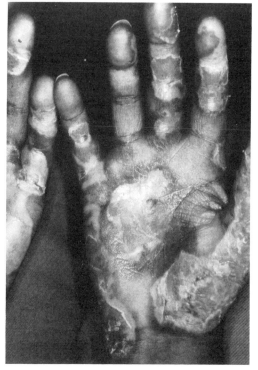

Figure 1–3. Erosive lesions of discoid lupus erythematosus involving the palms. Typical discoid lupus erythematosus is present elsewhere.

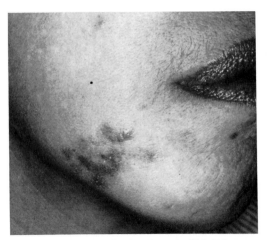

Figure 1–4. Lupus profundus (panniculitis). This young female has inflammatory, subcutaneous nodular lesions in coexistence with typical discoid lupus erythematosus in other areas of her body.

SLE or DLE to be classified as having LEP. LEP is often chronic, and it can lead to cutaneous and subcutaneous atrophy and to occasional ulceration. It occurs with or without systemic disease (1:2). It has been postulated that renal disease in the LEP patient is rarely present and, when present, is among the more benign forms.

The DLE-SLE subset defines a small group of patients (about 5–10%) who by the nature of their selection have systemic disease in association with scarring cutaneous disease. Patients who progress from pure cutaneous disease into this group are characterized by widespread DLE, the presence of clinically appreciable periungual telangiectasias, persistent elevated sedimentation rates, leukopenia, and positive antinuclear antibody (ANA). The patients in this group may have DLE alone at the onset, or DLE with other symptoms or signs, or they may have systemic disease without skin lesions. The time frame is variable, but most of the patients in this group develop the criteria for SLE within 1–3 years of diagnosis. These patients with DLE-SLE rarely have renal disease, and even when they do, it is most often transient and mild. DLE-SLE is a distinct LE subset because of its relatively benign, albeit chronic, course.

SUBACUTE CUTANEOUS LUPUS ERYTHEMATOSUS (SCLE)

SCLE is a skin lesion that has all the features of DLE without the scarring or atro-

phy. Also, follicular plugging is quite rare in the SCLE lesion. Patients with SCLE lesions as their major cutaneous manifestation have been classified as having a subset called SCLE. It is important to understand, however, that the patient in the SCLE subset can have scarring lesions of DLE, or can have lesions generally associated with SLE, such as a malar rash or vasculitic lesions. Many of the SCLE patients fulfill 4 or more of the ARA criteria for SLE; thus, some authorities have not recognized these patients as forming a distinct subset. However, they do differ from DLE patients and are still on the benign end of the LE spectrum. Therefore, it is our feeling that SCLE should be considered a distinct LE subset.

SCLE skin lesions are of at least two types: annular or papulosquamous. Annular SCLE (SCLE-A) lesions are characterized by erythematous rings with central clearing (Fig. 1–5; Plate IA). Often there is a slight scale. These lesions of SCLE-A must be differentiated from other figurate erythemas, such as erythema annular centrifugum, or from erythema multiforme. Papulosquamous SCLE

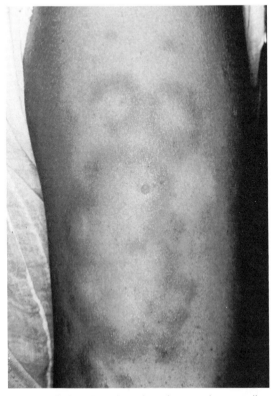

Figure 1–5. Annular subacute cutaneous lupus erythematosus. This erythematous, annular lesion lacks scarring or atrophy, yet represents a histologically specific pattern of lupus erythematosus (see also Plate IA).

(SCLE-P) lesions are characterized by plaques and papules with scale (Figs. 1–6 and 1–7; Plate IB). The differential diagnosis of SCLE-P lesions includes psoriasis and lichen planus. Several patients with presumed psoriasis who have shown flaring with ultraviolet light therapy have really had SCLE. Lesions of both SCLE-A and those of SCLE-P begin as small, erythematous papules that must be differentiated from polymorphous light eruption (Fig. 1–8; Plate IC). The usual patient has only one type of SCLE lesion, but in about 10% both annular and papulosquamous lesions can be present. DLE skin lesions, generally limited in their number, can occur in up to 35% of patients in the SCLE subset.

About 50% of the patients with SCLE have 4 or more of the ARA criteria for SLE. This takes into account the skin lesion as one criterion, and photosensitivity as a second (>90% of SCLE patients have these two criteria). SCLE patients also frequently have serologic abnormalities, in particular, the presence of anti-Ro (SS-A) antibody. Ap-

proximately 40–50% have severe arthralgias or a non-deforming arthritis. Serositis, central nervous system (CNS) disease, and renal disease are possible but are uncommon in SCLE. The type of clinical skin lesions (annular versus papulosquamous) has not been related to specific organ system involvement.

SCLE patients have been described in association with other conditions. SCLE patients may have Sjögren's syndrome, idiopathic thrombocytopenic purpura, urticarial vasculitis, other cutaneous vasculitic syndromes, and/or deficiency of the second component of complement (C2d). A group of anti-Ro positive SCLE patients, whose disease was induced by hydrochlorothiazide, has been described.

Laboratory abnormalities in the SCLE patient have focused on the finding of anti-Ro (SS-A) and anti-La (SS-B) antibodies in many of these patients. These antibody systems are poorly represented in rodent tissue substrates, and thus many of these patients were felt to have "ANA-negative lupus erythematosus." However, with the widespread use of HEp-2 (human epithelium) as a substrate, it has become apparent that many of the anti-Ro positive patients are not ANA-negative. On one examination of the SCLE patient, anti-Ro is present in 35–60% of the cases. There is some controversy regarding the special relationship of anti-Ro (SS-A) with annular SCLE, with several studies suggesting a stronger relationship than with papulosquamous SCLE. Repeated testing will demonstrate a positive anti-Ro in 60–95% of the SCLE patients. Despite this high percentage, one must keep in mind that the marker of the disease is not this serological test, but rather the clinical skin lesion. Also, anti-Ro (SS-A) is found in many non-SCLE situations; thus, it is not a sensitive or specific marker of SCLE. Another presumed marker in SCLE is the presence of HLA-DR3.

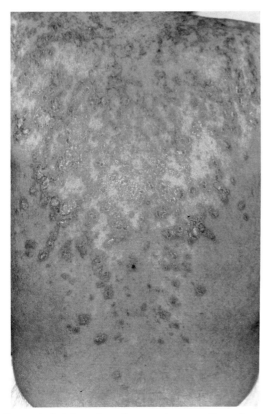

Figure 1–6. Subacute cutaneous lupus erythematosus, papulosquamous variant. This patient developed an exquisitely photosensitive eruption with minimal sun exposure (see also Plate IB).

NEONATAL LUPUS ERYTHEMATOSUS (NLE)

NLE is a syndrome in which cutaneous disease is frequently present. In addition, and in contradistinction to most other LE subsets, NLE can also be manifested as a congenital heart block. For unknown reasons, patients rarely have both skin disease and heart block. However, families in which one baby has had heart block can subse-

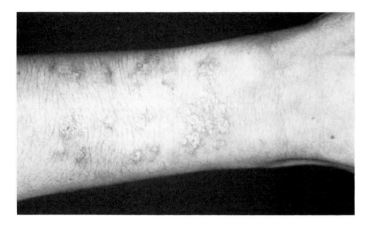

Figure 1–7. Lichen planus–like lesions of subacute cutaneous lupus erythematosus.

quently have normal infants, or infants with heart block or with skin disease. These neonates have photosensitive skin disease, which spontaneously resolves over a period of 4–6 months. The heart block is usually permanent. NLE has been linked to the presence of anti-Ro (SS-A) in the mother and infant, and to the presence of HLA-DR3 in the mother. However, babies with anti-Ro can be normal; thus, the presence of this antibody is not the only determining factor. The mother of an NLE baby can be asymptomatic or can have a connective tissue disease (LE, rheumatoid arthritis, Sjögren's syndrome, etc.). In one study, at the time of follow-up, one half of those mothers who had initially been asymptomatic developed a connective tissue disease (usually SCLE or SLE).

ACUTE CUTANEOUS LUPUS ERYTHEMATOSUS (ACLE)

Most cutaneous lesions characterized within the ACLE group are often not histologically LE-specific, in contrast to those of DLE and SCLE, which both have the LE pattern. Lesions such as those of vasculitis or urticaria may be present in patients with SLE, and many correlate with active systemic disease.

Malar erythema is the classic "butterfly" rash from which the name lupus erythema-

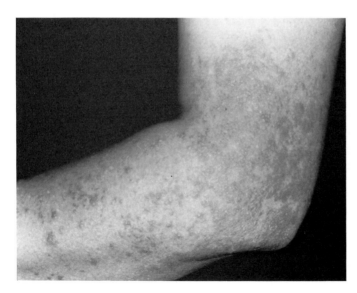

Figure 1–8. Erythematous papular lesion of polymorphous light eruption representing a clinical picture similar to that seen in subacute cutaneous lupus erythematosus (see also Plate IC).

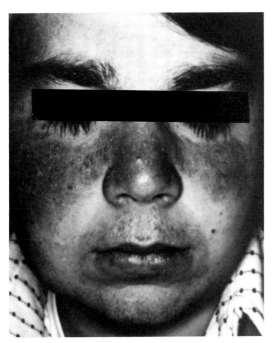

Figure 1–9. Systemic lupus erythematosus. This young man has a very typical butterfly eruption of systemic lupus erythematosus.

tosus (wolf-like redness) was coined (Fig. 1–9). The rash is induced by sun exposure and is usually induced by the ultraviolet B light (UVB; 290–320 nm). Patients with an active malar "butterfly" rash usually have active systemic disease, but there is no specific organ system involved.

Photosensitivity is a major factor in all types of cutaneous LE. It is one of the 11 ARA criteria for classification of SLE. Photosensitivity implies that there is an abnormal reaction to sunlight. An abnormal reaction to sunlight occurs in all LE patients; however, in general most DLE patients are not considered to have "true" photosensitivity despite a worsening of their clinical disease in the spring and summer. Almost all SCLE patients are photosensitive, and about 60–75% of SLE patients demonstrate photosensitivity. As with the malar rash, this reaction is induced by UVB light, but in some rare individuals UVA light (320–360 nm) can be involved as well.

Several cutaneous abnormalities had been part of the ARA criteria but have been found to be less specific than photosensitivity. Diffuse hair loss (alopecia) was in the original criteria. Patients with SLE can develop a diffuse hair thinning, but this is most likely related to the presence of a severe episode of systemic illness. This type of hair loss is seen with major surgery or can follow systemic infections or pregnancy. It is known as telogen effluvium, since the trauma of the associated disease forces most hairs to cycle into the same phase and then they all go through the telogen (resting) phase 3–6 months later, and hair loss occurs. This hair loss is different from the alopecic lesion of DLE.

Raynaud's phenomenon (RP) was part of the original 14 ARA criteria but has been removed. RP occurs in otherwise healthy patients and in those with scleroderma, cold-associated disorders, or other collagen-vascular diseases. There has been some suggestion that the presence of RP is associated with a more benign SLE course, but this is controversial.

Palmar erythema and periungual telangiectasias occur as non-specific signs of SLE. Periungual telangiectasias are important in the DLE patient, since their presence occurs only in those patients who are likely to have or develop SLE. Nailfold capillaroscopy has also demonstrated abnormalities, but the use of this procedure to differentiate LE from other collagen-vascular diseases is controversial.

Cutaneous vasculitis can complicate LE. It can be manifested as urticaria-like lesions, nailfold infarcts, or palpable purpura. The presence of vasculitis in the SCLE patient has been correlated with a positive anti-Ro (SS-A), but not with active systemic disease. However, the presence of vasculitis in the SLE patient correlates with active disease and a poor prognosis. In particular, active renal disease or CNS disease has been reported in the patient with vasculitis.

Bullous (or vesicular) lesions can complicate LE. Often these lesions are present in the patient with active systemic disease. The lesions are often grouped and can simulate a cutaneous disease known as dermatitis herpetiformis both clinically and histopathologically.

LABORATORY PHENOMENA IN PATIENTS WITH CUTANEOUS LUPUS ERYTHEMATOSUS

The full gamut of systemic disease manifestations of SLE can occur in patients with

Table 1–2. ANTIBODY SUBSETS IN LUPUS
ERYTHEMATOSUS

Test	Clinical Disorder
Antinuclear antibody (ANA)	Wide array of collagen vascular diseases, some normals
HEp-2 (substrate)	Less specific
Mouse liver	More specific
Peripheral pattern	Correlates with anti-nDNA
Homogeneous pattern	Non-specific
Speckled pattern	May be of several types
Nucleolar pattern	Scleroderma
Antibodies to DNA	
Single stranded DNA (ssDNA)	Non-specific presence in patients with cutaneous LE is suggestive of systemic disease
Double stranded DNA (nDNA)	SLE, active nephritis
Anti-histone antibody	Drug-induced LE
Anti-RNP (U₁RNP)	Mixed connective tissue disease (MCTD)
Anti-Sm	SLE
Anti-Ro (SS-A)	SCLE, neonatal LE, Sjögren's syndrome, vasculitis, C2 deficiency
Anti-La (SS-B)	Sjögren's syndrome

cutaneous disease, and thus these individuals can have any or all of the laboratory associations of the disorder. Serologic abnormalities are a common occurrence in LE. They are rarer in patients with "pure" cutaneous disease, such as DLE or HLE. The presence of abnormalities in these patients correlates with progressive disease, or with the criteria for SLE.

The antinuclear antibody (ANA) is a system that represents many antibodies to multiple substrates. The frequency of a positive ANA correlates with the substrate used. The reported pattern of the ANA may also correlate with specific antibodies; however, except when interpreted by experts the ANA pattern is not specific. Table 1–2 lists the antibody subsets and their clinical correlates. Table 1–3 represents the frequency of these antibodies in the subsets discussed. Anti-native DNA (double stranded) correlates with active SLE and in particular active renal disease. However, one must be certain that the testing method used does not detect anti-single stranded (ss) DNA, which is not SLE specific. Anti-Ro (SS-A) was initially described in ANA negative LE and Sjögren's syndrome. However, it is also present in neonatal LE, vasculitic patients, SCLE, and C2 deficient LE syndromes. Thus it is not specific for any one subset. Antibody testing must be carefully correlated with other laboratory findings and with clinical abnormalities. Therapy should *not* be based solely on these laboratory abnormalities.

Immunogenetic analyses have led to a better understanding of the pathogenesis of LE, and at times they are useful in separating the various LE subsets. Human leukocyte antigen (HLA) system (the major histocompatibility system), in particular the DR loci, seems to correlate with specific subsets of LE. HLA-DR3 has been linked to SCLE, to mothers of neonates with LE, and to production of anti-Ro (SS-A) antibodies. HLA-DR2 is present in C2 deficient LE patients. HLA-DR6 has been related to chronic cutaneous LE. Thus, these abnormalities suggest that the subset theory may have validity. In the future, these abnormalities may also be prognostically helpful as investigators further define subsets.

Circulating immune complexes (CIC) can be found often in SLE and SCLE patients, but rarely in patients with purely cutaneous disease. CIC tend to correlate with vasculitis, active renal disease, arthritis, or serositis. They may be pathogenetically important in vasculitis and renal involvement, but they are probably not involved in the pathogenesis of the non-vasculitic cutaneous lesion.

Table 1–3. FREQUENCY OF ANA AND OTHER ANTIBODIES IN VARIOUS CLINICAL SUBSETS OF LE (%)

Test	DLE	HLE	DLE/SLE	SCLE	NLE	ACLE
ANA	5–10	5	75	50–75	60–90	95
Anti-ssDNA	35	25	75	20–50	?	90
Anti-nDNA	5	5	10	10	10–50	70
Anti-RNP (U₁RNP)	5	25	?	10	?	40
Anti-Sm	5	5	5	10	?	25
Anti-Ro (SS-A)	5	5–10	5	40–95	90	30
Anti-La (SS-B)	5	5	5	15	15–20	10

Complement activation is also a feature of SLE, and hypocomplementemia correlates with active systemic disease. Those patients with persistent hypocomplementia should be evaluated for complement component deficiencies, of which C2 deficiency is the most common.

Cutaneous immunofluorescence was applied as a diagnostic and prognostic tool that led to a better understanding of LE. Lesional immunofluorescence may be helpful when the clinical and histopathologic diagnosis is in question. However, one must realize that normal facial skin can demonstrate 10–20% false positive reactions. The use of non-involved, "non-exposed" skin in the lupus band test (LBT) is believed to correlate with active renal disease. Refined antibody testing has reduced the need for this somewhat subjective and cumbersome test.

THERAPY OF CUTANEOUS LUPUS ERYTHEMATOSUS

Before therapy is begun, it is necessary to evaluate the patient thoroughly to note the extent of disease and to be able to reassure the patient of the benignity of the process. Table 1–4 lists the testing that should be ordered. This testing is not inexpensive, but if all results are negative the value of the reassurance that can be given is inestimable.

The most important therapeutic manipulation (Table 1–5) is the use of sunscreens

Table 1–4. EVALUATION OF THE PATIENT WITH CUTANEOUS LE

Standard Testing
Careful history and physical examination
Skin biopsy for routine histology
CBC with differential and platelet count
Serum multiphasic analysis
Anti-nuclear antibody
Serological Tests
Anti-nDNA
Anti-RNP (U₁RNP)
Anti-Ro (SS-A)
Erythrocyte sedimentation rate (ESR)
Urinalysis
Total hemolytic complement (if abnormal, C3, C2, C4 levels)
Serum protein electrophoresis
Optional Tests
Circulating immune complexes
Immunofluorescence skin biopsy
  Lesional
  Non-lesional, non-exposed (lupus band test)
Creatinine clearance

Table 1–5. THERAPEUTIC AGENTS USEFUL FOR CUTANEOUS LE

Standard Therapy
Sunscreens
Topical corticosteroids
Intralesional corticosteroids (avoid atrophy)
Antimalarials
  Hydroxychloroquine (H): potential ocular toxicity
  Chloroquine (C): potential ocular toxicity
  Quinacrine (Q): no ocular toxicity, bone marrow toxicity (may combine Q with either H or C)
Alternatives
Dapsone (best for bullous LE, vasculitis)
Auranofin (oral gold)
Accutane (13-cis-retinoic acid)
Clofazamine
Low dose cytotoxic agents: azathioprine or methotrexate
Systemic corticosteroids (poorly effective for chronic lesions)

and sun avoidance. This is a basic aspect of therapy that is frequently overlooked, particularly in the SCLE patient in whom the photosensitivity is exquisite. Sunscreens with a sun protective factor (SPF) of at least 15 are to be used every day. The patient should be encouraged to apply the sunscreen each morning and then again prior to sun exposure. Sunbathing, whether active or passive, is strongly discouraged. Protective clothing and intelligent planning (e.g., early morning or late afternoon) of sun exposure are encouraged.

Although topical corticosteroids have been shown under experimental conditions to be effective, in the clinic or office they may not be highly effective. Probably because of their expense, messiness, and time involved in application, they are not always used as directed. Despite these failures, topical corticosteroids should be prescribed in conjunction with other agents. The specific agent used is chosen based upon the clinical lesion and area of the body that is affected. The prescribing physician must keep in mind that these agents can produce atrophy, which is also a sign of the disease.

Lesions that do not respond to topical agents can be injected intralesionally with a corticosteroid such as triamcinolone acetonide (3–4 mg/ml). Hypertrophic lesions, scalp lesions, palmar lesions, and recalcitrant DLE lesions are well suited to therapy with intralesional corticosteroids. Again, it is important to recognize that atrophy is dose-related and that there is a fine line between effectiveness and this complication. Secondary infection can occur within the injection site.

Antimalarials form a mainstay of systemic therapy of cutaneous LE. The mechanism of action of these agents is unknown, but it may relate to photoprotection and/or to immunomodulation. The agents available include hydroxychloroquine HCl, chloroquine phosphate, and quinacrine HCl. Chloroquine and hydroxychloroquine may be associated with a retinopathy, whereas quinacrine's major side-effect is bone marrow suppression, and the patient's skin often turns yellow. Our first choice is hydroxychloroquine; despite possibly being less efficacious, it has less ocular toxicity than chloroquine. Hydroxychloroquine is given by mouth in a dose of 200–400 mg per day. Regular ophthalmologic examinations are scheduled. When this regimen is less effective than desired, either quinacrine 100 mg once or twice daily can be added, or the patient can be switched to chloroquine (250–500 mg per day). Antimalarials are effective for DLE, SCLE, LEP, and arthritis associated with LE, but they are poorly effective in hypertrophic or palmar lesions or vasculitis. Patients with the DLE-SLE subset respond less well to antimalarials than those without systemic manifestations.

Many other systemic agents have been used for cutaneous LE syndromes. Systemic corticosteroids are rarely effective for the cutaneous disease, despite their dramatic effect on systemic symptoms and signs. Immunosuppressives are rarely indicated for cutaneous LE, and furthermore, in our limited experience, are not very beneficial. Dapsone 100–200 mg daily has been reported to be effective. It may be helpful in the rare SCLE patient, LE patients with cutaneous vasculitis syndromes, and individuals with bullous LE. Retinoids are among the newest agents for cutaneous therapy. They may be effective for cutaneous LE, but further study is needed. Lastly, one report from England has suggested that oral gold therapy may be efficacious for cutaneous LE.

SUMMARY

Cutaneous LE has a myriad of presentations, which can be fitted into several subsets. The usefulness of a subset approach is in the ability to predict prognosis adequately. Systemic disease is possible in all subsets, but in general most patients with cutaneous DLE or SCLE have a benign form of disease. Effective therapy involves sunscreens, topical and intralesional corticosteroids, and oral antimalarials.

Suggested Readings

Callen JP: Chronic cutaneous LE. Arch Dermatol 118:412–416, 1982.
Callen JP (ed): Lupus erythematosus. Clin Dermatol 3:1–146, 1985.
Callen JP, Kulick KB, Stelzer G, Fowler JF: Subacute cutaneous lupus erythematosus. J Am Acad Dermatol 15:1227–1237, 1986.
Prystowsky SD, Herndon JH Jr, Gilliam JN: Chronic cutaneous lupus erythematosus (DLE): A clinical and laboratory investigation of 80 patients. Medicine 55:183–191, 1976.
Sontheimer RD, Maddison PJ, Reichlin M, et al: Serological and HLA associations in subacute cutaneous lupus erythematosus: A clinical subset of lupus erythematosus. Ann Intern Med 97:664–671, 1982.
Tuffanelli DL, Dubois EL: Cutaneous manifestation of systemic lupus erythematosus. Arch Dermatol 90:377–385, 1964.

2

Dermatomyositis

JEFFREY P. CALLEN

DEFINITION AND CLASSIFICATION

Dermatomyositis is a condition that combines an inflammatory myopathy with a characteristic cutaneous disease. This disorder is closely related to polymyositis, which has all the features of the muscle disease of dermatomyositis but lacks the characteristic cutaneous findings. Both of these disorders are of unknown etiology, but immune-mediated muscle damage is believed to be important as a pathogenetic mechanism. Both polymyositis and dermatomyositis may occur in the presence of other collagen vascular diseases, such as lupus erythematosus, scleroderma, Sjögren's syndrome, and various vasculitides. Dermatomyositis appears to be characterized by an increased frequency of internal malignancy, whereas the association with malignancy in patients with polymyositis is less well resolved. Both dermatomyositis and polymyositis may occur in children. Both disorders are associated with morbidity and occasional mortality; therefore, a prompt and aggressive approach to therapy is indicated.

Bohan and Peter first suggested the use of five criteria to define the entities of polymyositis and dermatomyositis. The criteria include (1) proximal symmetrical muscle weakness that progresses over a period of weeks to months, (2) elevated serum levels of muscle derived enzymes, (3) abnormal electromyogram, (4) abnormal muscle biopsy, and (5) the presence of cutaneous disease compatible with dermatomyositis. These criteria are useful for evaluation of a patient but should not be used in a dogmatic fashion.

Dermatomyositis and polymyositis may occur in several clinical circumstances; thus, the system of classification has been useful in differentiating groups of patients in their prognosis and therapy. The most widely accepted classification system separates five categories: (1) patients with dermatomyositis, (2) patients with polymyositis, (3) patients who have myositis with malignant disease, (4) patients who are children, and (5) patients with overlapping syndromes of other collagen vascular disease and myositis.

PATHOGENESIS

The pathogenesis of dermatomyositis and polymyositis is still not well understood. The pathogenetic mechanisms involved in the muscle disease are better understood than those involved in the induction of skin disease. Possibly multiple types of insults can lead to muscle damage. Multiple agents have been associated with the appearance of dermatomyositis and/or polymyositis, including various infections (particularly viral infections) post-vaccination, neoplasms, drug-induced disease, various types of stress, and trauma. In addition, dermatomyositis and polymyositis have been linked with various diseases associated with immunologic phenomena. Similarities of polymyositis and inclusion body myositis have led to theories involving a viral cause for the inflammatory myopathy. In addition, demonstration of the Jo-1 antibody in patients with polymyositis has further supported a viral cause, since the antigen for the Jo-1 antibody has similar characteristics with viral and muscle proteins. Dermatomyositis has on numerous occasions been linked to penicillamine therapy for other conditions. Genetic predisposition has been suggested, particularly in patients with childhood disease. Thus, under appropriate circumstances in a possibly immunogenetically predisposed individual, an infection, a drug, trauma, or a neoplasm may be able to initiate an inflammatory reaction in muscle and in skin. Through a complex set of reactions involving both humoral and cellular immunologic phenomena, muscle damage and cutaneous disease may occur.

CUTANEOUS MANIFESTATIONS

The characteristic and possibly pathognomonic cutaneous features of dermatomyositis are the heliotrope rash and Gottron's papules. Several other cutaneous features occur in patients who have dermatomyositis, and their presence allows for the confirmation of the diagnosis of dermatomyositis despite there not being pathognomonic signs. These other features include malar erythema, poikiloderma in a photosensitive dis-

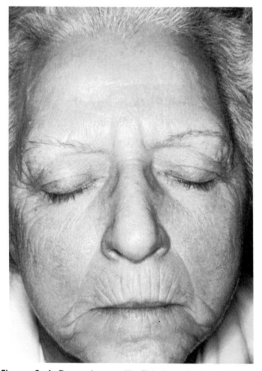

Figure 2–1. Dermatomyositis. This female has a history of uterine carcinoma and has developed inflammatory myopathy in conjunction with a very typical heliotrope eruption around the eyelids and typical lesions elsewhere on her body (see also Plate ID).

tribution, and periungual and cuticular changes. These signs can also occur in other connective tissue diseases and, thus, are not pathognomonic for dermatomyositis; however, they are important in differentiating dermatomyositis from polymyositis.

The heliotrope rash usually consists of a lilac discoloration or a violaceous to dusky erythematous rash with or without edema in a symmetrical distribution involving periorbital skin (Fig. 2–1; Plate ID). Often only the upper lid is involved. Sometimes this sign is quite subtle and may involve only a mild discoloration along the eyelid margin. The heliotrope rash can follow the course of myositis, or it can wax and wane in discordance with the disease activity. However, reactivation of this rash in a patient otherwise considered to be in remission has generally signified a relapse of the myositis as well.

Gottron's papules are found over bony prominences, particularly over the metacarpal-phalangeal joints, the proximal interphalangeal joints, and/or the distal interphalangeal joints. They may also be found over bony prominences such as the elbows, knees, and feet. The lesions consist of slightly elevated, violaceous papules and plaques (Figs. 2–2 and 2–3; Plate IE). Within the lesions there are often telangiectasias, and there may be hyper- and/or hypopigmentation. Usually the activity of the muscle disease is not reflected by the skin disease. These lesions can be clinically confused with those of lupus erythematosus or at times with papulosquamous disorders such as psoriasis or lichen planus. In instances in which differentiation is difficult, biopsy for routine histologic examination as well as for immunofluorescence microscopy may be helpful.

Nailfold changes consist of periungual telangiectasias and a characteristic cuticular change with hypertrophy of the cuticle and small, hemorrhagic infarcts within this hypertrophic area (Fig. 2–4). The periungual telangiectasias seen may be clinically apparent or may be appreciated only by capillary microscopy. Clinically the periungual telangiectasias are indistinguishable from those seen in other connective tissue diseases. The cuticular overgrowth that occurs may be similar to that seen in scleroderma.

Poikiloderma can occur within Gottron's papules or can occur on exposed skin (Fig.

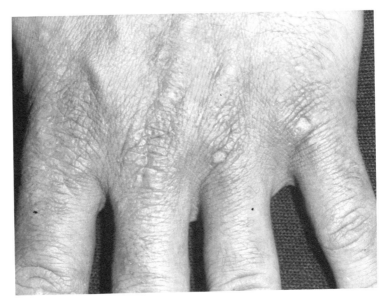

Figure 2–2. Gottron's papules. Typical erythematous to violaceous lesions over the bony prominences on the extensor surfaces of the hand.

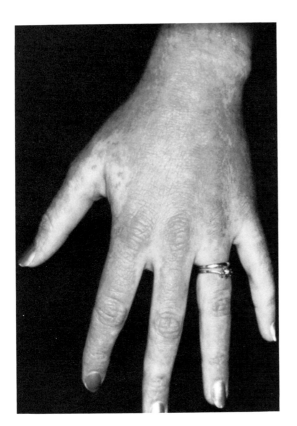

Figure 2–3. Photosensitivity dermatitis found in dermatomyositis. Note the sparing of the interdigital webs and the prominence of the lesions occurring over the joints (see also Plate I*E*).

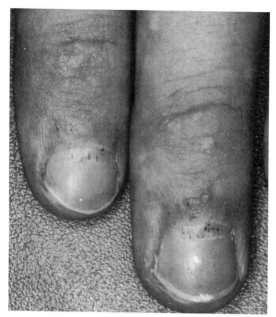

Figure 2–4. Cuticular hypertrophy, splinter hemorrhages, and periungual telangiectasias are present in this patient with dermatomyositis.

2–5; Plate IF). These changes are seen in about one third to one half of the patients with dermatomyositis but do not occur in patients with polymyositis. The patients rarely notice photosensitivity despite the prominent distribution of the rash. This photosensitive, poikilodermatous eruption must be differentiated from lupus erythematosus as well as from other diseases that cause poikilodermatous skin changes.

Patients with myositis can also develop lesions of other connective tissue diseases. The presence of these types of lesions allows physicians to classify the patients into an overlap category. In general, sclerodermatous skin changes have been the most frequently seen change in patients with an overlap syndrome. However, vasculitis, discoid lupus erythematosus, and rheumatoid nodules have also been known to complicate dermatomyositis.

MUSCLE DISEASE

Clinical and laboratory abnormalities suggestive of muscle disease are characteristic features of dermatomyositis and polymyositis. Even in those patients who initially have only skin disease, myositis usually follows at some point in time. The myositis occurring in dermatomyositis is indistinguishable from that occurring in polymyositis as assessed by clinical, histopathologic, or laboratory features. Also, when considered alone the individual features of myositis are not diagnostic of dermatomyositis or polymyositis; rather, the diagnosis is one of exclusion.

Clinically the myopathy affects mainly proximal muscle groups of the shoulder and pelvic girdle muscles. In severe progressive disease, all the muscles may become involved. The disease is usually symmetrical. Initial complaints include weakness, fatigue,

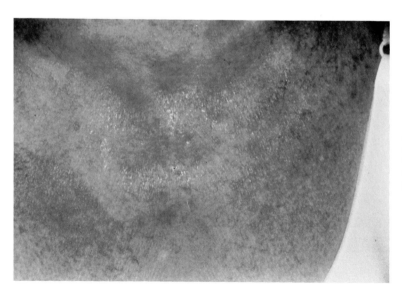

Figure 2–5. Poikilodermatous eruption in the photosensitive distribution is present in this woman with malignancy and dermatomyositis (see also Plate I F).

an inability to climb stairs, an inability to raise the arms for actions like hair grooming or shaving, an inability to rise from a squatting or sitting position, or a combination of these features. The progression of disease is variable but usually occurs over a period of weeks to months. Muscle aching is a common complaint, but frank tenderness upon palpation is variable. An inability to swallow and symptoms of aspiration may reflect the involvement of striated muscle of the pharynx or upper esophagus. Dysphagia often signifies a rapidly progressive course and may be associated with a poor prognosis.

The laboratory abnormalities are enzyme elevations, disturbances of electrical action, and/or histopathologic changes. Muscle enzyme levels are frequently elevated in patients with inflammatory myopathy. The enzymes that are commonly elevated are creatine kinase, aldolase, lactic dehydrogenase, and/or serum glutamic oxalate transaminase (SGOT). Creatine kinase determination seems to be the most practically available test for measuring activity of muscle disease. On occasion patients may have normal muscle enzymes, and in these individuals the measurement of creatine excretion in the urine may be reflective of active muscle disease.

Electromyography characteristically shows sharp or positive waves, insertional irritability, fibrillation, and short polyphasic motor units. Innervation remains intact; thus, there is a lack of neuropathic changes. Muscle biopsy shows typical features, including type II fiber atrophy, necrosis, regeneration, a centralization of the nuclei, and a lymphocytic infiltrate in a perifascicular and/or perivascular region.

SYSTEMIC FEATURES

Dermatomyositis and polymyositis are multisystem disorders. This is reflected by the high frequency of other clinical features in patients with these diseases.

Arthralgias and/or arthritis may be present in up to one fourth of the patients with inflammatory myopathy. This percentage rises in patients with overlap syndromes. The usual picture is one of generalized arthralgias accompanied by morning stiffness. The small joints of the hands, wrists, and ankles may be involved with a symmetrical non-deforming arthritis. Patients with arthritis may have a lower frequency of malignancy than those patients who do not have arthritis.

Esophageal disease as manifested by dysphagia is estimated to be present in 15–50% of patients with inflammatory myopathy. The dysphagia can be of two types: proximal dysphagia or distal dysphagia. Proximal dysphagia is caused by involvement of striated muscle in the pharynx or proximal esophagus. This involvement may be manifested by aspiration while attempting to swallow. This involvement correlates well with the severity of the muscle disease and is steroid-responsive. Distal dysphagia is related to involvement of non-striated muscle and appears to be more frequent in patients who have overlap syndromes. This may also be accompanied by symptoms of reflux esophagitis. Dysphagia in general portends a poor prognosis and is often associated with pulmonary involvement.

Pulmonary disease occurs in dermatomyositis and polymyositis in approximately 15–30% of patients. It can be characterized by a primary diffuse interstitial fibrosis (DIF) that may be manifested radiologically or by abnormalities seen on pulmonary function testing. Lung disease may also occur as a direct complication of the muscle disease, such as by hypoventilation or by aspiration in patients with dysphagia, or may be a result of treatment, as with opportunistic infections or drug-induced hypersensitivity pneumonitis. Pulmonary complications have been associated with a poor prognosis. Data have suggested that patients with polymyositis who possess the Jo-1 antibody are at a greater risk for pulmonary involvement than those who do not have Jo-1 antibodies.

Cardiac disease may also occur in patients with polymyositis, as manifested by a myocarditis or a pericarditis. Pericarditis appears to be more common in patients with overlapping features of other connective tissue diseases. Myocarditis can result in conduction defects, arrhythmias, or, when severe, congestive heart failure.

Calcinosis of the skin or muscle is unusual in adults but may occur in up to 40% of children with dermatomyositis. Calcinosis cutis is manifested by firm, yellow or flesh-colored nodules, often over bony prominences. Occasionally these nodules can extrude through the surface of the skin, in which case secondary infection may occur.

Calcification of the muscles is often asymptomatic and may be seen only on radiologic examination. In severe forms the calcinosis can cause loss of function, and rarely bone formation is possible.

Pregnancy has been shown to have an effect on the inflammatory myopathy. In addition, the inflammatory myopathy may produce profound effects upon the neonate and/or the mother. Studies have suggested that dermatomyositis and/or polymyositis may be activated during pregnancy or that the initial manifestations may be appreciated during pregnancy. In addition, in a large group of women with multiple pregnancies, premature delivery, spontaneous abortions, perinatal deaths, and fetal loss were more common in patients with active myositis.

MYOSITIS AND MALIGNANCY

One of the great controversies of medicine relates to the problem of dermatomyositis-polymyositis and its relationship to malignancy. The frequency of malignancy in dermatomyositis has varied from 6 to 60% in various studies. This variation is probably related to differing methodology. Even within the last few years, multiple published studies have reported varying incidence of malignancy. Malignancies may occur prior to the onset of myositis, concurrently with myositis, or after the onset of dermatomyositis. In addition, the myositis may follow the course of the malignancy or may follow its own course independent of the treatment of the malignancy. Studies supporting the relationship of myositis and malignancy, as well as those purporting to demonstrate a non-relationship, have been reported. In addition, studies demonstrating benefits of cancer surgery on myositis as well as those showing no relationship to the myositis or malignancy have been reported.

A wide variety of malignancies have been reported in patients with dermatomyositis and polymyositis. It had been suggested that gynecologic malignancy, in particular ovarian carcinoma, was overrepresented in published reports. Furthermore, in an Asian population, it seems that carcinoma of the nasopharynx is overrepresented. To date, studies have not convincingly demonstrated that there is overrepresentation of any one tumor.

Another issue is whether or not age is a factor in the frequency of malignancy in patients with myositis. Reports of young adults and children have appeared suggesting that age alone is not a factor in the presence of an underlying malignancy. Data relating the frequency of malignancy in patients with or without cutaneous findings have also been controversial. It has been our contention that dermatomyositis patients have more frequent associations with neoplasms than polymyositis patients. Further studies are required in order to substantiate this belief.

EVALUATION OF THE MYOSITIS PATIENT

The diagnosis of myositis is one of exclusion (Table 2–1). A complete history should be conducted, with particular attention to drugs or toxins that may be involved. It should include a history of previous malignancies, previous travel, changes in the diet, and any symptoms of associated phenomena such as dysphagia or dyspnea or arthritis. A thorough review of systems is necessary,

Table 2–1. EVALUATION OF THE PATIENT WITH MYOSITIS

1. *Careful history*
   a. Previous malignancy
   b. Associated symptoms
   c. History of toxins, infections, travel, drug intake
2. *Complete physical examination, including:*
   a. Female: pelvic and breast examinations
   b. Male: rectal examination
3. *Evaluation of muscle disease*
   a. Muscle biopsy
   b. EMG
   c. Creatine kinase (CK or CPK), aldolase, urinary creatine
4. *Routine laboratory studies*
   a. CBC, serum multiphasic analysis, urinalysis
   b. Chest x-ray
   c. Thyroid function
   d. Stool Hematest
   e. Electrocardiogram
   f. Female: Pap smear, mammography
5. *Pulmonary function tests*
6. *Esophageal studies:* manometry or cineradiography
7. *Optional*
   a. Holter monitor
   b. Echocardiogram
   c. Antibody studies: Jo-1, PM-1, Mi-2, 3
   d. Viral serologies
8. Further testing is based on abnormalities discovered in above tests (1–4).

which will aid in the evaluation of patients with dermatomyositis for malignancies.

A complete history and physical examination should be conducted, even if the examining physician is a specialist. The examination should include a careful breast and pelvic examination in women. These examinations should *not* be deferred. If the examiner does not feel confident in these areas, it is necessary to obtain gynecologic consultation. Similarly, in men, a rectal and prostate examination is necessary.

Routine laboratory evaluation includes a complete blood count and serum multiphasic analysis, urinalysis, chest roentgenogram, stool for Hematest, tests for thyroid function, an electrocardiogram, and, in women, mammography and a Pap smear. Pulmonary function tests (PFT) should be performed, including diffusion studies, regardless of whether there are symptoms or abnormalities on chest x-ray. An esophageal study is necessary to evaluate the possibility of dysmotility. Optional studies include a Holter monitor and echocardiography and serologic tests. Tests of antinuclear antibody (ANA), although they may be positive in pure cases of dermatomyositis-polymyositis, have not been shown to influence the prediction of the course of the disease or its therapy. Newer serologic studies such as the Jo-1 antibody may give physicians insights on pathogenesis, but at present they are still only useful for investigators. The correlation of Jo-1 with pulmonary disease has been reported, but whether the findings are positive or negative, pulmonary function testing should be ordered. Immunogenetic (HLA) testing has been of no value in the therapy of patients.

Subsequent evaluation is necessary following the initiation of therapy. Repeat testing of each abnormality is advised. Following the myositis generally includes a combination of the clinical examination with muscle enzyme determinations. Repeat muscle biopsy or electromyography are reserved for unusual circumstances. The use of biomechanical assessment to quantitate muscle strength may be of benefit in following patients' courses. Careful questioning for new symptoms should occur at each follow-up visit, and if a symptom develops, careful evaluation is necessary. On at least a yearly basis a repeat chest x-ray; urinalysis; CBC; serum multiphasic analysis; stool guaiac; rectal, pelvic, and breast examinations; mammography; and a Pap smear should be conducted.

COURSE AND THERAPY

Several general measures are helpful in treating patients with dermatomyositis and polymyositis. Bedrest is often valuable in the individual with progressive weakness; however, this must be combined with an aggressive but passive range of motion exercise program to prevent contractures. Nutrition is important because of a negative nitrogen balance that exists in inflammatory myopathy. Patients who have evidence of dysphagia should have the head of their bed elevated and should avoid eating meals before retiring.

The mainstay of therapy for dermatomyositis is the use of systemic corticosteroids. Debate over low-dose therapy versus high dose therapy and alternate day therapy has occurred. Traditionally, prednisone is given in a dose of 40–60 mg daily as the initial therapy. The treatment should continue for at least 1 month after the myositis has become clinically and enzymatically inactive. At this point the dose is slowly tapered, generally over a period lasting $1\frac{1}{2}$ to 2 times as long as the period of active treatment. Approximately 25 to 30% of patients with dermatomyositis and/or polymyositis will not respond to systemic corticosteroids or will develop significant steroid-related side-effects. In these patients, immunosuppressive agents may be an effective means of inducing or maintaining a remission. Roughly one half to three fourths of the patients treated with an immunosuppressive agent will respond with an increase in strength, a decrease in enzyme levels, or a reduction in steroid dosage.

Methotrexate can be used on a weekly basis, given either by mouth or intravenously. Methotrexate is administered in an empiric dose of 25–50 mg per week. The drug usually becomes effective in 4–8 weeks and, therefore, is not recommended for rapid control of a fulminant disease process.

Azathioprine has been used in a double-blind controlled trial with prednisone versus a group with prednisone and placebo. In a short term analysis of 3 months, there were no differences between these two groups.

However, in the open follow-up study 3 years later, there was a significantly lower steroid dosage and a significantly greater muscle strength in the patients who had been treated with azathioprine. Azathioprine is administered orally in a dose of 2 mg/kg/day.

The use of immunosuppressive agents is to be undertaken with caution. The usual measures of follow-up of these patients are necessary; a complete evaluation prior to prescribing immunosuppressive therapy is also necessary. The need for liver biopsy in patients being given methotrexate is controversial, but if chronic therapy is planned, liver biopsy should accompany this therapy.

Some patients will fail to respond to these agents as well, and in these individuals various other measures have been suggested. Anecdotal reports exist supporting the benefits of plasmapheresis, pulse methylprednisolone therapy, combination immunosuppressive therapy, cyclosporin-A, and total body irradiation. These methods all have multiple side-effects associated with their use, and they should be reserved for the most severe and non-responsive cases.

Therapy of cutaneous disease in patients with dermatomyositis is often difficult because even though the myositis may respond to treatment with corticosteroids and/or immunosuppressives, the cutaneous lesions often persist. Although cutaneous disease may be of minor importance in patients with serious fulminant myositis, in many patients cutaneous disease becomes a most important aspect of their disorder. Most patients with cutaneous lesions are photosensitive; thus, as in patients with lupus erythematosus, the daily use of a sunscreen with a sun protective factor (SPF) of at least 15 is recommended. Hydroxychloroquine in dosages of 200–400 mg per day is effective in approximately 80% of patients treated, as a means of partially controlling their cutaneous disease and allowing a decrease in the corticosteroid dosage. The patients who do not respond well or fully to hydroxychloroquine can be switched to chloroquine therapy, 250–500 mg per day, or can have quinacrine 100 mg twice daily added to their regimen. The usual precautions regarding antimalarial therapy should be undertaken, including careful ophthalmologic examination and follow-up.

The prognosis of dermatomyositis and polymyositis varies greatly, depending on the series of patients studied. Factors that affect the prognosis include the patient's age, the type and severity of myositis, the presence of dysphagia, the presence of an associated malignancy, and the response to corticosteroid therapy. That therapy alters prognosis seems to be well established by retrospective reports on the benefits of corticosteroids and immunosuppressives.

Suggested Readings

Bohan A, Peter JB, Bowman RL, et al: A computer-assisted analysis of 153 patients with polymyositis and dermatomyositis. Medicine 56:255, 1957.

Callen JP: Dermatomyositis and polymyositis. Disease-a-Month 33:239–305, 1987.

Callen JP, Hyla JF, Boles GG, et al: The relationship of dermatomyositis and polymyositis to internal malignancy. Arch Dermatol 116:295, 1980.

Lakhanpal S, Bunch TW, Melton LJ III: Polymyositis-dermatomyositis and malignant lesions: Does an association exist? Mayo Clin Proc 61:645–653, 1986.

Manchul L, Jin A, Pritchard KI, et al: The frequency of malignancy in patients with PM/DM. Arch Intern Med 145:1835, 1985.

Taieb A, Guichard C, Salamn R, et al: Prognosis in juvenile dermatopolymyositis: A cooperative retrospective study of 90 cases. Ped Dermatol 2:275–281, 1985.

Woo TY, Callen JP, Voorhees JJ, et al: Cutaneous lesions of dermatomyositis are improved by hydroxychloroquine. J Am Acad Dermatol 10:592–600, 1984.

3

Scleroderma, Raynaud's Phenomenon, and Related Conditions

KENNETH E. GREER

SCLERODERMA

Scleroderma is a cutaneous or multisystem disease of unknown cause and is classified into two major categories, localized or systemic (Table 3–1). Cutaneous sclerosis is the hallmark of the disease, although scleroderma-like changes occur in many diseases that are not part of the clinical spectrum of scleroderma. These disorders include porphyria cutanea tarda, graft versus host reaction, Werner's syndrome, vinyl chloride disease, carcinoid syndrome, Buschke's scleredema, and bleomycin toxicity.

Localized Scleroderma

Localized scleroderma can be divided into morphea and linear forms. Morphea is fur-

Table 3–1. CLASSIFICATION OF SCLERODERMA

Localized Scleroderma
  Morphea: plaque, guttate, generalized, and
    pansclerotic
  Linear (including en coup de sabre)

Systemic Scleroderma
  CREST syndrome (acrosclerosis)
  Diffuse scleroderma or progressive systemic sclerosis
    (PSS)

ther subdivided into plaque, guttate, generalized, and pansclerotic morphea. Plaque morphea, by far the most common form of localized scleroderma, occurs more frequently in females than males, develops primarily in children and young adults, and has no racial predilection. The lesions, which are usually single or few in number, begin as flesh-colored to erythematous edematous plaques. The center gradually becomes white and sclerotic, but, during the active growth phase, the border is often violaceous (Fig. 3–1). Hyperpigmentation and softening develop after a period of months to several years. Plaques on the trunk, the preferred site, are frequently oval in shape and vary from a few to many centimeters in diameter. However, lesions may be irregular and may occur on any site, including rarely the face.

The plaques are not bound to deeper structures and are rarely symptomatic. Guttate morphea refers to a rare variant that is characterized by multiple, 2–5 mm lesions. It is often confused with lichen sclerosis et atrophicus. The guttate lesions are not nearly as sclerotic as the plaques of morphea, but they may occur in combination with plaque disease. Speckled hypo/hyperpigmentation may persist for years after the lesions have resolved. Generalized morphea occurs rarely

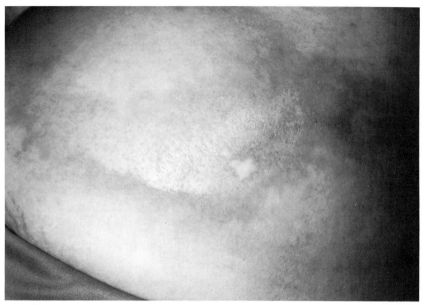

Figure 3–1. Sclerotic plaque of localized morphea with hyperemic border.

and can be divided into two forms. Adult generalized morphea resembles plaque disease with the exceptions of the large number of lesions, frequently coalescing on the trunk

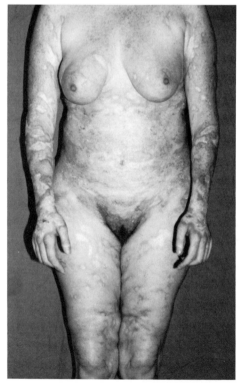

Figure 3–2. Generalized disabling pansclerotic morphea.

and extremities, and the morbidity, including pruritus and disability from the extensive sclerosis. Diaz-Perez and coworkers described a second form of generalized morphea, which they called disabling pansclerotic morphea of children. Although most common in young children, the disease can have its onset during late adolescence or early adulthood. Extensive and severe sclerosis is associated with musculoskeletal involvement and may produce cutaneous ulcers, contractures, and marked disability (Fig. 3–2). Bullae can occasionally occur in areas of extensive sclerosis (Fig. 3–3).

Linear scleroderma is classified as a form of localized scleroderma and is probably distinct from morphea. It can occur as a single lesion, usually on an extremity, can be widespread (Fig. 3–4), or can be limited to the forehead and scalp, where it is known classically as en coup de sabre (Fig. 3–5). Linear scleroderma occurs primarily in children and is seen most frequently on the lower extremity. It may produce contractures and limb shortening as a result of involvement of muscle and bone, distinguishing features from morphea. In addition, individuals with linear scleroderma are more likely to have antinuclear antibodies, hyperglobulinemia, eosinophilia, and antibodies to single-stranded DNA than patients with morphea. These findings have been correlated with contractures and with con-

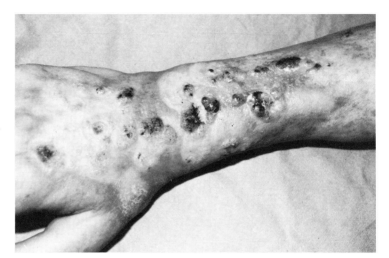

Figure 3–3. Bullae in severely scarred plaque of morphea.

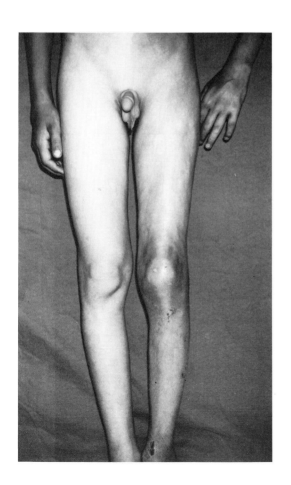

Figure 3–4. Unilateral linear morphea producing dystrophic changes of the arm and leg.

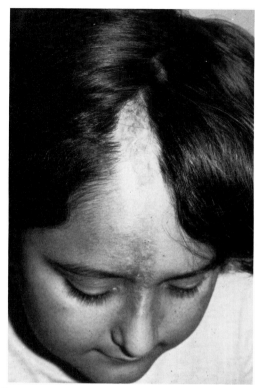

Figure 3–5. Linear scleroderma of the forehead (en coup de sabre).

tinued disease activity. Widespread linear scleroderma tends to be unilateral, and, since the onset most frequently occurs during the first two decades of life, severe deformities may result, including hemiatrophy of an extremity or severe distortion of the face, producing the changes of the Parry-Romberg syndrome, or facial hemiatrophy.

The diagnosis of morphea and other forms of localized scleroderma is based on the clinical appearance of the lesions and on the histopathologic findings. Biopsy specimens from well developed lesions reveal a normal epidermis, thickened and densely packed collagen bundles in the dermis, atrophy or absence of the skin appendages, and, not infrequently, replacement of the fat cells in the subcutaneous tissue by pale staining hyalinized collagen bundles. This histologic picture is identical to the changes seen in the skin in systemic scleroderma. In the early inflammatory stages of morphea, especially in specimens from the violaceous border, a predominantly lymphocytic infiltrate is seen between the collagen bundles and around the blood vessels. Rarely, subepidermal bullae, which probably result from lymphatic obstruction, are seen in severe generalized or pansclerotic morphea. The inflammatory and bullous changes are not seen in systemic scleroderma. The major disorder considered in the differential diagnosis of the plaque lesions of morphea is atrophoderma of Pasini and Pierini, and this disease may well be an end stage of morphea. Lichen sclerosis et atrophicus is the disease most often confused with guttate and, occasionally, generalized morphea (Fig. 3–6). Linear scleroderma, including en coup de sabre, is distinctive and rarely confused with other dermatological diseases. There is no effective treatment of localized scleroderma, although multiple therapies have been tried.

Eosinophilic fasciitis (also known as diffuse fasciitis with eosinophilia, or Shulman's syndrome) has features that are similar to those seen in scleroderma, especially the localized linear type. This disorder, which occurs most frequently on the proximal extremities, is characterized by pain, swelling, and, ultimately, induration. "Strenuous" exercise has been cited as a common trigger for the onset of this rare disease. Blood eosinophilia and hypergammaglobulinemia are common. Antinuclear antibodies (ANA) are rare. The patients have a good response to corticosteroid therapy, which certainly helps to distinguish them from those individuals with scleroderma.

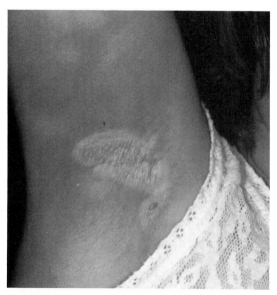

Figure 3–6. Localized hypopigmented lesions exhibiting features of both lichen sclerosus et atrophicus and morphea.

Systemic Scleroderma

Systemic scleroderma is divided into two subgroups: (1) acrosclerosis or the CREST syndrome, and (2) progressive systemic scleroderma with diffuse involvement. There is controversy concerning this division, as there may be considerable overlap between the two groups. The majority of patients, however, have a chronic or protracted course over a period of years, and they tend to have the clinical features characteristic of the CREST syndrome. A smaller group of patients have an aggressive and more diffuse form of scleroderma and shortened survival. The CREST syndrome is by no means benign in all patients, as it can cause severe morbidity. In addition to clinical differences, there is one laboratory test that may be helpful in separating systemic scleroderma into two groups. The speckled nuclear or centromere pattern of the ANA test appears to be a laboratory marker for the CREST subset.

CREST Syndrome

Winterbauer is credited for coining the term CRST syndrome in 1964 on the basis of subcutaneous calcinosis (C), Raynaud's phenomenon (R), sclerodactyly (S), and multiple telangiectasias (T). He differentiated this group of patients from both those with hereditary hemorrhagic telangiectasia and those with scleroderma. Rodnan and others added esophageal (E) involvement to include the syndrome as a definite subset of scleroderma. They also expanded the "S" to include more diffuse involvement than sclerodactyly (involvement of the digits). The expanded "S" included what was known as acrosclerosis, a much older term in the nomenclature of scleroderma.

The majority of patients with the CREST syndrome are female. Calcinosis cutis occurs late in the course of the disease and is not as disabling as it is in dermatomyositis. The calcium deposits are seen primarily as small foci on the fingers and about the joints (Fig. 3–7). Raynaud's phenomenon (RP) occurs in virtually 10% of patients with this form of the disease and may antedate the development of cutaneous sclerosis by several years. The RP varies from mild vasospasm to severe vascular insufficiency. It occurs primarily in the fingers but occasionally involves the toes and the nose. The patients with minimal disease frequently have small, pitted scars on the fingertips, whereas those with severe disease may develop painful ulcers and gangrene. Esophageal involvement occurs in the majority of patients with systemic scleroderma, producing dysphagia, reflux esophagitis, and, ultimately, fibrosis and obstruction. Severe esophageal disease may lead to emaciation, weight loss, and aspiration pneumonia. Loss of the normal peristaltic function of the distal portion of the esophagus and replacement of the smooth muscle by collagen produce the esophageal disease. Dysfunction of the stomach, small bowel, and, rarely, the colon, occurs very late in the course of the disorder and usually causes few symptoms. Persistent diarrhea can occur with small bowel disease. Patients with CREST syndrome may develop pulmonary

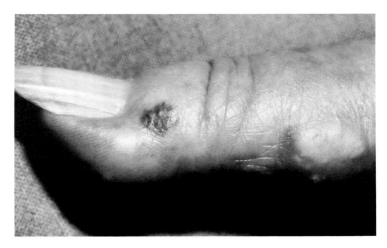

Figure 3–7. Telangiectatic mat and calcinosis cutis of the CREST syndrome.

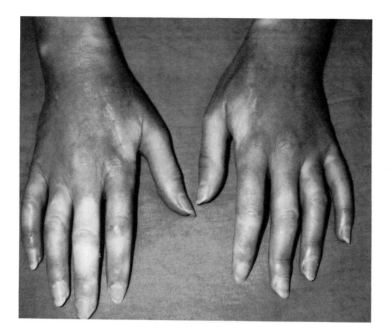

Figure 3–8. Taut, bound-down skin on the digits and hands in the CREST syndrome.

hypertension, but progressive fibrotic lung disease is rare.

The cutaneous sclerosis in the CREST group of patients typically is most severe on the fingers, producing taut, bound-down skin (Fig. 3–8). Ultimately, contractures and tapering of the distal portions of the fingers occur (Fig. 3–9). Late in the course of their disease, the majority of patients develop more widespread sclerosis, including on the face, upper trunk, and arms. This is more typical of the areas involved with progressive systemic sclerosis (PSS) and is evidence

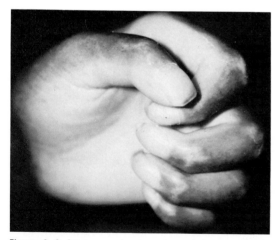

Figure 3–9. Severe contractures in end stage systemic scleroderma.

for the overlapping of CREST and PSS subsets. The vascular lesions, known as telangiectatic mats, occur on the hands (both dorsal and palmar aspects), central face, and oral mucous membranes and mimic the lesions of hereditary hemorrhagic telangiectasia. The telangiectasias cause no bleeding problems and are seen in the majority of patients with the CREST syndrome.

The prognosis for the CREST subset of patients with systemic scleroderma is superior to those with progressive systemic sclerosis. Eighty per cent of CREST patients in one large series survived over 20 years. Treatment is largely symptomatic and will be discussed with the treatment of progressive systemic scleroderma.

Progressive Systemic Sclerosis

Diffuse or progressive systemic scleroderma also occurs more frequently in females and may develop explosively or, more commonly, insidiously. The morbidity and mortality are related primarily to pulmonary, renal, and cardiac involvement and not to the cutaneous sclerosis, which typically begins in the chest and spreads to involve the head and extremities. The skin may be edematous and slightly erythematous at the onset, but pale, waxy, taut skin eventually ensues. Sclerodactyly may never develop, owing to the rapid course of the disease. Disturbance of the normal pigmentation of the skin is often remarkable in patients with systemic scleroderma, especially the diffuse form. Patients may develop widespread hyperpigmentation that simulates that of Addison's disease, but, more commonly, there is a patchy and often follicular hypo/hyperpigmentation that is most obvious in the areas of severe sclerosis (Fig. 3–10). This follicular pattern occurs late in the course of disease, can wax and wane in severity, and resembles repigmenting vitiligo. RP occurs frequently in progressive systemic scleroderma but is often insignificant in comparison with the problems produced by visceral disease. Telangiectatic mats and nailfold telangiectasias may be seen also.

Pulmonary System Involvement. Virtually all patients with progressive systemic scleroderma have abnormal pulmonary function tests, which may include reduced vital capacity, impaired carbon monoxide diffusion, and/or pulmonary hypertension. The pulmonary dysfunction is a result of actual parenchymal disease and not from restricted movement of the chest wall by the cutaneous sclerosis, as had originally been theorized. Roentgenograms of the chest are abnormal with chronic disease and may reveal fibrosis, cyst formation, and pulmonary calcification. There may be an increase in the incidence of alveolar cell carcinoma, as is seen in patients with extensive pulmonary fibrosis of any cause.

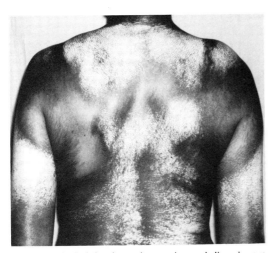

Figure 3–10. Patchy hypo-hyperpigmentation in systemic scleroderma.

Renal Involvement. Renal involvement occurs commonly in patients with diffuse systemic scleroderma, and renal failure is one of the leading causes of death in this disease. Proteinuria, hypertension, and azotemia may develop, especially late in the disease. Renal failure may be precipitated or aggravated by coexistent cardiac disease, manifesting as heart failure. Malignant hypertension may develop rapidly and, until successful intervention was achieved with potent antihypertensive drugs, dialysis, or renal transplantation, was uniformly fatal.

Cardiac Changes. Myocardial fibrosis as well as asymptomatic myocardial infarction from obliterative vascular changes may occur in patients with systemic scleroderma and can lead to a rapid downhill course and death. Congestive heart failure can also result from chronic pulmonary disease. Diagnostic studies for scleroderma heart disease include chest x-ray, electrocardiogram, and both invasive and non-invasive studies, such as cardiac catheterization and echocardiography.

Primary muscle, joint, and nervous system disease do occur in scleroderma, but they are relatively uncommon and may be seen more frequently in patients with overlap syndromes, such as sclerodermatomyositis, mixed connective tissue disease, or scleroderma and systemic lupus erythematosus.

Diagnosis, Course and Prognosis, and Treatment

The diagnosis of systemic scleroderma is primarily clinical, although there are laboratory studies that are helpful diagnostically and that may be important prognostically. These studies include baseline and follow-up tests for visceral involvement for pulmonary, renal, cardiac, and muscle disease. In addition, evaluation for antinuclear antibodies, including the anticentromere antibody, which may predict the likelihood of the more benign CREST form of the disease, is important. X-rays of the hands for calcification or of the teeth (widening of the periodontal space) have been used as confirmatory tests for the diagnosis in systemic disease. The barium swallow is more readily available than motility studies for evaluation of esophageal disease. The course of systemic scleroderma is largely unpredictable, but data from large series of patients suggest

Table 3–2. PHARMACOLOGIC AGENTS FOR SCLERODERMA

Hormones	Anti-inflammatory Agents	Lathyrogens	Immuno-suppressive Drugs	Vasoactive Agents	Miscellaneous Agents
Corticosteroids Cyclofenil	Potaba Nonsteroidal anti-inflammatory drugs	D-Penicillamine	Azathioprine Cyclo-phos-phamide	Captopril Nifedipine	Colchicine Dimethyl sulfoxide (DMSO)
Stanozolol				Prozosin	Phenytoin

that patients with CREST syndrome have prolonged survival when compared with patients with the progressive form of the disease. However, the morbidity may be severe with CREST syndrome, especially late in the course of the disease. Severe sclerodactyly limits hand function, as do the complications from RP. Esophagitis causes significant morbidity. Survival is greatly reduced by the presence of renal, cardiac, and pulmonary involvement, and these visceral changes occur earlier in the course of disease in patients with progressive scleroderma.

Owing largely to the fact that the cause of scleroderma is unknown, there is no cure and treatment is primarily directed toward complications. Pharmacologic agents that have been or are still frequently used in the treatment of scleroderma can be classified into various categories (Table 3–2). The two major groups of drugs that supposedly are directed toward what is believed to be the pathogenesis of scleroderma are the lathyrogens (D-penicillamine) and the immuno-suppressive agents (especially azathioprine and cyclophosphamide). The results of the treatment with these drugs are frequently disappointing, and side-effects are often substantial. To date there is no definite evidence that any one drug or group of drugs significantly affect the course of systemic scleroderma. Symptomatic treatment is essential to at least improve the quality of life and includes physical therapy, protection from the cold, and general skin care with proper hydration and lubrication. Medications are available for the symptomatic relief of RP (vasodilating agents primarily) and to treat esophagitis.

RAYNAUD'S PHENOMENON AND DISEASE

Raynaud's phenomenon (RP) and disease are due to paroxysmal vasospasm, primarily involving the digits, and are precipitated by an abrupt exposure to cooler temperature or by emotional stress. Raynaud's *disease* specifically refers to the idiopathic variety, and the *phenomenon* refers to identical clinical changes occurring with some other disease, especially a connective tissue disease. However, RP can occur as a result of constriction or obstruction of vessels from many causes, including vessel diseases such as atherosclerosis or thromboangiitis obliterans, neurovascular compression syndromes, and disorders of blood viscosity and agglutination, as well as from drugs (ergot, methylsergide, etc.) and as an occupational hazard (jackhammer operator classically). The majority of patients with RP will have an association with a connective tissue disease, especially systemic scleroderma. In scleroderma, the incidence of RP approaches 100%. RP is much more common in females than in males and occurs primarily in adult life.

Classic RP is a triphasic color reaction of pallor, followed by cyanosis and then a reactive hyperemia. The majority of patients, however, experience only one or two phases of the reaction, and the episodes usually occur over a period of a few minutes, at least initially. Each phase may be associated with specific symptoms. Arterial vasoconstriction produces the pallor, cold, and, often, numb digits. The cyanosis results from stagnation of venous blood as a result of a reduction in the vasospasm of the arterioles along with continued vasoconstriction of the venous outflow. Vasodilation produces the reactive hyperemia and may be accompanied by throbbing pain, burning, and swelling of the digits. RP initially appears on the digits of one or both hands and may eventually involve the feet, nose, ears, and tongue. Involvement of the digits is often splotchy or segmental. As the disorder progresses, vascular insufficiency frequently produces cutaneous ulcers, scars, and gangrenous lesions of the digits, causing significant morbidity.

The diagnosis is made clinically, but studies should be performed to differentiate Raynaud's disease from the phenomenon and its many causes. Angiography, thermography, and photoelectric plethysmography are primarily research tools and are rarely necessary to establish the diagnosis. Specific management is symptomatic for the disease and includes common sense (protection or avoidance from cold exposure), drugs (both those to be avoided, such as nicotine, ergot, and methylsergide, and those taken for protection, i.e., vasodilating drugs, such as nitroglycerin, nifedipine, prazosin, or reserpine), and, possibly, behavioral modification including biofeedback and relaxation techniques. The latter is helpful only in extremely motivated patients. Every attempt should be made to find a treatable cause for the Raynaud's phenomenon, but the therapeutic measures used for the disease are also employed. Avoidance of smoking and of smoke-filled rooms is essential for most patients with RP.

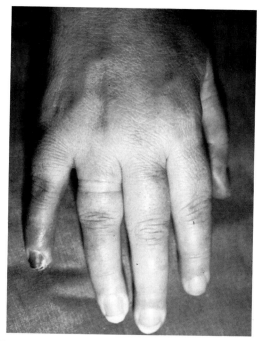

Figure 3–11. Puffy or edematous changes of the fingers in a patient with MCTD.

MIXED CONNECTIVE TISSUE DISEASE

Mixed connective tissue disease (MCTD) is classified as one of the overlap syndromes because it has features of several connective tissue disorders, especially lupus erythematosus and systemic scleroderma. Although somewhat controversial, MCTD is believed to be a distinct disorder that is defined by the presence of unusually high titers of a circulating antibody with specificity for a nuclear ribonucleoprotein antigen (U_1RNP) known as extractable nuclear antigen (ENA). In addition, anti-DNA antibodies are present only in a minority of patients and the positive antinuclear antibody in their sera produces a speckled immunofluorescence pattern. Overlap of two or three connective tissue disorders is not rare and is seen most frequently with systemic scleroderma and dermatomyositis and rarely with lupus erythematosus and dermatomyositis. Patients with such overlap syndromes do not have elevated titers of ENA and are not labeled as having MCTD. MCTD is much more common in women and has a mean age of onset of 37 years. The clinical features of MCTD include RP, swelling or puffiness of the fingers (Fig. 3–11) and hands, followed by sclerodactyly, arthralgias and arthritis, abnormal esophageal mobility, and polymyo-

sitis. Lupus erythematosus–like rashes, capillary dilatation of periungual vessels, Gottron's papules, and heliotrope discoloration of the eyelids are not infrequent cutaneous changes in MCTD, but widespread scleroderma and ulceration of the fingertips are rare.

The significance of separating MCTD from lupus erythematosus, systemic scleroderma, and dermatomyositis is based on studies of early series of patients that suggested that individuals with MCTD appeared to have a more benign course and a better response to prednisone than patients with these other connective tissue diseases. MCTD patients have a low incidence of renal and central nervous system disease, but not all patients have a benign course, especially those with early age onset of disease. Mild disease may be controlled with non-steroidal anti-inflammatory drugs or low doses of corticosteroids, but larger doses of prednisone, such as 1 mg/kg/day, are necessary in patients with more serious involvement of major organs. The changes least likely to respond to therapy appear to be the scleroderma-like features, especially pulmonary fibrosis. The ultimate prognosis in this relatively recently described disease is not known, and large series with prolonged follow-up are needed to determine this.

Suggested Readings

Braverman IM: Skin Signs of Systemic disease, 2nd ed. Philadelphia, WB Saunders Co., 1981, pp. 314–359.

Diaz-Perez JL, Connally SM, Winkelmann RK: Disabling pansclerotic morphea of children. Arch Dermatol 116:169–173, 1980.

Greer KE: Newer therapies of the sclerodermas. Derm Clin 1(4):505–515, 1983.

Lemmer JP, Curry NH, Mallory JH, et al: Clinical characteristics and course in patients with high titer anti-RNP antibodies. J Rheumatol 9:536–542, 1982.

McDonald CJ: Raynaud's syndrome. Derm Clin 1(4):493–504, 1983.

Rodnan GP, Medsger TA, Buckingham RB: Progressive systemic sclerosis–CREST syndrome: Observations on natural history and late complications in 90 patients. Arthritis Rheum 18:423, 1975.

Rodnan GP, Schumacher HR, Zvaifler NJ: Mixed connective tissue disease. In Primer on the Rheumatic Diseases, 8th ed. Atlanta, Arthritis Foundation, 1983, pp. 65–66.

Steen VD, Medsger TA, Rodnan GP: D-Penicillamine therapy in progressive systemic sclerosis (scleroderma). A retrospective analysis. Ann Intern Med 97:652, 1982.

Surwit RS, Gilgor RS, Allen LM, Duvic M: A double-blind study of prazosin in the treatment of Raynaud's phenomenon in scleroderma. Arch Dermatol 120:329–331, 1984.

4

Vasculitis

JEFFREY P. CALLEN

Vasculitis is a multisystem disorder with frequent involvement of the skin. The organs with the richest vascular supply are those most commonly affected by the disease process. There is evidence suggesting that the vasculitides are a reflection of an immune complex disease. In addition, local factors such as trauma, temperature, and pressure are involved in the clinical manifestations of the disease.

The understanding of the vasculitides has been difficult, owing to their many manifestations and the multitude of classifications that have been proposed. Part of the problem relates to descriptions by subspecialists, each with their own bias. This is similar to the story of the scientists examining an elephant while blindfolded. Each feels a different part, and the result is that there are multiple different descriptions of the same animal. In this chapter, we will discuss only cutaneous disease, and how it relates to the whole patient.

CLASSIFICATION

In 1952, Zeek offered a classification of vasculitis, which with modifications is still the one used today (Table 4–1). It is important to subclassify patients because of possible differences in etiopathogenesis, prognostic differences, associations with specific diseases or involvement in a certain organ,

Table 4–1. CLASSIFICATION OF VASCULITIS

Hypersensitivity vasculitis
Rheumatic vasculitis
Granulomatous vasculitis
Polyarteritis nodosa
Large vessel vasculitis

or because the therapeutic approach would be altered, Most of these features are not satisfied by this classification system. However, few, if any, of the other classification schemas have offered a better way to separate the disease into important subsets.

Another method of subclassifying these disorders separates the diseases by vessel size involved (Table 4–2). Capillaries are involved in capillaritis. Small vessels, usually the post-capillary venule, are involved in what is traditionally known as leukocytoclastic vasculitis (LV). Small arteries or arterioles can be involved in the panniculitides or polyarteritis nodosa (PAN). Medium-sized arteries are involved in PAN, particularly near their bifurcations, and in the granulomatous vasculitides. Lastly, large-sized vessels are involved in giant cell arteritis and its variants. The problem with this subclassification system lies with the fact that for the cutaneous disease even when it is associated with PAN or granulomatous vasculitis, the vessel involved is most often the post-capillary venule. Thus, palpable purpura, a common clinical correlate of vasculitis, can be seen as a manifestation of disease in several categories.

For the patient with cutaneous disease as a manifestation of vasculitis, it is necessary to perform a thorough systemic evaluation in order to offer reliable prognostic advice to the patient. The pitfalls of viewing a multisystem disorder through a specialist's eye is self-evident. Also, the problem of meaningful labeling and classification arises. Usually the label of PAN implies a poorer prognosis than that of cutaneous LV. However, as discussed previously and illustrated in the following discussion, these subclassifications are imperfect.

Table 4–2. CLASSIFICATION OF SYSTEMIC VASCULITIDES

Vessel Size	Clinical Picture	Systemic Symptoms	Therapy	Prognosis
Small vessel (venules)	Urticarial lesions, palpable purpura	Minimal	Symptomatic	Good
Small artery	Erythema nodosum	Mild, unless associated with systemic disorders	Symptomatic	Good
Medium-sized artery	Necrosis of major organs, livedo reticularis, purpura, mononeuritis multiplex	Severe	Steroids, cytotoxic drugs	Guarded
Large vessel	Claudication, necrosis	Moderate	Steroids, cytotoxic drugs	Poor

Probably our variation of these classifications can simplify and offer meaningful prognostication. We would divide these entities into those characterized by a small vessel vasculitis (necrotizing venulitis) versus those characterized by a large vessel vasculitis. The traditional leukocytoclastic vasculitis that could be due to unknown factors (idiopathic), infections, drugs, abnormal proteins, or an associated systemic disease is within the small vessel vasculitis category. In order to prognosticate within this group of patients, it is important to define the presence of and type of systemic involvement. Large vessel vasculitis includes PAN, granulomatous vasculitides, and giant cell arteritis. These patients generally have systemic disease, but they can have cutaneous disease. The cutaneous lesions can consist of those of typical LV, but claudication, ischemic changes, necrosis, and livedo reticularis may be more common.

PATHOGENESIS AND ETIOLOGIC ASSOCIATIONS

There is strong experimental and clinical evidence suggesting that cutaneous LV is an immune complex disease (Type III hypersensitivity reaction). Although there are multiple causes or associated conditions that are possible, and there are many clinical expressions, the linkage between the injury (etiology) and the manifestation is probably immune complex disease that leads to the inflammatory reaction.

Figure 4–1 is a schematic representation of the pathogenesis of LV. After antigenic exposure, soluble antigen-antibody complexes (circulating immune complexes— CIC) are formed. In the presence of antigen excess, these complexes can lodge in the vessel wall. Following the deposition of the CIC, a complex series of events are initiated that ultimately can lead to vessel wall dam-

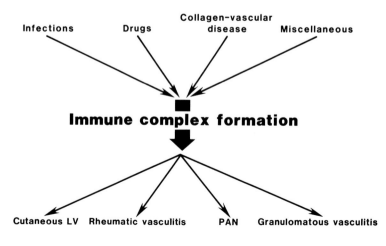

ANTIGENIC STIMULI

Infections   Drugs   Collagen–vascular disease   Miscellaneous

■ Immune complex formation

Cutaneous LV   Rheumatic vasculitis   PAN   Granulomatous vasculitis

Figure 4–1. A schematic representation of multiple antigenic exposures leading through the mechanisms of immune complex formation and deposition to the varying manifestations of vasculitis. LV = leukocytoclastic vasculitis; PAN = polyarteritis nodosa.

age, leakage of fluid, urticarial lesions, and leakage of red blood cells (purpura). With enough compromise, ischemia can occur and result in necrosis or ulceration of the skin.

In addition to the immunologic events, several non-immunologic factors may play a role in disease expression. Vasoactive amines, in particular histamine, can lead to deposition of immune complexes. This fact is clinically useful in identifying circulating immune complexes. Also, local factors such as anatomic location and viscosity may help explain the clinical manifestations of the vasculitic syndrome.

Multiple etiologic agents have been implicated in the various vasculitic syndromes. In general, the lists of etiologic factors or associated conditions are similar for all the syndromes and involve infections, drugs, protein abnormalities, and rheumatologic disease. Also, no matter which clinical syndrome appears, about half of the patients do not have an associated condition or an obvious etiologic agent (idiopathic). Table 4–3

Table 4–3. ETIOLOGIC FACTORS INVOLVED IN VASCULITIC SYNDROMES

A. *Infections*
  1. Hepatitis B (rarely hepatitis A)
  2. Acute respiratory infections (viral or bacterial)
  3. Streptococcal infections and post-streptococcal diseases
  4. Bacterial endocarditis
  5. Intestinal bypass syndrome
  6. Mycobacterial diseases
B. *Drugs:* Any drug can cause vasculitis, but particularly:
  1. Aspirin
  2. Sulfonamides
  3. Penicillins
  4. Barbiturates
  5. Amphetamines
  6. Propylthiouracil
C. *Genetic:* Deficiency of a component of complement
D. *Abnormal globulins*
  1. Cryoglobulinemia: essential or secondary
  2. Multiple myeloma
  3. Macroglobulinemia
E. *Rheumatic diseases*
  1. Systemic lupus erythematosus
  2. Rheumatoid vasculitis
  3. Dermatopolymyositis
F. *Other diseases*
  1. Ulcerative colitis
  2. Lymphomas
  3. Colonic carcinoma
  4. Hairy cell leukemia
  5. Serous otitis media
G. *Idiopathic*

lists the commonly found etiologic factors and associated conditions.

Several issues regarding etiologic associations are worthy of special mention. Although almost any drug can cause vasculitis, several as listed seem to be reported more frequently. Occasionally it becomes difficult to distinguish between an infection and an antibiotic as the etiologic agent. Rheumatic syndromes can be associated with the full gamut of vasculitic syndromes, and a small vessel cutaneous LV with a benign prognosis can and does occcur in rheumatoid arthritis. Therefore, the term rheumatoid vasculitis is insufficient to make prognostic statements. Similarly, urticarial lesions, palpable purpura, or large vessel vasculitis can complicate lupus erythematosus. Lastly, a host of unusual associations exist, including hairy cell leukemia, inflammatory bowel disease, and various solid tumors.

In reviewing the frequency of associations in our community (Louisville, Kentucky), it became evident that the experiences of practitioners are different from those seen in referral medical centers. There was a much lower incidence of paraproteinemias and malignancies. Subsequently, within a group of referred LV patients, I have found some individuals with hyperglobulinemia, some with complement component (C2) deficiencies, and a few with a malignancy.

CLINICAL MANIFESTATIONS

Small vessel vasculitis involves the postcapillary venules, and as such the lesions represented are most often urticaria-like lesions or palpable purpura (Fig. 4–2; Plate IG). Additionally, vesiculobullous lesions (Fig. 4–3), pustules, necrosis, and ulceration can occur but are much less commonly seen. The purpuric lesions occur most frequently on the legs or dependent areas, whereas the urticaria-like lesions are usually generalized. The urticarial lesions are different from "garden-variety" urticaria; they tend to resolve over a prolonged period of time, may leave a bruised appearance, and are not as pruritic.

About 40–50% of patients with small vessel cutaneous LV do not have any systemic manifestations. The most common problems occur in patients with rheumatic syndromes and involve the joints. In patients with Henoch-Schönlein purpura (HSP), symptoms of

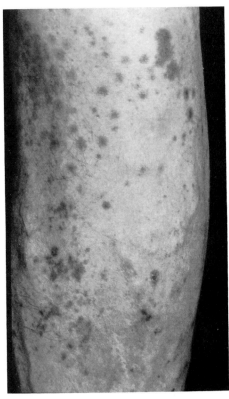

Figure 4–2. Typical palpable purpuric lesions seen in a patient with a hypersensitivity angiitis (cutaneous leukocytoclastic vasculitis) (see also Plate I*G*).

abdominal pain, arthritis, and signs of renal involvement are frequent. HSP is more common in children, but it can occur in adults as well. It may be different in some respects, since it is associated in most cases with IgA circulating complexes. Patients with abnormal proteins generally have additional symptoms. In addition to the aforementioned problems, almost any organ system can be involved in patients with small vessel vasculitis. Gastrointestinal symptoms include colicky pain, hemorrhage, ulceration, and perforation. Pulmonary involvement includes pleuritis and effusions (particularly in lupus erythematosus patients), nodules, infiltrates, or cavitation. Nervous system involvement can be manifested by neuropathy, cephalalagia, or intracranial hemorrhage. Lastly, rare patients can have pancreatitis or myocarditis. Fortunately, signs and symptoms of major organ involvement are rare in cutaneous LV when seen in the general population.

An unusual cutaneous vasculitic syndrome known as erythema elevatum diutinum (EED) is worthy of special mention. It is rare, but its major manifestation is skin disease. The lesions begin as red-purple papules that coalesce to form red-yellow plaques (Fig. 4–4; Plate I*H*). The lesions are most prominent over points of trauma such as the elbows, knees, dorsum of the hands, and buttocks. Systemic disease is rare. EED is said to be responsive to the antileprosy agent dapsone, whereas most cases of the other cutaneous vasculitides may be dapsone resistant.

The prognosis of cutaneous LV is directly dependent on the presence or absence of major organ involvement, and thus is generally good. Most patients with drugs or infections as an etiologic association will have a self-limited course. Some patients will have recurrent disease, whereas about one fourth will have chronic cutaneous LV that lasts more than 3 months. Among our patients with chronic cutaneous LV, there appears to be a higher incidence of associated rheumatic diseases and abnormal circulating proteins.

Large vessel vasculitis involves arterioles and arteries. Patients with large vessel disease can also have small vessel cutaneous

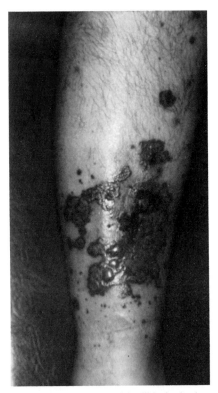

Figure 4–3. Bullous lesions exist within typical areas of palpable purpura in this patient with leukocytoclastic vasculitis and cancer of the colon.

Systemic signs and symptoms are common in large vessel vasculitis and include those mentioned previously for small vessel disease. The types of "large" vessel vasculitis include classic polyarteritis nodosa (PAN), Wegener's granulomatosis, allergic granulomatosis of Churg-Strauss, and giant cell arteritis. With the exception of the last syndrome, all of these have similar clinical manifestations on the skin.

PAN is in general a systemic vasculitis. Rarely patients have disease limited to the skin (cutaneous PAN). PAN is associated with multisystem involvement, and patients with it have significant morbidity and potentially fatal outcomes. The skin is involved in 40–50% of patients with PAN. This involvement may be palpable purpura, livedo reticularis (Fig. 4–6), nodules, necrosis, or ulcerations (Fig. 4–7). Urticarial lesions have been described early in PAN associated with hepatitis B antigen-antibody complexes. Systemic disease frequently involves the kidneys and may result in renal failure and/or hypertension. Peripheral neuropathy, arthritis, and/or muscle weakness are also very common. The lungs are not commonly involved, which helps to distinguish PAN from Churg-Strauss allergic granulomatous angiitis.

Wegener's granulomatosis (WG) occurs in limited and generalized forms. The limited form usually involves only the respiratory tract, whereas the generalized form is characterized by respiratory tract involvement, glomerulonephritis, and eye disease. Cutaneous involvement in WG is generally manifested by a small vessel vasculitis, and the

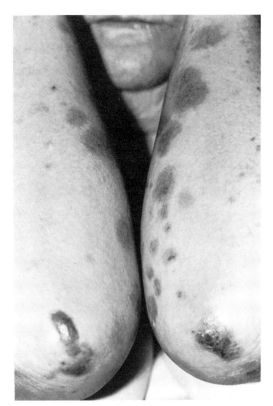

Figure 4–4. Erythema elevatum diutinum. These violaceous nodular lesions on the extensor surfaces and over bone prominences represent a localized leukocytoclastic vasculitis (see also Plate I*H*). (Courtesy of Dr. Neil A. Fenske, Tampa, FL.)

vasculitis (Fig. 4–5), which complicates the classification. Involvement of the larger vessels may result in livedo reticularis, purpura, necrosis, ulceration of the skin, Raynaud's phenomenon, and/or small nailfold infarcts.

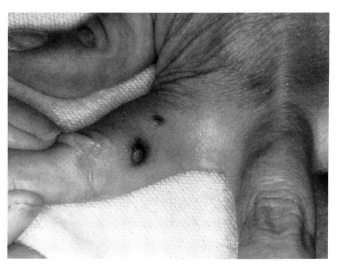

Figure 4–5. Cutaneous leukocytoclastic vasculitis was the first evidence of recurrence of this patient's Wegener's granulomatosis.

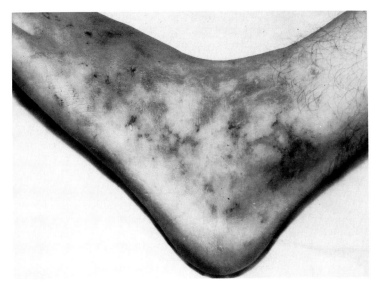

Figure 4–6. Cutaneous polyarteritis nodosa as manifested by a livedo pattern with purpuric and necrotic lesions.

skin biopsy rarely demonstrates granulomatous vasculitis. The skin disease may or may not correlate with active systemic disease. WG is associated with progressive, life-threatening disease; thus, aggressive therapy is indicated.

Allergic granulomatous angiitis (AGA) of Churg-Strauss combines features of PAN with asthma, eosinophilia (circulating and tissue bound), granuloma formation, and frequent pulmonary involvement. Renal involvement occurs less frequently than in PAN or WG. Skin disease occurs in 50–60% of patients with AGA and can involve a palpable purpura (small vessel vasculitis) or nodules. The nodular skin lesions are representative of a necrotizing palisading granuloma with eosinophils. The skin disease does not always correlate with active systemic involvement.

Giant cell arteritis is characterized by involvement of the largest vessels and includes temporal arteritis (TA), polymyalgia rheumatica, and Takayasu's aortitis within its classification. Cutaneous disease is rare, but an occasional patient with TA will have scalp necrosis as a result of ischemia.

Rheumatic vasculitis refers to any of the vasculitides in a patient with one of the collagen-vascular diseases such as rheumatoid arthritis, lupus erythematosus, Sjögren's syndrome, scleroderma (progressive systemic sclerosis [PSS]), or dermatomyositis-polymyositis. As referred to previously, in

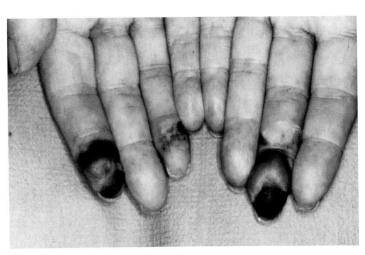

Figure 4–7. Ischemic necrosis of the fingertips in a patient with polyarteritis nodosa secondary to hepatitis B antigenemia. (Courtesy of Dr. Neil A. Fenske, Tampa, FL.)

both small and large vessel vasculitis, collagen-vascular syndromes are listed among the associated conditions. Thus, rheumatic vasculitis becomes a very confusing concept. Several developments in this area, however, are worthy of consideration.

Patients with lupus erythematosus can have various vasculitic syndromes. Urticarial vasculitis has been reported on numerous occasions in systemic lupus erythematosus (SLE). These patients have been said to have active clinical disease, often with renal involvement. Our group has reported that 25% of patients with subacute cutaneous lupus erythematosus who were anti-Ro (SS-A) positive had cutaneous vasculitis. One of these patients had urticarial lesions, whereas three had palpable purpura and one had palpable purpura and nailfold infarcts. The vasculitis in these patients has been associated with active joint disease in 4 patients and with active renal disease in 1 patient, but other serious systemic sequelae have not occurred. In contrast, when vasculitis is manifested by nailfold infarcts or livedo reticularis in the general SLE population, our experience has been that it is associated with active progressive renal and/or central nervous system involvement.

Rheumatoid arthritis may be complicated by vasculitis. In addition, capillaritis has been reported as a complication of rheumatoid arthritis. Rheumatoid vasculitis (RV) is usually characterized by palpable purpura, digital infarcts, nodules, ulcerations (Fig. 4–8), or necrosis. RV has been correlated with high titers of rheumatoid factor and with the presence of rheumatoid nodules. The role of corticosteroids in the induction of RV is controversial, and it seems doubtful to us that corticosteroid therapy will cause this complication. In a large study, Scott and colleagues reported that cutaneous lesions complicated RV in 88% of the 50 patients. RV is frequently a systemic vasculitis with an associated mortality rate of 30–40%. The prognosis appears to be worse in RV when neuropathy is present or when the vasculitis is an early manifestation of systemic disease.

Inflammatory vascular disease (vasculitis) has been recognized as a complication of Sjögren's syndrome. Provost and his coworkers have characterized two varieties, one with predominant neutrophilic vasculitis, and one in which mononuclear cells predominate. These patients with leukocytoclastic vasculitis (LV) have high titers of anti-Ro (SS-A) antibodies, rheumatoid factor, hyperglobulinemia, and hypocomplementemia. Those with mononuclear inflammatory vasculopathy do not have these features. However, both types of vasculopathy are associated with frequent peripheral and/or central nervous system disease.

DIFFERENTIAL DIAGNOSIS AND PATIENT EVALUATION

Palpable purpura is the most common finding in cutaneous vasculitis, and the differential diagnosis of purpura is dealt with in Chapter 12. Several steps are necessary in the differential considerations of purpura. The first step is deciding whether the lesions are palpable or macular. Macular purpura may be representative of thrombocytopenia, disseminated intravascular coagulation, Rocky Mountain spotted fever, or hemorrhagic disorders (see Chapter 12). In addition, if pustules are present, the differential diagnosis must be expanded to include infections such as disseminated gonorrhea and bacterial or fungal endocarditis. Palpable purpura can occur in embolic disorders such as endocarditis, artheromatous emboli (Fig. 4–9), or left atrial myxoma, as well as in leukocytoclastic vasculitis.

After the diagnosis has been confirmed, considerations of whether the process is systemic in nature and its severity become im-

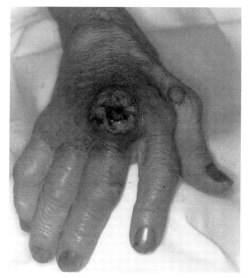

Figure 4–8. Nodular leukocytoclastic vasculitis in a patient with rheumatoid arthritis.

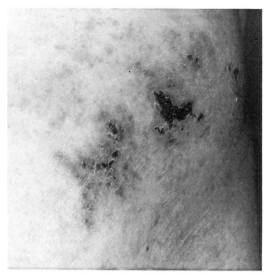

Figure 4–9. Livedo reticularis with cutaneous necrosis is present in this patient with atheromatous emboli.

portant. It becomes necessary to evaluate whether the small vessel vasculitis seen on the skin is a manifestation of a large vessel vasculitis. Also, all of the potential associations, particularly those that might alter the therapeutic approach or prognosis, must be sought. The basic evaluation is thorough and comprehensive (Table 4–4). A thorough

Table 4–4. EVALUATION OF PATIENTS WITH VASCULITIS

1. *History*
   a. Infections
   b. Drugs
   c. Other symptoms: Raynaud's phenomenon, musculoskeletal, neurologic, cardiorespiratory, etc.
   d. Previous history of associated disorders
2. *Physical examination*
   a. General appearance
   b. Type of cutaneous lesion
3. *Skin biopsy*
4. *Laboratory studies*
   a. *Necessary*
      i. Complete blood count
      ii. Sedimentation rate
      iii. Urinalysis
      iv. Cryoglobulin, serum protein electrophoresis
      v. Hepatitis B antigen
      vi. Antinuclear antibody, anti-Ro (SS-A)
      vii. Chest x-ray
      viii. Serum multiphasic analysis, which includes test of renal and hepatic function
   b. *Optional*
      i. Total hemolytic complement
      ii. Circulating immune complexes
      iii. Skin biopsy for direct immunofluorescence

evaluation will be helpful in determining the prognosis.

THERAPY

The therapy of vasculitis is based on the organs involved and on the severity of disease. All the agents used in treating vasculitides have anti-inflammatory effects as part of their mode of action. Certain of the vasculitides have specific therapies, such as dapsone (diaminodiphenylsulfone [DDS]) for EED.

Any factor causing or exacerbating vasculitis should be treated or removed. This may occur in the vasculitis complicating drug therapy, treatable infections, drug abuse, or tumors. Often the patient has recognized drugs as a cause and has stopped them. Other factors are more difficult to remove. Factors such as dependency or a cool environment can be altered by local measures that may be beneficial.

In limited cutaneous disease, whether palpable purpura of LV or cutaneous polyarteritis nodosa, little therapy may be required. Often antihistaminic agents are sufficient. In more persistent cases, salicylates and other non-steroidal anti-inflammatory agents may be effective. Colchicine has been shown to be effective in controlling chronic cutaneous vasculitis. In non-responsive patients, low doses of systemic corticosteroids can be used or, rarely, immunosuppressives may be added.

In urticarial vasculitis, the first line of therapy is antihistamines. Our experience suggests that usually therapy with systemic corticosteroids is necessary to control symptoms in these patients. Indomethacin has been reported to be an effective therapy, but our experience has not demonstrated it to be corticosteroid-sparing or to have other beneficial effects in urticarial vasculitis.

Systemic disease is treated with a variety of anti-inflammatory agents. Arthralgias, arthritis, serositis, and other musculoskeletal symptoms often respond to local measures and/or non-steroidal anti-inflammatory agents. Ophthalmologic disease is treated locally unless the optic nerve is involved.

Corticosteroid therapy is a first line of treatment for many patients. Although corticosteroids are used widely and are of short-term benefit for symptoms, there have been no published studies that confirm their efficacy by reduced morbidity or mortality. In patients with chronic disease, the continued use of corticosteroids may be fraught with multiple side-effects. Therefore, I usually attempt some form of adjuvant therapy in patients being given long-term corticosteroids. Agents with possible use are indomethacin, hydroxychloroquine, D-penicillamine, dapsone, colchicine, and immunosuppressive drugs. With the exception of the immunosuppressive drugs and colchicine, we have not found these other agents to be steroid-sparing or effective.

Many immunosuppressive and cytotoxic agents have been used in the treatment of vasculitis. The agents used most frequently are the alkylating agents such as cyclophosphamide or chlorambucil, the antimetabolite azathioprine, and the folic acid antagonist methotrexate. Cupps and Fauci have written that, of these agents, cyclophosphamide is the best in treating severe vasculitis. The other agents, in particular azathioprine, also can be beneficial in various vasculitides. Studies by Fauci and others have led to the conclusion that cyclophosphamide is the agent of choice in treating Wegener's granulomatosis and severe necrotizing vasculitis, which is steroid resistant. Cyclophosphamide produces lymphopenia and monocytopenia and a decrease in both T and B cells. The greatest decrease is in the level of circulating B cells. In this manner, the drug is believed to exert its immunosuppressive effects at doses that are not cytotoxic. Cyclophosphamide is used in a dosage of 2 mg/kg/day. Several weeks of therapy are necessary before benefits are seen and the corticosteroid dosage is lowered. This same induction period occurs with the other agents mentioned. When using cyclophosphamide, the physician must monitor carefully for leukopenia and bladder complications. Hemorrhagic cystitis can be avoided by the administration of cyclophosphamide early in the day and by proper hydration. Long-term sequelae are not usually problematic. However, patients on these drugs combined with corticosteroids are susceptible to infections, and viral infections may disseminate.

Chlorambucil is similar in its effects to cyclophosphamide but does not cause the bladder complications. It may be useful in patients with bladder problems from cyclophosphamide. Also, it has been used successfully in limited Wegener's granulomatosis.

Azathioprine, which is used extensively in renal transplantation, is believed by Cupps and Fauci to be less effective in vasculitis than is cyclophosphamide. It is complicated less often by leukopenia, and can be used as a corticosteroid-sparing agent.

Several other therapeutic modalities might be useful in the vasculitides. Plasmapheresis has been used to remove circulating agents such as immune complexes or antigens, so improvement is short-term and other therapeutic agents must be begun simultaneously. Complications include protein loss, volume reduction, and depletion of clotting factors. The use of plasmapheresis is best in acute situations in which a stopgap measure is necessary.

Suggested Readings

af Ekenstam E, Callen JP: Cutaneous leukocytoclastic vasculitis. Arch Dermatol 118:412–416, 1984.

Callen JP: Cutaneous vasculitis and its relationship to internal disease. Disease-a-Month 28:1–48, 1981 (Oct).

Callen JP: Colchicine is effective in controlling chronic cutaneous leukocytoclastic vasculitis. J Am Acad Dermatol 13:193–200, 1985.

Cupps TR, Fauci AS: The Vasculitides (Major Problems in Internal Medicine, No. 21). Philadelphia, WB Saunders Co., 1981.

Provost TT, Vasily D, Alexander E: Sjögren's syndrome: Cutaneous, immunologic, and nervous system manifestations. Neurol Clin, 5:405–426, 1987.

Sams WM Jr, Thorne EG, Small P, et al: Leukocytoclastic vasculitis. Arch Dermatol 112:219–226, 1976.

Scott DGI, Bacon PA, Tribe CR: Systemic rheumatoid vasculitis: A clinical and laboratory study of 50 cases. Medicine 60:288–297, 1981.

5

Cutaneous Disease and Arthritis

KENNETH E. GREER

RHEUMATOID ARTHRITIS

Definition, Diagnosis, and Epidemiologic Data

Rheumatoid arthritis (RA), defined classically by Garrod in 1858, is a multisystem disease of unknown etiology characterized primarily by its destructive attack on multiple joints, producing typical deformity in many cases. The clinical and pathologic findings result from chronic inflammation of synovial membranes. There is a remarkable heterogeneity from patient to patient with respect to the clinical manifestations and course of RA. Extra-articular activity commonly involves the skin and/or the lungs, but may also involve the hematologic, cardiovascular, and neurologic systems. Occasionally the extra-articular manifestations dominate the clinical picture, but most often RA is a disease of the joints. It has a worldwide distribution, affects females 2–3 times more often than males, and occurs at all ages, but especially between the fourth and sixth decade.

The diagnosis is relatively easy in advanced stages but is challenging early in the course of the disease. Criteria have been developed by the American Rheumatism Association (ARA) for diagnosis of classic, definite, probable, and possible RA, as well as criteria for clinical remission, disease progression, and functional capacity of patients with the disease. These criteria are available from the Arthritis Foundation, Atlanta, Georgia, and have been established primarily to classify large groups of patients for inclusion in epidemiologic surveys, drug trials, and studies of the natural history of RA. The diagnosis is made using a combination of clinical, roentgenographic, and laboratory findings, including the rheumatoid factor. Histologic changes of the synovium and the presence of skin nodules are additional criteria. The rheumatoid factor, measured primarily as IgM immunoglobulin with specificity against altered IgG, is positive in approximately 75% of patients with RA, but it is not specific for the disease, occurring in 1–5% of normal subjects. However, high titers of rheumatoid factor are generally associated with more severe forms of the disease, patients with rheumatoid nodules, and a higher incidence of systemic complications.

Cutaneous Features

There are a number of cutaneous findings reported in patients with RA, but there are no pathognomonic manifestations (Table 5–1). Very few of the conditions are characteristic for the disease, with the notable exception of the rheumatoid nodule. Pyoderma gangrenosum and a wide spectrum of vasculitic lesions are not uncommon in patients with RA, but they occur more commonly in association with other disorders. The rash of juvenile RA is very helpful in establishing the diagnosis of the disease, but it is certainly not specific. There is a large group of miscellaneous changes, most of them quite

Table 5–1. CUTANEOUS FINDINGS IN
RHEUMATOID ARTHRITIS

Rheumatoid nodules and superficial ulcerating
rheumatoid necrobiosis
Vasculitic lesions: petechiae and purpura to large
gangrenous plaques and ulcerations
Pyoderma gangrenosum
Urticaria-like lesions of Still's disease
Miscellaneous changes include palmar erythema,
nailfold capillary dilatation, atrophic or transparent
skin over bone prominences, patchy
hyperpigmentation, and red lunulae
Associated conditions: amyloidosis and bullous
diseases
Cutaneous changes associated with therapeutic
agents
Capillaritis

minor, that may be noted in patients with RA, and there are several distinct disorders that may be associated with RA on a statistical basis. Finally, there are a wide variety of cutaneous changes associated with various therapeutic agents for the disease.

Rheumatoid Nodules

Rheumatoid nodules are firm, non-tender, freely movable subcutaneous masses that occur in approximately 20–25% of adult patients with RA. They are the most characteristic extra-articular manifestations of the disease and are more common in patients with severe arthritis, high titer rheumatoid factor, or rheumatoid vasculitis. The dome-shaped, flesh-colored nodules usually vary from 0.5 cm to several cm in diameter and tend to arise in areas subject to trauma, particularly over bone prominences and especially near the elbows (Figs. 5–1 and 5–2). Any subcutaneous site can be affected, however, and histologically identical lesions have been found in the sclera, larynx, heart, lungs, and abdominal wall. The lesions develop insidiously and are usually persistent, although they may regress spontaneously. The clinical differential diagnosis of rheumatoid nodules includes gouty tophi, xanthomas, deep or nodular granuloma annulare, ganglions, and epidermal inclusion cysts. Histologically, 3 distinct zones are found in well-developed rheumatoid nodules: (1) a central zone of fibrinoid necrosis; (2) a middle zone of palisading histiocytes; and (3) a peripheral zone of highly vascularized granulation tissue with a chronic, mononuclear inflammatory cell infiltrate. Early lesions are composed primarily of the granulation tissue but with focal areas of leukocytoclastic vasculitis that are felt to be important in the pathogenesis of the nodules. The differential diagnosis histologically includes the transient nodules seen in acute rheumatic fever, granuloma annulare, and necrobiosis lipoidica diabeticorum.

Rheumatoid nodules have been seen in disorders other than RA, including systemic lupus erythematosus and scleroderma. They may also occur independently of other diseases and in a disorder reported as benign rheumatoid nodulosis. The nodules in this latter disorder are now believed to be the subcutaneous or nodular lesions of granuloma annulare and not those of RA. An additional necrobiotic but also ulcerative process reported extremely rarely in patients with RA has been called superficial ulcerating rheumatoid necrobiosis. Patients with

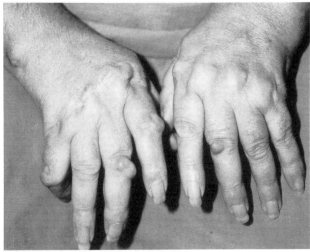

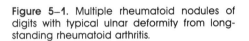
Figure 5–1. Multiple rheumatoid nodules of digits with typical ulnar deformity from long-standing rheumatoid arthritis.

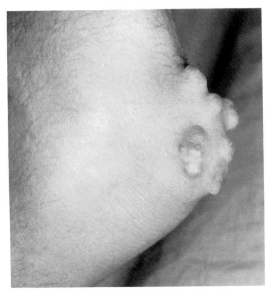

Figure 5–2. Rheumatoid nodules of the elbow.

this disorder have RA and superficial ulcerations of the legs, with histologic features resembling those of rheumatoid nodules (Fig. 5–3).

Rheumatoid Vasculitis

The spectrum of clinical lesions reported as those of rheumatoid vasculitis is wide and varies with the size and location of the vessels involved as well as with the extent of the disease. Leukocytoclastic changes can occur in the small arterioles and venules of the skin most commonly, but this same necrotizing process may rarely occur in larger vessels of the mesentery, heart, and central nervous system. Cutaneous lesions include petechiae, palpable purpura, gangrenous plaques, digital infarcts, and large ischemic ulcerations of the lower extremities, especially over the malleoli. The cutaneous vasculitis is usually found in patients with chronic and severe forms of RA and has been classified as mild, moderate, or severe. The cutaneous lesions of mild rheumatoid vasculitis include small digital infarcts, especially of the nailfolds and digital pulp, as well as petechiae and livedo reticularis. Palpable purpura of the lower extremities and buttocks are typical findings in moderate disease (Fig. 5–4). Severe disease can occa-

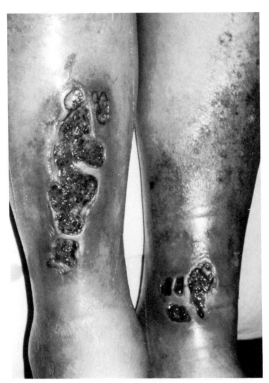

Figure 5–3. Bilateral ulcerations with granulomatous features histologically consistent with those of ulcerating rheumatoid necrobiosis.

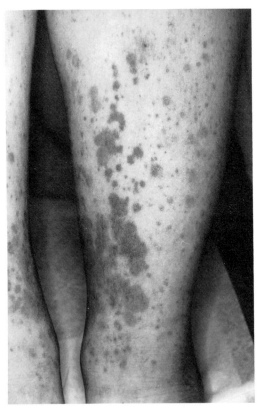

Figure 5–4. Multiple palpable purpuric lesions typical of cutaneous vasculitis in a patient with circulating immune complexes and high titer rheumatoid factor.

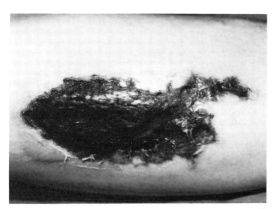

Figure 5–5. Large necrotic hemorrhagic plaque, with biopsy revealing leukocytoclastic vasculitis.

sionally occur in an explosive fashion, involving cutaneous as well as systemic organs and with a mortality rate approaching 30%. The cutaneous lesions may include the changes seen in mild or moderate rheumatoid vasculitis in addition to large necrotic ulcers (Fig. 5–5). The majority of evidence suggests that the vasculitic lesions are related to circulating immune complexes. A small percentage of patients may have the vascular lesions on the basis of an associated cryoglobulinemia.

Pyoderma Gangrenosum

Pyoderma gangrenosum is a distinctive ulcerative disease of the skin that historically has been associated with inflammatory bowel disease but that may occur with a rheumatoid-like arthritis as well as with a number of other systemic diseases. The diagnosis is made on the basis of historical and morphologic characteristics rather than histopathologic changes, but the diagnosis is one of exclusion of other processes. Lesions usually begin as painful, furuncle-like nodules that rapidly expand, become fluctuant, and ulcerate. The ulcer is covered by a purulent exudate and the border is undermined, often irregular, and purple or violaceous in color (Fig. 5–6). Lesions are often multiple, occur especially on the lower extremities and trunk, and heal with atrophic and hyperpigmented scars (Fig. 5–7). The ulcers of pyoderma gangrenosum frequently begin following trauma, the so-called pathergy phenomenon. The disease is usually chronic and is characterized by remissions and exacerbations. The histopathologic find-

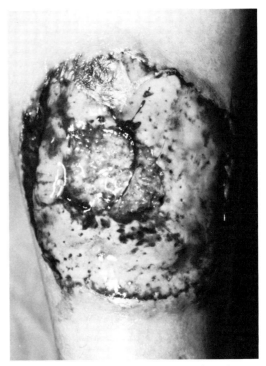

Figure 5–6. Large necrotic ulcer with overhanging purple border typical of pyoderma gangrenosum.

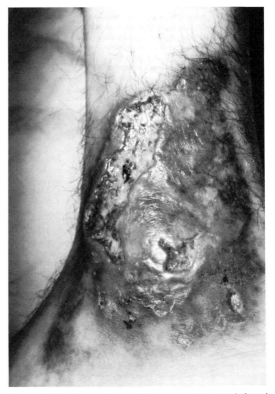

Figure 5–7. Hyperpigmentalism, scarring, and focal ulcers in a patient with recurrent pyoderma gangrenosum of the ankle.

ings of this inflammatory and necrotic process are not diagnostic and vary with the site of biopsy as well as with the stage of the disease. There are no specific abnormal laboratory findings. The pathogenesis is unknown. The differential diagnosis is exhaustive, including numerous infectious diseases, as is the list of therapeutic agents used in the management of the disease. Treatment is challenging and should include the management of the associated disorder, although frequently there is no direct correlation between control of the ulcers of pyoderma gangrenosum and the associated disease.

Miscellaneous Dermatological Conditions

There are several non-specific cutaneous lesions that have been reported in patients with RA, including such changes as palmar erythema, focal or generalized hyperpigmentation, thinning of the skin (especially over the joints), Raynaud's phenomenon, yellow skin as well as the yellow nail syndrome, and nails with dusky red lunulae (Fig. 5–8).

Patients with so-called juvenile rheumatoid arthritis (JRA), which is being reported more and more frequently in older patients as adult onset Still's disease, often have a characteristic pink- to salmon-colored, urticarial or measles-like rash associated with high, spiking fever. The rash and fever peak in the late afternoon. The rash is minimally pruritic to asymptomatic and is most ob-

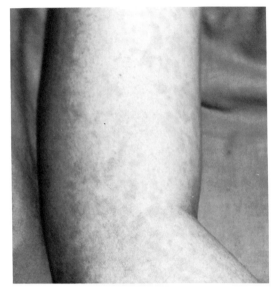

Figure 5–9. Patchy urticaria-like lesions in an adult with Still's disease.

vious on the chest, abdomen, and extensor upper arms (Fig. 5–9). Although not pathognomonic for the disease, the eruption, which is usually transitory but which may persist for several days, is very helpful diagnostically when considering a patient with arthralgias, fever, and negative laboratory parameters, including the rheumatoid factor.

There are numerous reports linking RA to several of the autoimmune blistering diseases of the skin, especially bullous pemphigoid, but the incidence or significance of this association is unknown. Finally, one must be aware of the many cutaneous changes that result from the myriad of therapeutic agents used in the management of patients with RA.

PSORIATIC ARTHRITIS

Historical and Epidemiologic Data

Psoriatic arthritis is a distinctive inflammatory joint disease with widely variable clinical manifestations that occur in approximately 6% of psoriatics and in 0.02–0.1% of the general population. The association of psoriasis with arthritis is attributed to the Frenchman Alibert in 1822, and the disease was named in 1860 by Bazin, another Frenchman. Many physicians have regarded the association of psoriasis and arthritis as a chance occurrence. However, epidemio-

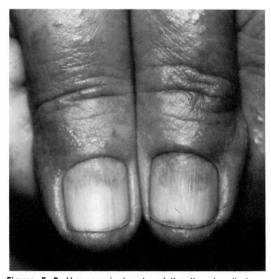

Figure 5–8. Hyperemic lunule of the thumbnails in a patient with rheumatoid arthritis.

logic, genetic, clinical, serologic, and radio-logic data have established that psoriatic arthritis is a distinctive disease. The overall sex ratio is equal. The male predominance reported in some studies is probably based on series dealing with specific clinical sub-types, such as distal joint psoriatic arthritis, which appears to be more common in men. Psoriatic arthritis is typically an adult onset disease with a peak age of onset between 35 and 45 years. It may occur in childhood, however, and it may be difficult to distin-guish from JRA. The pathogenesis is un-known, but genetic factors are important. The genetic marker HLA-B27 has a high incidence in patients with psoriatic spon-dylitis but not in individuals with the other subtypes of psoriatic arthritis.

Classification and Clinical Features

Owing to the wide spectrum of disease activity of psoriatic arthritis, several classi-fication systems have been proposed. The classification that appears to be inclusive defines 5 patterns of joint involvement (Ta-ble 5–2). All 5 types of arthritis in this classification, however, can occur independ-ently of psoriasis. At least 70% of the pa-tients are classified as having the "asymmet-rical oligoarticular pattern," in which the arthritis is restricted to one or a few small joints of the hands and feet (Figs. 5–10 and 5–11). The metatarsophalangeal joints and the interphalangeal joints are affected most

Table 5–2. CLASSIFICATION OF PSORIATIC ARTHRITIS

Types	Incidence (%)	Major Characteristics
Asymmetrical oligoarthritis	70	Usually one or a few small joints of hands and feet
Symmetrical polyarthritis	15	Clinically indistinguish-able from rheuma-toid arthritis, yet more benign
Primarily distal in-terphalangeal joints	5	So-called classic pat-tern; marked nail in-volvement and "sausage digits"
Arthritis mutilans	5	Severe, rapid devel-opment; destructive, telescoping
Psoriatic spondylitis	5	Not an uncommon accompaniment of other forms; uncom-mon alone (5%)

frequently, and the disease develops acutely in 50% of these cases. Fifteen per cent of patients with psoriatic arthritis develop a pattern of arthritis that is clinically indistin-guishable from RA, the so-called symmetri-cal polyarthritis. The distal interphalangeal joints may be involved along with the prox-imal interphalangeal joints, but the rheu-matoid factor is negative. Patients with pso-riasis who have arthritis, rheumatoid nodules, and positive tests for rheumatoid factor are said to have RA and coincidental psoriasis and are not classified as having psoriatic arthritis. Rheumatoid nodules are

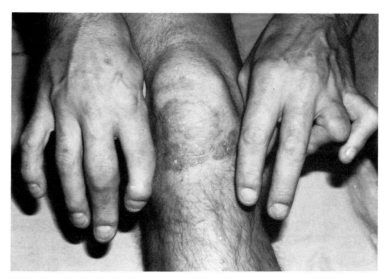

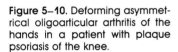
Figure 5–10. Deforming asymmet-rical oligoarticular arthritis of the hands in a patient with plaque psoriasis of the knee.

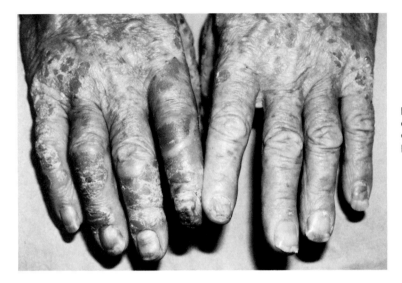

Figure 5–11. Psoriasis of the hands and nails with swelling of the digits and radiographic evidence of psoriatic arthritis of several fingers.

never considered to be part of the clinical spectrum of psoriatic arthritis.

The 3 remaining types, "arthritis mutilans," "psoriatic spondylitis," and "classic distal interphalangeal arthritis," each account for approximately 5% of cases. Arthritis mutilans is the most destructive and disabling type of psoriatic arthritis (Fig. 5–12). There may be overlap in those patterns, especially with psoriatic spondylitis, which has been estimated to occur in some degree in as many as 40% of patients with psoriatic arthritis. However, the spondylitis occurring in psoriatics differs from ankylosing spondylitis in several respects and is more akin to the spondylitis that occurs in Reiter's syndrome.

At least 75% of patients with psoriatic arthritis will have cutaneous psoriasis before the onset of the arthritis. Dystrophic nails eventually develop in at least 85% of cases, a higher frequency than in psoriasis without arthritis. The nail dystrophy appears to be especially common in patients with distal joint disease.

Diagnosis and Differential Diagnosis

The diagnosis of psoriatic arthritis is based on clinical, laboratory, and radiologic findings. The major laboratory finding is the negative test for rheumatoid factor in a psoriatic patient with arthritis that fits the clinical definition of psoriatic arthritis. Many of the radiologic changes occur in both rheumatoid and psoriatic arthritis. There are several radiologic features, however, that appear to be more characteristic but not specific for psoriatic arthritis, and they include the following: (1) destructive changes of isolated small joints, especially the interphalangeal joints of fingers and toes, with erosion and expansion of the base of the terminal phalanx; (2) arthritis mutilans, producing the so-called pencil-in-cup changes; (3) terminal phalangeal osteolysis, predominantly of the hallux; (4) periostitis, periostosis, and ankylosis of the small bones of the hands and feet; and (5) atypical spon-

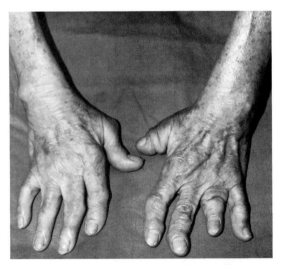

Figure 5–12. Severe psoriatic arthritis mutilans.

dylitis or sacroiliitis. In addition, a resorbtive osteolysis with soft tissue atrophy of the digits has been seen in association with acral pustular psoriasis and is to be distinguished from psoriatic arthritis mutilans.

Early in the course of psoriatic arthritis, the radiographic appearance is usually normal or shows non-specific changes such as soft-tissue swelling. The destructive changes, which result from more severe joint inflammation, appear with time. The differential diagnosis includes Reiter's syndrome (which shares many features with psoriatic arthritis), RA, acute gouty arthritis, and osteoarthritis.

Treatment and Prognosis

The majority of patients with psoriatic arthritis will have mild disease characterized by periods of remission and exacerbation and a more benign course than that seen in patients with RA. Aspirin and other nonsteroidal anti-inflammatory drugs are often sufficient to control the disease. Systemic corticosteroids are best avoided, owing to their adverse effects, which in some patients include a marked "rebound" exacerbation of their cutaneous disease. Improvement of the skin lesions, especially with non-systemic forms of therapy, is not generally associated with improvement in the joint disease. The oral retinoids, including isotretinoin and, more recently, etretinate, have been used successfully to control both the cutaneous disease and the arthritis. Adverse effects from the long-term administration of the retinoids, especially the production of bone hyperostoses, may well limit the usefulness of these drugs for chronic diseases, including psoriatic arthritis. In severe or progressive forms of the disease, oral methotrexate, 6-mercaptopurine, or azathioprine may be very beneficial for both skin and joint disease. Studies support the use of low dose methotrexate as the drug of choice for crippling psoriatic arthritis. Gold salts and antimalarials, commonly used in the treatment of RA, are often avoided because of reports of exacerbation of the skin disease, but the arthritis in some patients responds very well to these agents. They must be used very cautiously, however. Physical or occupational therapy, including rest, splinting, range of motion exercises, adaptive devices, and so forth, are essential aspects of patient care. In patients with severe disease producing functional limitation, reconstructive surgery, similar to that used in RA, can be remarkably effective.

The long-term prognosis of psoriatic arthritis is unpredictable, and there may be periods of acute inflammation followed by months or years of disease inactivity. Recurrence of joint disease occurs spontaneously and without any known provoking stimulus. Fortunately, only a small percentage of patients with psoriatic arthritis develop severe crippling disease.

Suggested Readings

Eccles JT, Wright V: Psoriatic arthritis. Clinical aspects and management. Dermatol Clin 2:477–491, 1984.

Jorizzo JL, Daniels JC: Dermatologic conditions reported in patients with rheumatoid arthritis. J Am Acad Dermatol 8:439–453, 1983.

Jorizzo JL, Olansky AJ, Stanley RJ: Superficial ulcerating necrobiosis rheumatoid arthritis. Arch Dermatol 118:255–259, 1982.

Kaplan R, Russell D, Lowe N: Etretinate therapy for psoriasis: Clinical responses, remission times, epidermal DNA and polyamino responses. J Am Acad Derm 8:95–102, 1983.

Kragballe K, Zachariae E, Zachariae H: Methotrexate in psoriatic arthritis: A retrospective study. Acta Derm Venereol 63:165, 1983.

Rodnan GP, Schumacher HR (eds): Rheumatoid arthritis. In Primer on the Rheumatic Diseases, 8th ed. Atlanta, Arthritis Foundation, 1983, pp. 38–48.

Sibbitt WL Jr, Williams RC Jr: Cutaneous manifestations of rheumatois arthritis. Int J Dermatol 21:563–572, 1982.

6

Miscellaneous Rheumatologic/ Dermatological Disorders

JOSEPH L. JORIZZO

There are a number of important conditions that warrant at least brief review in any overview of cutaneous rheumatology. Behçet's disease and other pustular vasculitides, Reiter's syndrome and the HLA-B27 spectrum, Kawasaki's disease, gout, and graft versus host disease are reviewed in this chapter.

BEHÇET'S DISEASE

Behçet's disease is a complex multisystem disorder described by the Turkish dermatologist Hulusi Behçet in the late 1930s. As there is no pathognomonic laboratory test, the diagnosis is based on clinical criteria. Several sets of criteria have been published. One system of diagnosis is based on the presence of recurrent oral aphthosis (canker sores) and at least two of the following five additional features: recurrent genital aphthosis, uveitis, synovitis, cutaneous pustular vasculitis (pathergy), and meningoencephalitis. Inflammatory bowel disease, which can be associated with recurrent oral aphthosis and synovitis, and other autoimmune diseases must be excluded.

Pathogenesis

The pathogenesis of Behçet's disease remains unknown. Disease susceptibility genes studied in large, independent Japanese and British surveys are HLA-B51 and HLA-DRW52. Genetic predisposition that triggers immunologic disease in response to viral or other infection is one theory of disease pathogenesis. No strong evidence, however, supports a role for any infectious agent in Behçet's disease.

Cellular immunity has been extensively evaluated in patients with Behçet's disease because the histologic appearance of late, established lesions is dominated by a lymphocytic infiltrate in various tissues. No consistent abnormality of cellular immunity has been described.

More recent evidence suggests that the earliest mucocutaneous lesions in Behçet's disease represent a neutrophilic vascular reaction or fully developed leukocytoclastic vasculitis. Both standard in vitro assays for circulating immune complexes and in vivo immunopathologic assessment of histamine-induced pathergy lesions support a role for immune complex–mediated vessel damage in lesion pathogenesis. Furthermore, studies of neutrophil function show that a heat stable serum factor (present in the serum of patients with Behçet's disease) dramatically enhances the migration of patient and control neutrophils. The characteristic pustular vasculitic lesions, the aphthae, and possibly the systemic lesions in this disease may well result from enhanced accumulation of neutrophils in sites of immune complex–mediated vasculitis.

Clinical Features

Behçet's disease occurs in both sexes and is primarily a disease of young adults. Although relatively common in the Middle East and in Asia, it is uncommon in Northern Europe, Great Britain, and the United States.

The oral aphthae experienced by these patients are like those seen in patients with simple aphthosis (i.e., canker sores). They are usually multiple and occur in crops (Fig. 6–1). The genital aphthae are similar, with the exception that they occur less frequently (Fig. 6–2). Pathergy, the development of cutaneous papulopustular lesions 24 hours after cutaneous trauma (e.g., by needle prick or intradermal injection), is a characteristic feature seen in many patients with Behçet's disease. The term pustular vasculitis excludes the often confused acneiform or follicle-based lesions from diagnostic consideration (Fig. 6–3). Deeper lesions, occurring in subcutaneous fat, may mimic those of erythema nodosum or superficial migratory thrombophlebitis.

Posterior uveitis (i.e., a retinal vasculitis) is the most classic ocular lesion in Behçet's disease. This is the common cause of blindness in patients with Behçet's disease who have that complication.

The arthritis seen in patients with Behçet's disease is non-erosive and inflammatory and affects both large and small joints. Patients with HLA-B27 positive sacroiliitis should be

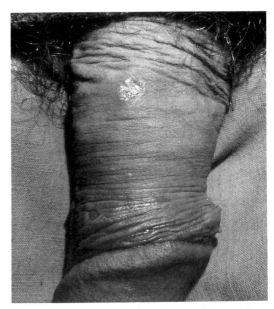

Figure 6–2. Aphthosis-like ulcerations on the penis in a patient with Behçet's disease.

considered as part of the Reiter's/HLA-B27 spectrum of diseases.

Meningoencephalitis may be more common in patients with Behçet's disease than previously appreciated. Neurologic manifestations have a late onset in patients with Behçet's disease and are remarkably variable in their presentation.

A thrombotic tendency, with a propensity to affect large arteries and veins, can be a

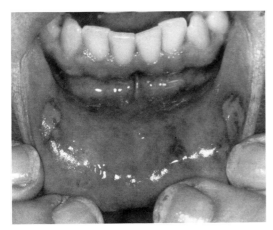

Figure 6–1. Recurrent severe oral aphthous lesions in a patient with Behçet's disease.

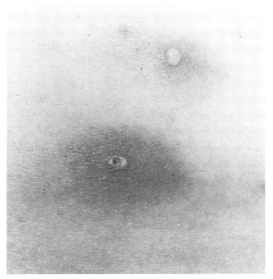

Figure 6–3. Pustular vasculitis on an erythematous base is present in this patient with Behçet's disease. This lesion can be induced by minor trauma.

cause of death in patients with Behçet's disease. The kidney may be relatively spared in these patients.

Histopathology

Most studies of lesions of internal organs in Behçet's disease are of autopsy material. It is not surprising that the major finding reported is a lymphocytic "perivasculitis." This same type of picture is seen in late mucocutaneous lesions. Earlier lesions (more accessible to study in the skin) show leukocytoclastic vasculitis or a milder, neutrophilic vascular reaction.

Course and Treatment

The clinical course of Behçet's disease is extremely variable. Many patients suffer frequent, painful bouts of oral and genital aphthae and arthritis for years. The progression of posterior uveitis to ultimate blindness is the major cause of morbidity. Death in Behçet's disease is usually due to central nervous system involvement, bowel perforation, or large arterial or venous occlusion.

Therapy for mucosal lesions may be supportive, with topical viscous lidocaine and potent topical corticosteroids. Oral colchicine therapy may be associated with reduced severity and frequency of aphthae. Oral thalidomide therapy was extremely effective for mucocutaneous involvement, but the drug is now unavailable. Oral dapsone may be substituted. Systemic corticosteroid therapy, alone or with azathioprine, is a mainstay of treatment for more severe ocular and systemic disease. Oral chlorambucil therapy and cyclosporin A are more toxic therapies for patients with resistant ocular or neurologic disease.

BOWEL BYPASS–BOWEL-ASSOCIATED DERMATOSIS-ARTHRITIS SYNDROME

Approximately 20% of patients who undergo jejunoileal bypass surgery for morbid obesity develop a serum sickness–like illness characterized by a cutaneous pustular vasculitis, synovitis, fever, and flu-like symptoms. An identical syndrome has been reported in patients who have not had bypass surgery but who have had Billroth II surgery for peptic ulcer disease or who have

had inflammatory bowel disease. The concept of pustular vasculitis has been proposed to link the similar clinicopathologic features with the proposed immunopathogenetic features seen in patients with Behçet's disease, bowel bypass–bowel-associated dermatosis-arthritis syndrome, and an idiopathic cutaneous pustular vasculitis.

Pathogenesis

The pathomechanism of lesions in bowel bypass syndrome may involve circulating immune complexes that contain bacterial peptidoglycans of presumed bowel origin as the circulating antigens. Bacterial overgrowth in the blind loop of bowel could result in the formation of immune complexes that enter the circulation and deposit in target tissues such as skin and synovium, producing the clinical features of this syndrome.

In a small group of patients with bowel-associated dermatosis-arthritis syndrome, preliminary immunofluorescence and routine microscopic evidence for circulating immune complex–mediated vessel damage was demonstrated. In addition, there is a preliminary suggestion that a serum factor is present, like that seen in patients with the pustular vasculitis in Behçet's disease, that is capable of enhancing neutrophil migration.

Clinical Aspects

Patients experience the onset of serum sickness–like signs and symptoms 2–3 months or later after bypass surgery or after Billroth II surgery or at some point in the course of their inflammatory bowel disease. Increased frequency of diarrhea and gastrointestinal disturbance accompanies the systemic disease. Polyarticular arthralgias, myalgias, and a non-erosive arthritis that effects peripheral joints are frequent findings. Cutaneous pustular vasculitis occurs in a truncal distribution (Figs. 6–4 and 6–5). Erythema nodosum–like lesions may also occur. Bouts may recur every 4–8 weeks.

Histopathology

Early reports of the histopathology of cutaneous lesions in bowel bypass syndrome described leukocytoclastic vasculitis. Sub-

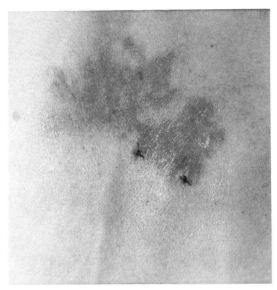

Figure 6–4. Erythematous, plaque-like lesions with small vesicles present are representative of a pustular vasculitis in this patient with a bowel-associated dermatosis-arthritis syndrome that was due to Billroth II surgery for peptic ulcer disease.

sequent reports have corrected this to a neutrophilic vascular reaction indistinguishable from the vessel changes seen in cutaneous lesions of Behçet's disease. We prefer the designation "neutrophilic vascular reaction" to "Sweet-like vasculitis."

Course and Treatment

Systemic corticosteroid therapy controls the signs and symptoms of bowel-associated dermatosis-arthritis syndrome. The bowel bypass patients can be cured by restoration of normal bowel anatomy. Systemic antibiotics (e.g., tetracycline, metronidazole, erythromycin) are efficacious, perhaps owing to an effect on reduction of bowel bacterial overgrowth. The beneficial effects of thalidomide (no longer available) suggest that the related compound oral dapsone might also be beneficial.

REITER'S SYNDROME AND THE HLA-B27 SPECTRUM

Reiter's syndrome is a multisystem disease of uncertain pathogenesis that is clinically characterized by the triad of non-gonococcal urethritis, arthritis, and conjunctivitis. The psoriasis-like skin lesions are called keratoderma blennorrhagicum and circinate bal-

anitis. The oral lesions are pustular psoriasis-like and not aphthae, as in Behçet's disease. The association of ankylosing spondylitis with the histocompatibility antigen (HLA-B27) has expanded the concept of HLA-B27 spondyloarthropathy to a spectrum of diseases that include Reiter's syndrome, ankylosing spondylitis, enteropathic arthritis, and psoriasis with spondyloarthritis.

Pathogenesis

The evidence for a genetic predisposition to Reiter's syndrome and the HLA-B27 spectrum of diseases is strong, with the convincing HLA association. Reiter's syndrome has been well known to develop following nongonococcal urethritis (venereal form with *Chlamydia* or *Ureaplasma urealyticum*) or following dysentery (dysenteric form after shigellosis or infection with other enteric pathogens). It has been proposed that complex multisystem disease results from an abnormal immunologic response to the infections mentioned, in genetically predisposed individuals.

Clinical Aspects

The post-venereal form of Reiter's syndrome is a disease primarily of young men, with women very infrequently affected. The disease process usually occurs in bouts that often last from 1 to 12 months and that recur in about one half of patients. Fever, malaise, weight loss, and gastrointestinal distress are

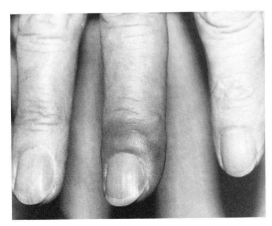

Figure 6–5. The same individual as in Figure 6–4, who has an erythematous periungual lesion representative of this syndrome.

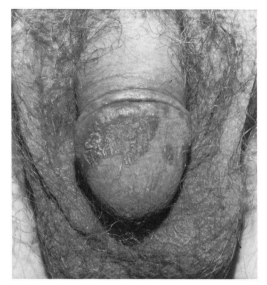

Figure 6–6. Circinate balanitis present in a patient with Reiter's syndrome.

almost always accompanied by the seronegative, erosive, axial arthropathy. Achilles tendinitis and plantar fasciitis are prototypic manifestations that occur in about one fifth of patients. The urethritis is non-specific and is a feature of the post-venereal form. The

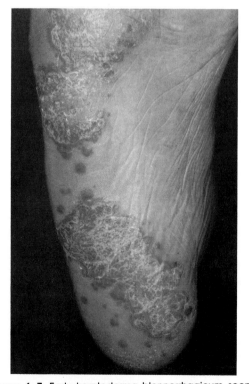

Figure 6–7. Early keratoderma blennorrhagicum seen in a patient with Reiter's syndrome.

eye findings include conjunctivitis, iritis, and keratitis. Neurologic manifestations are varied and include meningoencephalitis, psychotic episodes, seizures, or cranial or peripheral neuropathies. Cardiac conduction abnormalities may occur.

The mucocutaneous manifestations of Reiter's syndrome and the HLA-B27 spectrum of disease are clinicopathologically similar to those of psoriasis. Characteristic patterns of cutaneous disease exist in patients with Reiter's syndrome. Circinate balanitis is a psoriasiform dermatitis of the head of the penis (Fig. 6–6). Keratoderma blennorrhagicum is the name given to the psoriasiform lesions, which may be particularly thick (i.e., oyster shell–like) on the soles (Fig. 6–7). The oral lesions resemble the pustular, geographic tongue–like lesions of acute pustular psoriasis. Patients with HLA-B27 positive enteropathic arthritis may also have aphthae, creating confusion with Behçet's disease. These patients are best considered with the HLA-B27 spectrum of disease.

Pathology

The histopathologic findings of cutaneous lesions from patients with Reiter's syndrome are indistinguishable from those of lesions of psoriasis. The hallmark of these lesions is the intraepidermal spongiform pustule. Neutrophils migrate into the epidermis to form these pustules. The epidermis is thickened (acanthosis), and nuclei are retained in the stratum corneum (i.e., parakeratosis).

Course and Treatment

More than 50% of patients with Reiter's syndrome may experience a relapsing course of the disease. Death occurs in less than 1% of patients; however, a significant percentage (about one third of patients) acquire some disability.

Although not curable, the disease is quite treatable. Non-steroidal anti-inflammatory agents and topical regimens (corticosteroids/tar derivative/ultraviolet light, as for psoriasis) are the mainstays of treatment for the mild musculoskeletal and cutaneous manifestations of Reiter's syndrome. Systemic methotrexate given in low weekly doses is an important therapeutic option for severe disease. Systemic corticosteroids are beneficial, but, as in psoriasis, they may produce severe pustular flares of the cutaneous disease when tapered.

KAWASAKI'S DISEASE (MUCOCUTANEOUS LYMPH NODE SYNDROME)

Kawasaki, a Japanese pediatrician, first described an acute febrile mucocutaneous syndrome with striking lymphadenopathy occurring in Japanese children in the late 1960s. This syndrome has now been described worldwide. Diagnostic criteria have been described, which include fever unresponsive to antibiotics; conjunctival congestion; oral changes (e.g., strawberry tongue; dry, red lips or oral cavity, etc.); red, edematous hands and feet; an exanthem, and cervical lymphadenitis. Five or six of these criteria must be present for the diagnosis to be made.

Pathogenesis

The etiology of Kawasaki's disease remains unknown. Epidemiological factors suggest an infectious cause, but no rickettsial, viral, or toxic agent has been identified.

Clinical Aspects

Kawasaki's disease is most common in children between 6 months and 4 years of age. Asian ancestry is a high risk factor, although the syndrome occurs in whites and blacks. There is no clear HLA association.

High fevers (up to 40.5°C) are described as being "hectic," and fever may last for up to 3 weeks. Within the first week of fever, edema and erythema develop on the hands and feet, a macular erythematous eruption begins, and oral erythema and conjunctival congestion occur (Fig. 6–8). A strawberry tongue may develop. During the resolution stage, brawny change and desquamation occur acrally (Fig. 6–9). Cervical lymphadenopathy may be dramatic.

The most important clinical complication is the development of coronary aneurysms, which may even result in death from myocardial infarction. These may result from a form of juvenile polyarteritis nodosa.

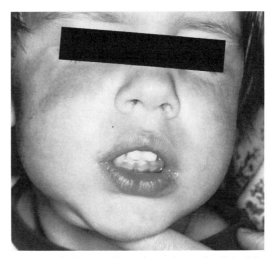

Figure 6–8. Kawasaki's syndrome (see also Plate IIA).

A number of other acute syndromes may mimic some features of Kawasaki's syndrome. The differential diagnosis includes Stevens-Johnson syndrome, scarlet fever, infantile polyarteritis nodosa, Rocky Mountain spotted fever, leptospirosis, mononucleosis, viral exanthems, the phenytoin (Dilantin) syndrome, and collagen vascular diseases.

Pathology

The cutaneous lesions may show simple vasodilation and perivascular lymphocytic reaction. They may resemble lesions of erythema multiforme. Cardiac changes are indistinguishable from the changes seen in juvenile polyarteritis nodosa.

Course and Treatment

The patients usually recover spontaneously in 1–3 weeks. Up to one third of patients may have coronary artery involvement. The mortality rate in Kawasaki's syndrome may be as high as 1–2%. Studies suggest that high dose salicylate treatment (80–180 mg/kg/day) may be efficacious in reducing coronary involvement in this syndrome. Data suggest that systemic corticosteroid therapy should be avoided.

GOUT

A detailed discussion of gout, which is a systemic disorder characterized by recurrent

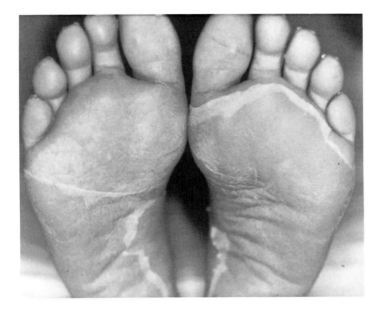

Figure 6–9. Acral desquamation seen in a patient with Kawasaki's syndrome.

arthritis and hyperuricemia with urate deposition in synovial and non-articular tissues, is beyond the scope of this chapter. The cutaneous manifestations of gout are intradermal or subcutaneous nodules called tophi. They occur in avascular tissue over the ears, olecranon, and pre-patellar bursae or in acral sites, often associated with tendons (Fig. 6–10; Plate IIB). They may discharge a chalky material. Microscopic examination of this material reveals the typical crystals, which can also be seen in biopsy specimens fixed in alcohol, but not in formalin. Therapy includes oral colchicine, allopurinol as

a preventative, and indomethacin for acute attacks.

HUMAN GRAFT VERSUS HOST DISEASE

Graft versus host disease may occur when a graft containing immunocompetent cells is placed in a host that is different enough from the graft that the graft is perceived as being foreign, and the host is unable to reject the graft effectively. Although classically described after allogeneic bone marrow transplantation, this reaction may also occur after

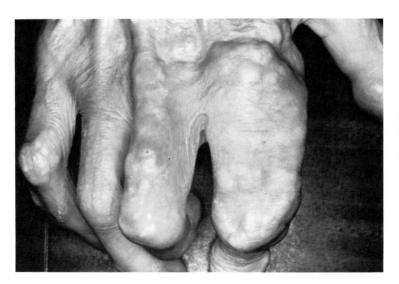

Figure 6–10. In this patient, multiple yellowish nodular lesions are seen, which are representative of tophi (see also Plate IIB).

maternofetal cell transfer in immunodeficient children, or even after transfusion of non-irradiated blood products into immunodeficient patients.

Pathogenesis

A detailed discussion of the pathomechanism of graft versus host disease is beyond the scope of this section. There appears to be a complex interplay between cell-mediated cytotoxic reactions and recruited effector systems such as complement, antibody, and macrophages.

Clinical Aspects

Acute graft versus host disease occurs in up to 80% of patients receiving allogeneic bone marrow transplants. Although the disease may be mild in one quarter of these patients, it may be life-threatening, with multisystem involvement and risk of sepsis. The skin, liver, and gastrointestinal systems are the most affected. The cutaneous reaction may begin with a truncal macular and papular eruption that may generalize. In more severely affected patients, the skin becomes edematous and bullae and erythroderma may occur. A toxic epidermal necrolysis–like reaction is the most severe cutaneous manifestation of graft versus host disease.

Chronic graft versus host reactions may develop in about one third or more of long-term survivors of allogeneic bone marrow transplantation. Mortality is primarily from sepsis. Patients develop involvement of the skin and mucous membranes (Figs. 6–11 and 6–12; Plates IIC and D), liver, eyes, upper respiratory tract, esophagus, serosal surfaces, lower gastrointestinal tract, and skeletal muscles. Systemic disease manifestations are similar to those of scleroderma. Cutaneous lesions may resemble those of lichen planus (i.e., purple, pruritic, polygonal, flat-topped papules) or scleroderma.

Histopathology

The histopathologic changes of the skin in acute graft versus host disease are most helpful in the diagnosis and classification of the reaction. Skin biopsies have become a part of the follow-up of the bone marrow transplant patient. Changes range from focal or diffuse vacuolar alteration of basal cells to dyskeratosis and spongiosis of the epidermal cells to complete loss of the epidermis. The histopathologic changes seen in cutaneous lesions in chronic graft versus host disease resemble those of lichen planus (i.e., band-like infiltrate of mononuclear cells and vac-

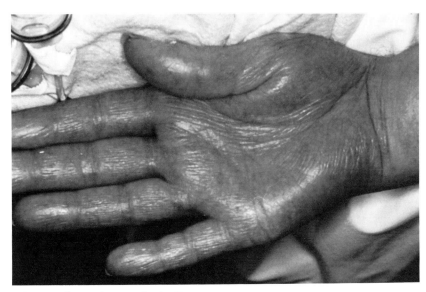

Figure 6–11. Palmar erythema in a patient with an acute graft versus host disease following bone marrow transplantation (see also Plate IIC). (Courtesy of Dr. Richard Sturm, Atlanta, GA.)

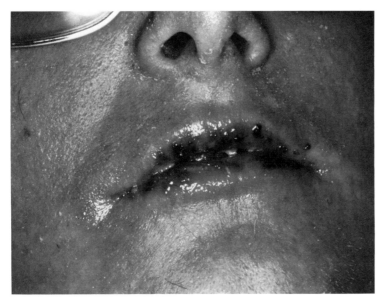

Figure 6–12. Same patient as in Figure 6–11, demonstrating mucosal surface lesions (see also Plate IID). (Courtesy of Dr. Richard Sturm, Atlanta, GA.)

uolar interface change) or scleroderma (i.e., dermal sclerosis with a patchy mononuclear cell infiltrate). The association of lymphocytes with degenerating or necrotic keratinocytes in the epidermis is called satellite cell necrosis and is a histopathologic hallmark of the graft versus host reaction.

Course and Treatment

Although a percentage of patients with significant acute or chronic graft versus host reactions die of the disease or from sepsis, milder forms of the disease may actually be associated with a reduced risk of relapse in leukemic patients treated with bone marrow transplantation. Cyclosporin A and systemic prednisone are the mainstays of treatment for both acute and chronic forms of the disease. Aggressive supportive care is required. Azathioprine and cyclophosphamide have been used, especially in chronic graft versus host disease. Psoralen and long wave ultraviolet light (PUVA) therapy is beneficial in the treatment of cutaneous manifestations.

Suggested Readings

DeCastro P, Jorizzo JL, Solomon AR, et al: Coexistent systemic lupus erythematosus and tophaceous gout. J Am Acad Dermatol 13:650–654, 1985.

James WD, Odom RB: Graft versus host disease. Arch Dermatol 119:683–689, 1983.

Jorizzo JL: Behçet's disease: An update based on the 1985 International Conference in London. Arch Dermatol 122:556–558, 1986.

Jorizzo JL, Schmalstieg FC, Solomon AR, et al: Thalidomide effects in Behçet's syndrome and pustular vasculitis. Arch Intern Med 146:878–881, 1986.

Khan MA, Khan MK: Diagnostic value of HLA-B27 testing in ankylosing spondylitis and Reiter's syndrome. Ann Intern Med 96:70–76, 1882.

McNeely MC, Jorizzo JL, Solomon AR, et al: Primary idiopathic cutaneous pustular vasculitis. J Am Acad Dermatol 14:939–944, 1986.

Weston WL, Huff JC: The mucocutaneous lymph node syndrome: A critical re-examination. Clin Exp Dermatol 6:167–178, 1981.

II

CUTANEOUS REACTIONS TO SYSTEMIC DISEASE

7

Urticaria

JOSEPH L. JORIZZO

Urticaria is a cutaneous vascular reaction pattern characterized by well-circumscribed areas of dermal edema and erythema (Fig. 7–1). By definition, lesions resolve within 24 hours. Lesions that simulate urticaria and that can be proved to last for greater than 24 hours (e.g., by drawing circles around individual lesions and observing their duration) are properly termed urticarial lesions. Angioedema is the name given to the identical clinicopathologic process as urticaria except that the subcutaneous tissue rather than the dermis is affected. As many as 1 in 5 people are affected by urticaria and/or angioedema at some point in their lives. Acute urticaria, which is urticaria that resolves spontaneously in less than 1 month, affects primarily young adults. Chronic urticaria, the occurrence of urticaria for more than 6 consecutive weeks, is most common in middle-aged women.

PATHOGENESIS

Urticaria and urticarial lesions may be a final common pathway for a number of immunologic or non-immunologic reactions that lead to cutaneous vasodilation with extravasation of edema fluid in response to perivascular inflammation. Although the mechanisms involved in the various types of urticaria are not completely understood, it is believed that the vascular reaction in most patients with urticaria results from release of mediators from cells such as mast cells and basophilic leukocytes. These mediators affect vascular permeability and result in extravasation of plasma into the dermis or subcutaneous tissue with resultant urticaria or angioedema, respectively.

One classic mechanism of mast cell activation with resultant mediator release that is involved in some cases of urticaria is IgE-mediated (i.e., type I reaction of Gell and Coombs, immediate hypersensitivity reaction) mast cell degranulation. IgE antibody is produced by B cells and plasma cells in response to an array of antigens. IgE then binds to mast cells or basophils via Fc receptors on those cells. Exposure to antigen results in antigen bridging of 2 IgE molecules. A calcium requiring process that ultimately leads to histamine release follows. Immunologically mediated urticaria may also occur via C3a- and C5a-mediated mast cell degranulation. This is most probably the mechanism involved in mast cell effects from circulating immune complexes (i.e., type III reaction of Gell and Coombs, serum sickness–like reaction) that activate complement after their deposition in cutaneous blood vessels.

Direct or indirect pharmacologic mechanisms (i.e., non-immunologic) may also lead to mast cell degranulation. Medications such as the opiate derivatives may have a direct effect on mast cells. Non-steroidal anti-inflammatory agents may have indirect effects on blood vessels, possibly via lipoxygenase pathway (of arachidonic acid metabolism) products.

Other inflammatory mediators, in addition to histamine, are most probably involved in urticaria. Some of these include eosinophil chemotactic factor of anaphylaxis, neutrophil chemotactic factor, serotonin, slow reacting substances of anaphylaxis, prostaglandins, proteases, thromboxanes, and others. Immediate sequelae include smooth muscle effects, vascular leakage, and pruritus. Delayed consequences of mast cell de-

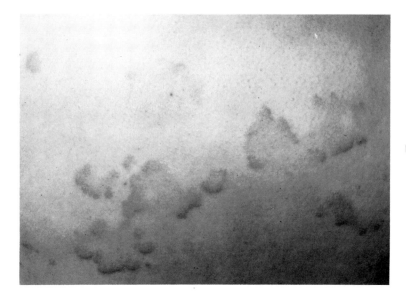

Figure 7–1. Acute urticaria.

granulation include infiltration with eosinophils, neutrophils, and mononuclear cells.

CLASSIFICATION

A personal method for the classification of urticarial reactions is presented in Table 7–1. The classification of urticarial lesions within one of these categories requires a combination of information obtained from the patient's history, physical examination, laboratory assessment, and, occasionally, histopathologic findings.

IgE-dependent urticaria and angioedema may occur in a number of different settings.

Unfortunately, a provable association between urticaria and a specific antigen can only be established in a minority of patients.

Patients with an atopic diathesis, possibly with a personal or family history of asthma, hay fever, allergic rhinitis, or atopic dermatitis, have an increased incidence of urticaria. Although scratch test evaluation and radioallergosorbent test results to specific antigens may correlate with asthma, hay fever, and allergic rhinitis, they seldom correlate with antigens producing urticaria. Urticaria seldom accompanies an exacerbation of the other atopic conditions, such as asthma. Categories of antigen that may produce urticaria by a presumed IgE-dependent

---

Table 7–1. CLASSIFICATION OF URTICARIAL REACTIONS

I. IgE-dependent urticaria and angioedema
   A. Specific antigen sensitivities
   B. Some physical urticarias in which an IgE-mediated pathogenesis is suspected
      1. Symptomatic dermatographism
      2. Cholinergic urticaria
      3. Solar urticaria
      4. Essential acquired cold urticaria
II. Non–IgE-dependent urticaria and angioedema
   A. Direct mast cell effects
   B. Effects via alteration of arachidonic acid pathways
III. Angioedema related to complement
   A. Hereditary angioedema
   B. Acquired angioedema
IV. Urticarial reactions probably related to circulating immune complexes
   A. Serum sickness–like reactions
   B. Urticarial vasculitis
V. Contact urticaria
VI. Idiopathic urticaria

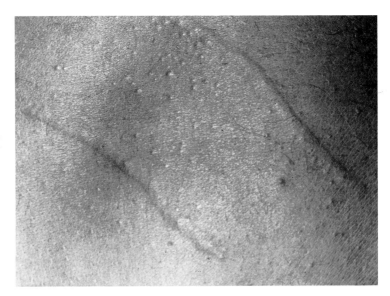

Figure 7–2. Dermatographism. Stroking of the skin leads to the urticarial reaction.

mechanism include foods (e.g., those that contain salicylate, tartrazine or azo dyes, nuts, seafood, fruits), infections (e.g., bacterial, fungal, viral), infestations (e.g., scabies, intestinal parasites), drugs and chemicals (e.g., penicillin, sulfa drugs), inhalants, physical stimuli, and systemic disease.

The physical urticarias are an important subgroup of the chronic urticarias that may account for as many as one tenth of all cases. Lesions of urticaria are induced by various physical stimuli. In several of these physical urticarias, an IgE-mediated pathogenesis has been strongly supported by clinical laboratory passive transfer experiments. The mechanisms involved in the other types of physical urticaria remain more speculative. Symptomatic dermatographism (Fig. 7–2), cholinergic urticaria, solar urticaria, and essential acquired cold urticaria are 4 well studied physical urticarias that may involve IgE-mediated immunologic reactions. The physical stimulus (e.g., stroking the skin, general increase in body temperature, sun exposure, and cold contact) may produce antigens that react with IgE and lead to release of mast cell–derived mediators with subsequent production of urticarial lesions.

Lesions of urticaria or angioedema that are otherwise indistinguishable from those produced by an IgE-mediated mechanism may be produced by non-immunologic mechanisms. Examples include urticaria from radiocontrast media, opiates, and tubocurarine, which have direct effects upon mast cells. Also, the non-steroidal anti-inflammatory agents, including aspirin, may exacerbate urticaria, possibly via increased generation of products of arachidonic acid metabolism such as leukotrienes.

Hereditary angioedema occurs as an autosomal dominant genodermatosis. Urticaria and angioedema may be associated with systemic histamine effects such as wheezing, diarrhea, and laryngeal edema that may even result in asphyxiation. Lesions result from a qualitative or quantitative C1 esterase inhibitor deficiency. Complement cascade activation results in mast cell degranulation by C3a and C5a; however, the episodic nature of the attacks remains unexplained.

A deficiency of C1 esterase inhibitor may also occur as an acquired defect in association with lymphomas, monoclonal gammopathies, or systemic lupus erythematosus. Family members are not affected in this acquired form.

In addition to typical urticaria, in which by definition individual lesions last less than 24 hours, urticarial lesions may occur in a serum sickness–like setting (Fig. 7–3). Urticarial vasculitis is one type of urticarial lesion associated with serum sickness–like signs and symptoms (Fig. 7–4). The clinical lesions are identical to those of urticaria but last for 24–72 hours. They often resolve with residual purpura. Arthralgias, arthritis, fever, lymphadenopathy, myalgias, and other serum sickness–like features may accompany the cutaneous lesions. Histologic eval-

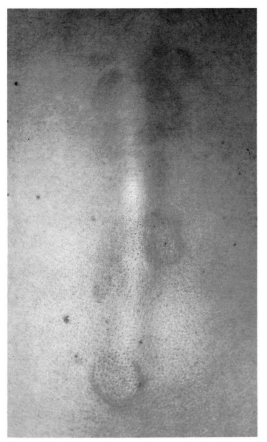

Figure 7–3. Urticarial lesions in a patient with serum sickness.

that occur 1–2 weeks after exposure to antigens such as heterologous serum (classic reaction) or certain infectious agents or drugs. Systemic signs and symptoms may include fever, arthralgias, arthritis, myalgias, lymphadenopathy, elevated liver function tests, and possibly proteinuria.

In general, urticaria should be viewed as a cutaneous reaction to substances that are systemically distributed, often after oral intake or inhalation. Contact urticaria is the term applied to urticarial lesions occurring on skin or mucous membranes after simple contact with eliciting substances. The reaction occurs within 30–60 minutes and resolves within 24 hours (Fig. 7–5). This reaction may occur by immunologic or non-immunologic mechanisms, depending on the offending agent.

Unfortunately, the cause of urticaria may never be found in up to one quarter of patients with acute urticaria and in up to 90–95% of patients with chronic urticaria. These patients with idiopathic urticaria appear well despite their cutaneous malady. Of patients with chronic urticaria that lasts

uation may reveal leukocytoclastic vasculitis, which is considered to be a marker for circulating immune complex–mediated vessel damage. Urticarial vasculitis was originally reported as a lupus erythematosus–like syndrome and as hypocomplementemic vasculitis. The normocomplementemic end of the urticarial vasculitis spectrum may be associated with less systemic disease. The severe end of the spectrum may feature patients with fully developed systemic lupus erythematosus. It is important to distinguish urticarial vasculitis from usual urticaria because of these systemic implications and because therapy involves systemic corticosteroids rather than antihistamines.

Urticarial lesions that do not show leukocytoclastic vasculitis histologically but that last for greater than 24 hours are features of classic serum sickness and serum sickness–like reactions. These reactions are circulating immune complex–mediated (i.e., Gell and Coombs type III) immunologic reactions

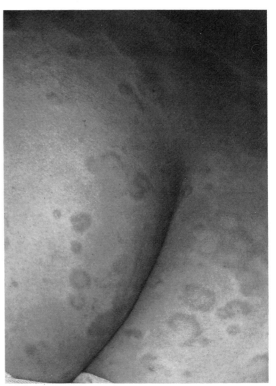

Figure 7–4. Urticarial lesions present in a patient with urticarial vasculitis. These lesions would resolve in 18–24 hours.

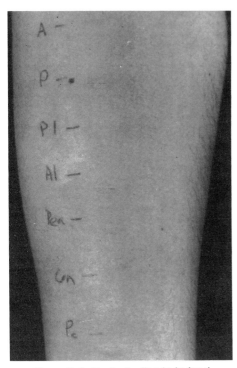

Figure 7–5. Contact urticaria to food.

for 6 months, almost one half will have active disease 10 years later, indicating the chronic frustration that some of these patients experience.

DIFFERENTIAL DIAGNOSIS

Diagnosis of a cutaneous eruption as urticaria is not usually difficult, owing to the characteristic appearance and short duration of the urticarial lesions. Other dermatological diseases may have diagnostic lesions that occur in association with or superimposed on urticarial eruptions (i.e., urticaria-like lesions that last more than 24 hours), such as bullous pemphigoid with tense blisters and urticarial eruptions, and erythema multiforme with target lesions and urticarial lesions. Insect bites often appear urticarial but last for several days, and close examination usually discloses a central punctum. Lesions of mast cell disease, such as urticaria pigmentosum lesions, are persistent dermal mast cell infiltrates that urticate when firmly stroked.

The cutaneous lesion in urticaria results from infiltration of the dermis with fluid, giving the tissue an orange peel appearance like that produced by intradermal injection (e.g., intradermal skin tests). Unless a history is taken showing that the lesions have lasted for greater than the 24 hours allowed by definition for urticaria, other dermal infiltrates can be confused with urticaria on cursory cutaneous examination. These long-standing infiltrative conditions include granulomatous infiltrates (e.g., sarcoidosis, leprosy, cutaneous tuberculosis), malignant infiltrates (e.g., cutaneous T cell lymphoma, metastatic disease), fibrous processes (e.g., morphea), metabolic deposits (e.g., amyloidosis, mucinoses), and non-urticaria inflammatory infiltrates (e.g., polymorphic light eruption, lymphocytoma cutis).

EVALUATION OF THE PATIENT WITH URTICARIA

Once a diagnosis of urticaria is made, the further evaluation of the urticaria patient begins with a thorough history, including details of the present illness; past medical history, including medications and social and family history; and review of systems. The patient must understand that urticaria may result from a newly developed allergy to a medication or other substance to which the patient has been exposed for years. With this in mind, the patient should relate possibly relevant exposures for the 12–24 hours prior to each outbreak of hives. Are clues provided by the time of onset, association with work, with meals, with medications, or with environmental exposures? The clinician should inquire specifically about certain typical exposures associated with urticaria (Table 7–2).

In addition to questions directed at exposures possibly related to urticaria, the clinician must also ask questions aimed at separating urticaria from urticarial lesions resulting from circulating immune complex–mediated vessel damage (i.e., urticarial vasculitis and the urticarial lesions of serum sickness–like reactions). To this end, the clinician should inquire about the duration of individual lesions (i.e., less than or greater than 24 hours) and about the presence of serum sickness–like signs and symptoms. These signs, symptoms, and findings may include fever, arthralgias, arthritis, myalgias, lymphadenopathy, proteinuria, or elevated liver function tests.

Table 7–2. SOME CAUSES OF URTICARIA

Infections	Bacterial
	  Dental abscess
	  Sinusitis
	  Otitis
	  Cholecystitis
	  Pneumonitis
	  Cystitis
	  Hepatitis
	  Vaginitis
	Fungal
	  Tinea
	  Candida
	Other
	  Scabies
	  Helminth
	  Protozoa
	  Trichomonas
		Inhalants
		
		Contactants
			Animal danders
			Pollen
			
			Wool
			Silk
			Occupational exposure
			Potatoes
			Antibiotics
			Cosmetics
			  Dyes
			  Hair spray
			  Nail polish
			  Mouthwash
			  Toothpaste
			  Perfumes
			  Hand cream
			  Soap
			  Insect repellent

Drugs and chemicals	Salicylates Indomethacin and other, newer nonsteroidal anti-inflammatory agents Opiates Radiocontrast material Penicillin (medication, milk, blue cheese) Sulfonamides Sodium benzoate Cosmetics Douches Ear or eye drops Insulin Menthol (cigarettes, toothpaste, iced tea, hand cream, lozenges, candy) Tartrazine (vitamins, birth control pills, antibiotics, TDC yellow #5)	Endocrinopathies Physical stimuli Systemic diseases Familial disorders	Hyperthyroidism Menstruation Hormones Dermatographism Light Pressure Heat Cold Water Vibration Rheumatic fever Juvenile rheumatoid arthritis Leukemia Lymphoma Collagen vascular disease Hereditary angioedema Muckle-Wells syndrome
Foods	Nuts Berries Fish Seafood Bananas Grapes Tomatoes Eggs Cheese		

(From Archer ME, Jorizzo JL: Chronic urticaria. *In* Taylor RB: Difficult Diagnosis. Philadelphia, WB Saunders Co, 1985, p 533.)

The patient may be encouraged to keep a personal diary. If the patient records possibly relevant exposures occurring during the 24 hours prior to the onset of each outbreak of lesions, a pattern may emerge that would provide clues as to the cause of the urticaria.

A comprehensive physical examination is mandatory in all cases of chronic urticaria. Not only might systemic signs associated with the urticaria be revealed, but also clues as to etiologic systemic disease might be unveiled. During the cutaneous examination, the clinician might draw a circle with a pen around a new lesion and ask the patient to report later on the duration of that individual lesion. As mentioned, a lesion that lasts for more than 24 hours is urticarial, not urticaria. Also on cutaneous examination, the clinician can assess for dermatographism by firmly stroking the skin on the patient's back. Although this test is positive in 5% of normal individuals, it is a useful test in patients with urticaria as a way to assess patient compliance in taking and effectiveness of antihistamine therapy. If the dermatographic response is not blocked, the antihistamine dose must be increased if the urticaria itself is to be controlled. Urticarial lesions should also be examined for purpura. If purpura is present on the lower legs it may be of no significance, but if it is present on non-excoriated truncal lesions it may be a sign of urticarial vasculitis.

Histopathologic examination of lesional skin is not required in the patient with routine urticaria. If examination is performed, a mixed cellular dermal, perivascular infiltrate is usually observed. An identical reaction occurring in the deep dermis and subcutaneous tissue is a sign of angioedema. When urticarial vasculitis is suspected, a biopsy of a lesion is indicated. The characteristic histologic finding is leukocytoclastic vasculitis with the following features: fibrinoid necrosis of blood vessel walls, infiltrate of vessel walls with neutrophils showing karyorrhexis (breaking up of nuclei), extravasation of erythrocytes, and endothelial swelling.

Although the clinical laboratory can be an invaluable adjunct to the evaluation of the urticaria patient, a cost effective approach is mandatory. As the list of associations of urticaria is vast, the "shotgun" approach to laboratory evaluation would not be complete even after many thousands of dollars of tests

Table 7-3. LABORATORY TESTS THAT MAY BE HELPFUL IN EVALUATION OF URTICARIA

Complete blood count with differential counts
Erythrocyte sedimentation rate
VDRL test
Hepatitis B surface antigen assay
Monospot test (mononucleosis-heterophile test)
T_3 resin uptake and T_4 level
Antinuclear antibody test
C3 and C4 tests
Antistreptolysin titer
Urinalysis
Vaginal smear
Stool specimen examination for ova and parasites
Sinus radiographs
Dental radiographs
Skin biopsy
Other specific tests as directed by history and
physical examination

(From Archer ME, Jorizzo JL: Chronic urticaria. *In* Taylor RB: Difficult Diagnosis. Philadelphia, WB Saunders Co, 1985, p 534.)

had been ordered. In general, tests should be ordered when suggested by the history and physical examination. A complete blood count with differential, Westergren's sedimentation rate, urinalysis, and chemistry profile might be a screening approach for the patient with urticaria of unknown cause that lasts for more than 1–2 weeks. These tests might point to leads that supplement information from history and physical examination and suggest additional evaluation. For example, an urticaria patient with intermittent diarrhea who shows peripheral blood eosinophilia should have multiple stool evaluations for ova and parasites. Table 7–3 suggests additional laboratory tests.

A detailed summary of the special evaluations required in the patient with suspected physical urticaria is beyond the scope of this chapter. However, Table 7–4 provides an overview of the physical urticarias.

TREATMENT

Treatment of acute or chronic urticaria consists of two aspects: removal of the cause and treatment of the signs and symptoms. Acute urticaria is, by definition, self-limiting. An evaluation aimed at uncovering the cause of acute urticaria is warranted to allow avoidance of the offending precipitant to prevent future attacks. Therapy of acute urticaria is aimed at relieving signs and symptoms.

Table 7–4. COMPARISON OF THE PHYSICAL URTICARIAS

Urticaria	Relative Frequency	Precipitant	Time of Onset	Duration	Local Symptoms	Systemic Symptoms	Tests	Mechanism	Treatment
Symptomatic dermatographism	Most frequent	Stroking skin	Minutes	2–3 hr	Irregular, pruritic wheals	None	Scratch skin	Passive transfer, IgE, histamine, possible role of adenosine triphosphate, substance P, possible direct pharmacologic mechanism	Continual hydroxyzine hydrochloride regimen, combined H_1 and H_2 blockers
Delayed dermatographism	Rare	Stroking skin	30 min–8 hr	≤ 48 hr	Burning; deep swelling	None	Scratch skin; observe early and late	Unknown	Avoidance of precipitants
Pressure urticaria	Frequent	Pressure	3–12 hr	8–24 hr	Diffuse, tender swelling	Flu-like symptoms	Apply weight	Unknown	Avoidance of precipitants; if severe, low dosages of corticosteroids given for systemic effect
Solar urticaria	Frequent	Various wavelengths of light	2–5 min	15 min–3 hr	Pruritic wheals	Wheezing; dizziness; syncope	Phototest	Passive transfer; reverse passive transfer; IgE; possible histamine	Avoidance of precipitants; antihistamines; sunscreens; chloroquine phosphate regimen for short time
Familial cold urticaria	Rare	Change in skin temperature from cold air	30 min–3 hr	≤ 48 hr	Burning wheals	Tremor; headache; arthralgia; fever	Expose skin to cold air	Unknown	Avoidance of precipitants

Essential acquired cold urticaria	Frequent	Cold contact	2–5 min	1–2 hr	Pruritic wheals	Wheezing; syncope; drowning	Apply ice-filled copper beaker to arm; immerse arm in cold water	Passive transfer; reverse passive transfer; IgE (IgM); histamine; vasculitis can be induced	Cyproheptadine hydrochloride regimen; other antihistamines; desensitization; avoidance of precipitants
Heat urticaria	Rare	Heat contact	2–5 min (rarely delayed)*	1 hr	Pruritic wheals	None	Apply hot water-filled cylinder to arm	Possibly histamine; possibly complement	Antihistamines; desensitization; avoidance of precipitants
Cholinergic urticaria	Very frequent	General overheating of body	2–20 min	30 min–1 hr	Papular, pruritic wheals	Syncope; diarrhea; vomiting; salivation; headaches	Bathe in hot water; exercise until perspiring; inject methacholine chloride	Passive transfer; possible immunoglobulin; product of sweat gland stimulation; histamine; reduced protease inhibitor	Application of cold water or ice to skin; hydroxyzine regimen; refractory period; anticholinergics
Aquagenic urticaria	Rare	Water contact	Several minutes–30 min	30–45 min	Papular, pruritic wheals	None reported	Apply water compresses to skin	Unknown	Avoidance of precipitants; antihistamines; application of inert oil
Vibratory angioedema	Very rare	Vibrating against skin	2–5 min	1 hr	Angioedema	None reported	Apply body of vibrating mixer to forearm	Unknown	Avoidance of precipitants

(From Jorizzo JL, Smith EB: The physical urticarias. Arch Dermatol *118*:194–201, 1982.)

The identification of causative factors in chronic urticaria is frustrating in many patients, and a reversible factor may be isolated in as few as 5–10% of patients. Most studies suggest poor correlation between positive scratch testing and antigens responsible for urticaria. As part of the treatment approach, many clinicians advocate empiric trials with elimination diets even if careful history excludes the common precipitants listed in Table 7–2. A group of chemicals contained in many foods that relatively commonly produce urticaria are azo dyes, tartrazine, and salicylates. Diets that exclude these substances are well known to nutritional consultants and are widely published. Diets excluding yeasts have also been well described. Another approach is to use a very restrictive diet such as rice and water for 2–3 days. If the patient has urticaria while eating only rice and water, the urticaria is almost certainly not food related. However, if the urticaria resolves on this diet, foods can be gradually reintroduced until the urticaria recurs. In this way, the offending substance may be identified. Other general points of therapy include the avoidance of dairy products in penicillin sensitive individuals (i.e., possibility of penicillin treated cattle with trace amounts in dairy products) and the avoidance of non-steroidal anti-inflammatory agents or opiate derivatives that may exacerbate urticaria of any cause by non-immunologic mechanisms.

The patient with acute urticaria and/or angioedema may present to the primary care physician or to the emergency room in acute distress with wheezing, anaphylactoid signs and symptoms, or laryngeal edema with airway obstruction. Emergency measures include administration of epinephrine (1:1000, 0.3–0.5 ml subcutaneously), which reduces histamine release from mast cells by increasing cyclic adenosine monophosphate levels within cells. Tracheotomy may rarely be required. Patients prone to develop laryngeal edema, such as those with hereditary angioedema, should be given commercially available kits containing pre-loaded epinephrine syringes with instructions for intramuscular injection.

Antihistamines with specificity for H1 receptors are the treatment of choice for almost all types of urticaria. These agents competitively inhibit histamine at the H1 receptor of blood vessels. Antihistamines do not prevent mast cell release of histamine; therefore, they must be given to the patient around the clock. Simply taking the antihistamine "When I get hives" is practically useless, as the histamine will have already bound to H1 receptors and induced its pathologic effects. In most studies, hydroxyzine, a piperazine class antihistamine, is the most effective traditional antihistamine. Dosage can be low initially (10 mg orally every six hours with 20–30 mg at bedtime), owing to sedative effects, with relatively prompt pushing to maximal dosages to control lesions (50–100 mg four times daily). The major side-effect is sedation. If hydroxyzine is ineffective, an H1 antihistamine from another class may be added. The non-piperazine classes include ethanolamines (e.g., diphenhydramine), ethylenediamine (e.g., tripelennamine), alkylamines (e.g., chlorpheniramine), phenothiazines (e.g., promethazine), and piperidines (e.g., cyproheptadine). Cyproheptadine is the treatment of choice for cold urticaria.

Newer treatments include new classes of antihistamines with less sedative effects, tricylic antidepressants, and combinations of H1 and H2 antihistamines or H1 antihistamines with beta-adrenergic agents. Two newer H1 antihistamines currently under clinical investigation are terfenadine and astemizole. Tricyclic antidepressant agents have long been known to have H1 antihistamine effects. Doxepin is a particularly potent agent that is being used to treat urticaria. Side-effects from doxepin are not insignificant, and examples include agranulocytosis, hallucinations, ataxia, and photosensitization. Reports of synergistic therapeutic benefits from combining oral cimetidine with H1 antihistamines have been balanced by reports showing no added benefit. The same controversy exists regarding adding the beta-adrenergic agent terbutaline.

Patients with hereditary angioedema may have a dramatic reduction in frequency and severity of attacks and benefit during acute attacks with systemic treatment with attenuated androgens such as danazole or stanozolol. These agents stimulate the synthesis of the deficient C1 esterase inhibitor.

Systemic corticosteroids have no place in the routine therapy of chronic urticaria, although they may be the treatment of choice for urticarial vasculitis or the urticarial lesions of serum sickness. High doses are required to benefit patients with chronic urticaria, and these doses cannot be maintained for the many years that numerous patients with chronic urticaria would require them. Once the chronic urticaria patient has experienced the relief provided by 50 mg of oral daily prednisone, he or she will not be satisfied with disease that recurs completely at lower doses. The patient may continue to change physicians, seeking one who will prescribe the higher doses. Inevitably, such patients may have many complications from long-term, high dose corticosteroid therapy.

Suggested Readings

Archer ME, Jorizzo JL: Chronic urticaria. *In* Taylor RB: Difficult Diagnosis. Philadelphia, WB Saunders Co, 1985, pp 531–539.

Champion RH, Highet AS: Investigation and management of chronic urticaria and angio-oedema. Clin Exp Dermatol 7:291–300, 1982.

Jorizzo JL (ed): Symposium on urticaria and the reactive inflammatory vascular dermatoses. Dermatol Clin 3:1–118, 1985.

Jorizzo JL, Smith EB: The physical urticarias. Arch Dermatol 118:194–201, 1982.

Soter NA, Wasserman SI: Urticaria and angioedema: A consideration of pathogenesis and clinical manifestations. Int J Dermatol 18:517–532, 1979.

Warin RP, Champion RH: Urticaria. London, WB Saunders Co, 1974.

8

Erythema Multiforme

JOSEPH L. JORIZZO

Erythema multiforme is an acute self-limited mucocutaneous syndrome with characteristic targetoid skin lesions that are often accompanied by systemic serum sickness–like signs and symptoms. Erythema multiforme, as the name implies, may be extremely variable as to the spectrum of cutaneous lesions present, the associated systemic signs and symptoms, the etiology, the specific cause, and the tendency for episodes to recur. Since Hebra's early coining of the title erythema multiforme, the concept of the disease has been confused such that there is little agreement among clinicians as to the exact boundaries of the syndrome. There is little disagreement that the relatively benign syndrome of classic, often acral, target lesions as described by Hebra should be called erythema multiforme. This end of the spectrum is often called erythema multiforme minor, to distinguish it from the more serious mucocutaneous illness described by Stevens and Johnson. The latter syndrome, called erythema multiforme major, is often characterized by less targetoid cutaneous lesions and by serum sickness–like signs and symptoms. The process, known as the Stevens-Johnson syndrome, may also be similar to drug-induced toxic epidermal necrolysis (TEN).

In general, erythema multiforme is a disease of young people with a male preponderance, but all ages are affected. Erythema multiforme minor particularly may be a recurrent illness in as many as 30% of patients.

PATHOGENESIS

An immunologically mediated pathogenesis has long been suspected for erythema multiforme. Patients with classic serum sickness may have targetoid lesions as well as urticarial lesions. Patients with erythema multiforme major have serum sickness–like signs and symptoms, often beginning 1–2 weeks after exposure to an offending substance, including fever, myalgias, arthralgias and arthritis, lymphadenopathy, and elevated liver function tests. These clinical aspects have led to studies aimed at uncovering a circulating immune complex–mediated (CIC) pathogenesis, the presumed mechanism of many serum sickness–like reactions. In fact, patients frequently do have detectable CIC on standard *in vitro* assays such as the Raji cell or C1q binding assay. Immunoglobulin and complement deposition in dermal blood vessels has been described on lesional immunofluorescence microscopy. However, these findings are not antigen specific and provide only indirect evidence for a CIC-mediated pathogenesis. Many investigators believe that only a neutrophil-dominated, vessel-based histologic finding is compatible with CIC-mediated vessel damage.

Some investigators believe that the lack in erythema multiforme lesions of neutrophils or of the leukocytoclastic vasculitis typical of CIC-mediated vessel damage and the dominant presence of lymphocytes, particularly T-cytotoxic-suppressor cells, are compatible with a delayed hypersensitivity reaction. Furthermore, other investigators point to the prominent epidermal injury and suggest that erythema multiforme may be a delayed hypersensitivity reaction whose primary target is the epidermis rather than dermal blood vessels.

Multiple possible etiologic agents have been implicated as causes of erythema multiforme (Table 8–1). These may be thought of as the antigens in an as yet unclassified

Table 8–1. SOME POSSIBLE CAUSES OF
ERYTHEMA MULTIFORME*

Infectious Agents
Infectious mononucleosis
Mycoplasma pneumoniae
Herpes simplex
Vaccinia
Yersinia infections
Tuberculosis
Deep mycoses (e.g., histoplasmosis)

Medications (only the most common)
Penicillins
Sulfonamides
Diphenylhydantoin
Trimethoprim-sulfamethoxazole
Phenylbutazone
Barbiturates

Other Conditions
Irradiation of tumors
Immunizations
Connective tissue diseases (e.g.,
    systemic lupus erythematosus)
Sarcoidosis
Inflammatory bowel disease
Pregnancy

*A partial list, including best-documented causes.

immunologic reaction. The best documented causes include recurrent herpes simplex infection and *Mycoplasma pneumoniae* infection, as these respective antigens have been identified in target tissue in selected patients. Reactions to many drugs have also been strongly implicated as causes of erythema multiforme. Interestingly, drug reactions and mycoplasmal infections are more likely to produce erythema multiforme major, and recurrent herpes simplex infection is the most common cause of erythema multiforme minor. In fact, the incidence of causative recurrent herpes simplex infection in recurrent erythema multiforme minor in young adults approaches 100% in series using modern identification techniques. Drugs most frequently associated with erythema multiforme include sulfa drugs, penicillins, phenytoin, phenobarbital, and trimethoprim-sulfamethoxazole. Other associations implicated in erythema multiforme include mononucleosis, other viral infections (such as mumps, poliomyelitis, orf, milkers' nodules, vaccinia), granuloma inguinale, psittacosis, histoplasmosis, syphilis, streptococcal infection, radiation therapy of tumors, sarcoidosis, pregnancy, carcinomas, reticuloses, leukemias, systemic lupus erythematosus, or other collagen vascular diseases. A significant percentage of cases remain idiopathic.

CLINICAL ASPECTS

Erythema Multiforme Minor

Typically, erythema multiforme minor begins with non-specific prodromal symptoms such as malaise, fever, and sore throat. The cutaneous eruption occurs as a primarily acral, symmetrical eruption of asymptomatic to burning or itching, erythematous macules. These lesions evolve into the characteristic dusky to purpuric, possibly vesiculobullous, target lesions (Fig. 8–1; Plate IIE). Individual lesions last from 1 to 2 weeks, but they may be replaced by succeeding waves of lesions. The entire episode may last 4–6 weeks. Erythematous macules, papules, and urticarial lesions may be associated with the more diagnostic target lesions. Sites of trauma (Koebner's, or isomorphic, phenomenon), especially physical trauma or sun-exposed sites, may be favored.

Erythema Multiforme Major

This end of the erythema multiforme spectrum is more likely to be characterized by

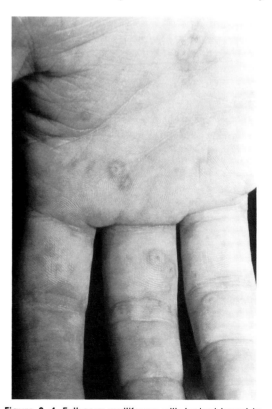

Figure 8–1. Eythema multiforme with typical target lesions (see also Plate II*E*).

generalized, especially truncal, lesions. Individual lesions are less typically targetoid and are more likely to be confluent areas of erythema with some purpura or urticarial lesions. Large bullae may be seen, at times giving the impression of subclinical toxic epidermal necrolysis (see following discussion). The proximal nailfold may be affected and result in nail matrix dystrophy. Mucosal lesions are more commonly seen than in erythema multiforme minor, being present in the vast majority of patients. These lesions present as superficial erosions anywhere in the oral cavity (Fig. 8–2), on the vaginal mucosa, or on the conjunctiva (Fig. 8–3; Plate IIF). The penile corona (Fig. 8–4) or the esophagus may also be affected. Mucosal complications may include keratitis, conjunctival scarring, uveitis or even scleral perforation, urethral stricture, or esophageal stricture. This more serious type of erythema multiforme is also referred to as the Stevens-Johnson syndrome. Patients often experience high fevers, arthralgias, arthritis, and myalgias, and may even experience hepatitis, bronchopulmonary disease, glomerulonephritis or acute renal tubular necrosis, and rarely severe prostration or even death.

Toxic Epidermal Necrolysis

Toxic epidermal necrolysis (TEN) was named by Alan Lyell in the mid 1950s to

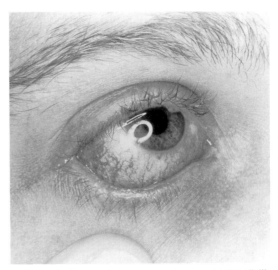

Figure 8–3. Stevens-Johnson syndrome—conjunctivitis (see also Plate IIF).

refer to a severe illness characterized by a generalized scalded appearance of the skin and by life threatening serum sickness–like features. Subsequently, the staphylococcal scalded skin syndrome has been separated as a distinct entity occurring primarily in children, with the scalded appearance resulting from an exfoliative toxin produced by a group 2 staphylococcus. TEN is thought by many investigators to represent the most severe end of the erythema multiforme spectrum. Patients usually report prodromal fea-

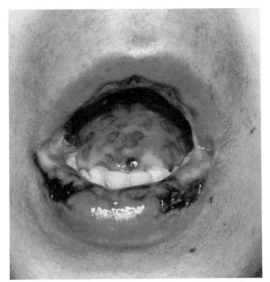

Figure 8–2. Stevens-Johnson syndrome. Erosive glossitis and erosive lesions on the lips in this patient with erythema multiforme and multiple mucosal surfaces involved.

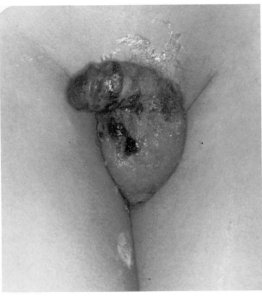

Figure 8–4. Stevens-Johnson syndrome with mucosal surfaces involved.

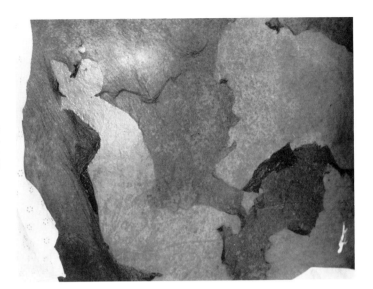

Figure 8–5. Toxic epidermal necrolysis as a result of phenytoin (Dilantin) therapy. This individual demonstrates loss of multiple sheets of skin with denuded areas below the loss (see also Plate IIG).

tures like those seen in erythema multiforme minor. This is rapidly followed by a generalized macular erythema that progresses to confluent erythema with skin tenderness and vesiculation. Targetoid lesions may also occur. Large, flaccid bullae with a positive Nikolsky sign (spread of blister with pressure to adjacent skin) follow shortly afterward (Fig. 8–5; Plate IIG). Mucosal involvement is like that of erythema multiforme major. The nails may be lost. Gastrointestinal, pulmonary, and renal involvement may be severe. Recovery may be slow, but may be complete without cutaneous or mucosal scarring if competent care is administered, usually in an intensive care unit setting. Mucosal, cutaneous, and nail scarring may result if secondary infection occurs. The mortality rate approaches 30%. The most common cause of TEN is drug-induced. The most common offenders include sulfa drugs, barbiturates, phenytoin, penicillins, tetracycline, and allopurinol. A number of cases remain idiopathic.

DIFFERENTIAL DIAGNOSIS

The differential diagnosis of erythema multiforme must be divided into two categories: a differential list for the cutaneous eruption and one for the mucosal lesions, which may at times occur alone. Other chronic erosive mucosal diseases include pemphigus vulgaris (diagnostic histopathology showing acantholysis and diagnostic direct and indirect immunopathology), herpetic gingivostomatitis (diagnostic histo-

pathology with multinucleated giant cells and diagnostic culture), recurrent aphthous stomatitis (morphology and time course of lesions suggestive of diagnosis), cicatricial pemphigoid (suggestive histopathology with dermal-epidermal junction blister and confirmatory direct immunofluorescence microscopy), and erosive lichen planus (diagnostic histopathology). The oral lesions of erythema multiforme are acute in onset; last about 2 weeks; and histopathologically show focal epidermal necrosis, a dermal-epidermal junction zone blister, and a perivascular lymphocytic infiltrate.

The differential diagnosis of the cutaneous lesions of erythema multiforme is extensive, particularly if the typical target lesions are not noticed. Patients with typical erythema multiforme with target lesions may have other cutaneous lesions that are clinicopathologically similar to those of simple erythema, urticaria, annular erythemas, viral exanthems, secondary syphilis, toxic shock or mucocutaneous lymph node syndromes, or the following vasculitides: necrotizing venulitis (leukocytoclastic vasculitis), pustular vasculitis (disseminated gonococcemia or meningococcemia, or lesions of Behçet's or bowel bypass syndromes), or vasculitis associated with collagen vascular diseases. Detection of the classic target lesions and typical histopathologic features facilitate diagnosis.

In typical cases, the explosive presentation and dramatic physical findings leave no confusion in the diagnosis of TEN. This end of the erythema multiforme spectrum may blend with erythema multiforme major. The

9

Erythema Nodosum

JOSEPH L. JORIZZO

Erythema nodosum is not an uncommon dermatosis, characterized by the occurrence of tender, non-ulcerative nodules on the legs resulting from primarily acute inflammation in the subcutaneous fat (i.e., panniculitis) (Fig. 9–1). It is a reactive process that is usually self-limited, lasting 3–6 weeks. Lesions are often symmetrical, and the anterior tibial surface is the most common site of involvement. Patients may have accompanying serum sickness–like signs and symptoms, such as fever, malaise, arthralgias, and arthritis. Mainly younger patients (ages 20–40) and primarily females are affected. Up to one third of patients may experience a recurrent bout. Erythema nodosum was first described in the English literature by Robert Willan in 1807. Patients with erythema nodosum often present to primary care physicians; therefore, it is a particularly important cutaneous entity for their awareness.

PATHOGENESIS

Although the pathogenesis of erythema nodosum remains unknown, several lines of evidence support a circulating immune complex–mediated pathogenesis. Clinically, the patients classically have serum sickness–like signs and symptoms such as fever, malaise, arthralgias and arthritis, and myalgias that are often associated with circulating immune complex–mediated disease. The histopathologic detection of a primarily neutrophilic, vessel-based, septal panniculitis is not inconsistent with this hypothesis. Non-specific in vitro assays (e.g., C1q binding assay) have been positive in a significant percentage of erythema nodosum patients,

especially those with sarcoidosis or streptococcal pharyngitis. In addition, immunoreactants (e.g., IgG and C3) have been demonstrated in subcutaneous septal blood vessels in early lesions from some patients with erythema nodosum. These findings only provide non-specific support for a circulating immune complex–mediated pathogenesis. These findings, plus the occurrence of erythema nodosum in patients with diseases with strong circulating immune complex associations such as inflammatory bowel disease, Behçet's syndrome, and bowel bypass syndrome, will no doubt prompt future investigators to apply modern immunoblot and immunoperoxidase techniques in the identification of specific antigen in circulating immune complexes and septal blood vessels, respectively, to assess a role for specific immune complexes in disease pathogenesis better.

Erythema nodosum has been associated with a host of underlying conditions. It may be postulated that the associations are responsible for antigens in circulating immune complexes that then deposit in septal blood vessels in the subcutaneous fat, producing the lesions of erythema nodosum.

An important etiologic category for erythema nodosum is bacterial infections. Streptococcal infection is a major cause of erythema nodosum. The onset of erythema nodosum may follow the acute streptococcal infection by 2–3 weeks. Other bacterial causes of erythema nodosum include tuberculosis, leprosy, brucellosis, lymphogranuloma venereum, leptospirosis, and yersinial infection. Chlamydial infections have also been associated with erythema nodosum. Tuberculosis was one of the leading causes

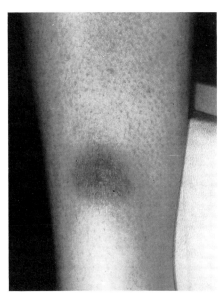

Figure 9–1. Erythema nodosum. This patient has a typical erythematous, tender nodule on the lower extremity.

of erythema nodosum earlier in this century. Erythema nodosum occurs during primary exposure to the tuberculous bacilli, possibly even before skin test conversion. Rather than occurring early in the course of leprosy, erythema nodosum leprosum occurs as a reactional form of leprosy, usually in patients with disease toward the lepromatous pole of the leprosy spectrum. Lesions may be atypical in location and in clinical appearance in erythema nodosum leprosum.

Erythema nodosum can also occur following primary exposure to deep fungal organisms. This is especially true for coccidioidomycosis (i.e., San Joaquin Valley fever) and for histoplasmosis. Erythema nodosum may less commonly be seen with other deep fungal infections, such as blastomycosis or sporotrichosis, and has even been attributed to severe dermatophytosis.

Viral infections may also be a cause of erythema nodosum. Although herpes simplex virus and hepatitis B virus infections are the principal viral culprits, milkers' nodules, measles, and other viruses have been occasionally implicated.

Erythema nodosum may be a manifestation of parasitosis, such as hookworm infestation. Other infections or infestations that are less commonly associated with erythema nodosum include toxoplasmosis and secondary syphilis.

Sarcoidosis is an important cause of ery-thema nodosum. Erythema nodosum lesions occur with serum sickness–like signs and symptoms and pulmonary hilar adenopathy in what is called Löfgren's syndrome. This represents stage I pulmonary sarcoidosis. These patients may have a more benign form of sarcoidosis that usually resolves; only rare patients who present this way may later develop other systemic pulmonary manifestations of sarcoidosis.

Drug allergy is another major etiologic group to be considered in the evaluation of patients with erythema nodosum. The most common drugs that cause erythema nodosum are oral contraceptives. All too frequently, these agents are overlooked as a cause of erythema nodosum as the physician embarks on a costly evaluation and a drug regimen modification approach to evaluate the patient with erythema nodosum. Sulfa drugs have also been implicated. Although drug allergy is difficult to prove in patients with erythema nodosum, the following drugs have been implicated as causes: trimethoprim-sulfamethoxazole, salicylates, phenacetin, and (historically) iodides and bromides.

Various underlying diseases have also been associated with erythema nodosum. Patients with inflammatory bowel diseases such as ulcerative colitis and Crohn's disease or infectious colitis such as from *Yersinia enterocolitica* infection may develop erythema nodosum. The onset of the cutaneous disease and serum sickness–like signs and symptoms often correlates with increasing bowel disease and high levels of circulating immune complexes. Patients with Behçet's disease and bowel bypass syndrome can have erythema nodosum lesions, perhaps by a similar mechanism. Patients with malignancy, especially of the lymphoreticular system, may have erythema nodosum. Erythema nodosum may also occur during pregnancy. A significant percentage (over half) of patients have idiopathic erythema nodosum.

CLINICAL FEATURES

Lesions of erythema nodosum usually begin suddenly as painful, red, round nodules. They range from 1 to 5 cm in size. Lesions are most commonly located bilaterally on extensor surfaces. The shins are the classic site of involvement. Lesions typically evolve over a 3-week period through a bruise-like cycle of discoloration. Other sites of reported involvement include the arms, trunk, and face. Lesions of erythema nodosum do not ulcerate, which is an important differential point. Arthralgias, arthritis, fever, and malaise may be associated serum sickness–like features. Lesions may resolve with a mild post-erythemal desquamation. Up to one third of patients may experience recurrent bouts of erythema nodosum, with each average episode lasting 2–4 weeks.

DIFFERENTIAL DIAGNOSIS

Clinicians are usually able to establish that erythema nodosum lesions are a panniculitis (i.e., inflammatory process of subcutaneous fat) based on clinical examination. Therefore, the differential diagnosis involves excluding other forms of panniculitis. Examples of other types of panniculitis are panniculitis that is due to pancreatic disease (this may be suppurative), lupus panniculitis, and nodular vasculitis (may be suppurative, chronic, and on the posterior leg). A review of other forms of panniculitis is beyond the scope of this chapter. Superficial migratory thrombophlebitis may be confused with panniculitis, despite occurring as a result of inflammation of larger veins, because the phlebitis spreads to involve surrounding fat. Lesions of thrombophlebitis tend to be arranged in a linear fashion along veins and last from days to 1 week, instead of several weeks like lesions of erythema nodosum. Erythema induratum, now termed nodular vasculitis, is a more chronic panniculitis that may produce suppurative, scarring lesions that affect primarily the calves. This form of vasculitis may also be circulating immune complex–mediated, but it is otherwise quite distinct from erythema nodosum. Disseminated bacterial, fungal, or tuberculous infections may rarely mimic erythema nodosum. Other forms of panniculitis, such as that associated with lupus erythematosus or with pancreatitis, can usually be separated on clinicopathologic grounds. Cellulitis, or other forms of vasculitis, rarely causes confusion. Panniculitis that is due to subcutaneous injections, to other exogenous factors such as cold exposure, or to factitial disease must also be considered.

HISTOPATHOLOGY

It must be emphasized that since erythema nodosum is a panniculitis, a punch biopsy specimen is inadequate for interpretation. The deepest punch biopsy will only sample superficial subcutaneous fat. A small, but deep, incisional biopsy is required. The histopathology of erythema nodosum is focused on the septal panniculus. Acute lesions show a primarily neutrophilic perivascular reaction. Fibrinoid degeneration may be seen in the septal collagen. Endothelial swelling of blood vessel walls is commonly seen. Necrosis of fat is not observed. Older lesions show a more mononuclear cellular reaction. In acute or chronic erythema nodosum, the centers of the fat lobules remain clear and the inflammation is focused on peripheral septal areas.

PATIENT EVALUATION

The evaluation of the patient with erythema nodosum proceeds in two directions—first the dermatosis must be confirmed as erythema nodosum, and then underlying disease must be excluded. The diagnosis of erythema nodosum is usually made on clinical grounds. If the diagnosis is not certain, a biopsy may be required. A portion of the biopsy specimen may be cultured for bacteria, fungi, and acid-fast bacilli.

Patients with erythema nodosum often have significant elevation of the Westergren erythrocyte sedimentation rate, peripheral leukocytosis, and elevated gammaglobulin levels as acute phase reactants associated with the serum sickness–like illness. A thorough history and review of systems as well as a physical examination looking for the etiologies reviewed previously are essential. A chest roentgenogram should also be a mandatory part of the evaluation of the erythema nodosum patient because of the possibility of detecting early changes of tuberculosis, sarcoidosis, or deep fungal infection. A purified protein derivative (PPD) test for tuberculosis should also be performed. The possibility of current or recent streptococcal infection can be assessed by a throat culture, antistreptolysin-O (ASO) titer, and anti-DNase B titer. A complete blood count and urinalysis should be performed as useful screening tests. In females of childbearing age, a pregnancy test may be performed.

Further evaluation can be performed in a cost effective manner if guided by the history, physical examination, and required laboratory screening tests. For example, the patient with gastrointestinal symptoms should be evaluated completely for inflammatory bowel disease and possibly for *Yersinia* enterocolitis. Geography is also a relevant factor, as tuberculosis and yersinial infections are less common in the United States and coccidioidomycosis and histoplasmosis are important etiologic considerations in the southwestern United States and Ohio River Valley, respectively. The use of oral contraceptives should not be ignored in obtaining a complete drug history, as dermatologists are often referred patients with erythema nodosum who have undergone expensive laboratory evaluation and changes in medications but who are still taking their oral contraceptives. Discontinuation of the oral contraceptive often is followed by prompt clinical remission. More than half of the patients with erythema nodosum do not have an underlying cause identified.

TREATMENT

If an underlying cause for the erythema nodosum is found, this should be addressed as a key to treatment. Most patients require symptomatic treatment for the erythema nodosum as well. Non-steroidal anti-inflammatory drugs, in particular aspirin and indomethacin, are useful, as they relieve fever and arthralgias and may also alleviate the painful cutaneous lesions. Potassium iodide is an important treatment advance for patients with more resistant disease. Potassium iodide can be given as an oral solution in daily doses of up to 900 mg for three to four weeks (0.3 ml equals 300 mg). This therapy is relatively safe except for occasional gastrointestinal upset or cutaneous eruptions; however, it is contraindicated in patients with hyperthyroidism. Systemic corticosteroid therapy is occasionally required. In these patients, cautious exclusion of infections that might be made worse by this treatment (e.g., tuberculosis, deep fungal infection) is required.

Suggested Readings

Kirby JF: Oral contraceptives and erythema nodosum. Ob Gyn *40*:409–410, 1972.

Sams WM, Winkelman RK: The association of erythema nodosum and ulcerative colitis. South Med J *61*:676–679, 1968.

Schultz EJ, Whiting DA: Treatment of erythema nodosum and nodular vasculitis with potassium iodide. Br J Dermatol *94*:75–78, 1976.

Soderstrom RM, Krull EA: Erythema nodosum: A review. Cutis *21*:806–810, 1978.

White JW: Erythema nodosum. Derm Clin *3*:119–127, 1985.

Winkelman RK, Forstrom L: New observations in the histopathology of erythema nodosum. J Invest Dermatol *65*:441–446, 1975.

10

Generalized Pruritus

JOSEPH L. JORIZZO

Generalized cutaneous pruritus (itch) is an important symptom. Scratching and rubbing, which are the natural sequelae to the pruritus, lead to cutaneous lesions such as excoriations or lichenification. The clinician's first task is to determine whether the pruritus in a given patient is due to a primary dermatological disorder with specific cutaneous changes (e.g., urticaria, eczema, scabies) or whether there is no primary dermatological disorder. In the first instance, the underlying dermatosis can be diagnosed using standard dermatopathologic principles and usually treated successfully. When cutaneous examination reveals only excoriations or lichenification but no evidence of a primary cutaneous disease, a vigilant search for possible underlying systemic disease becomes important.

EXCLUSION OF SUBTLE PRIMARY CUTANEOUS DISEASE

When confronted with a patient with generalized pruritus, the physician must exclude subtle as well as obvious primary cutaneous disease. Infestations such as scabies or pediculosis can result in pruritus with physical signs, such as finger web burrows, that require meticulous search to discover. Dermatitis herpetiformis is pruritic vesiculobullous dermatosis that can present with small, grouped vesicles that are rapidly excoriated and ruptured and thus will simulate secondary excoriations. Other dermatoses that produce generalized pruritus without an obvious primary eruption include bullous pemphigoid, cholinergic urticaria, miliaria rubra (prickly heat), fiberglass dermatitis, symptomatic dermatographism, and asteatotic (dry skin) eczema in the elderly.

CUTANEOUS LESIONS IN PATIENTS WITH GENERALIZED PRURITUS WITHOUT A PRIMARY CUTANEOUS DISEASE

Patients who have generalized pruritus in the absence of primary cutaneous disease often induce "secondary" cutaneous lesions by intense rubbing and/or scratching of their skin. The typical cutaneous sign of pruritus is an excoriation. This is an acute, reversible lesion produced by epidermal and dermal damage from tearing the skin with a fingernail or other sharp object. If the site is not scratched further, the lesion will resolve spontaneously. Chronic rubbing of one area of skin is followed by lichenification. Lichenification is the term applied to the thickening of epidermis with resultant increase in skin markings as a result of chronic friction. If the skin is chronically picked with a fingernail (as opposed to rubbed), a "picker's nodule," termed prurigo nodularis, results. Lesions of lichenification and prurigo nodularis are important signs to the clinician examining a patient with generalized pruritus. The clinician must realize that these lesions are secondary to chronic scratching or rubbing of the skin and are not a sign of a primary cutaneous disease. Occasionally, biopsy of these lesions is necessary to exclude subtle primary cutaneous disease that can masquerade as lichenification or prurigo nodularis.

PRURITUS SECONDARY TO SYSTEMIC DISEASE

Several published series have examined causes of generalized pruritus in patients without primary cutaneous disease. The most important causes are summarized in

Table 10–1. SOME IMPORTANT SYSTEMIC CAUSES OF GENERALIZED PRURITUS

Chronic renal failure
Obstructive biliary disease
Pregnancy
Lymphoma
Leukemia
Multiple myeloma
Polycythemia rubra vera
Iron deficiency
Carcinoid syndrome
Solid tumors
Endocrine disease
  Diabetes mellitus (localized pruritus)
  Hyper- or hypothyroidism
  Hypo- or secondary hyperparathyroidism
Parasitic infestations (occult)
Drug reaction (without primary cutaneous eruption)
Psychiatric disease
Other systemic disease
Idiopathic

Table 10–1. The reported incidence of diagnosable systemic disease in these patients ranges from 10 to 50%. The lower figure is the most realistic. This variability most probably relates to factors such as referral patterns from other specialists, length of follow-up, systemic evaluation performed, and criteria for accepting associated systemic disease as related to pruritus.

Chronic Renal Failure. The increased general availability of hemodialysis and renal transplantation has resulted in dramatic improvement in survival rates in chronic renal failure with a companion increase in the pruritus that accompanies this condition. It has long been appreciated that pruritus is not a feature of acute renal failure, but the cause of pruritus in chronic renal failure remains unknown. Although there is a rough correlation between blood urea nitrogen levels and uremic pruritus, some patients do not experience this symptom until dialysis is begun. Early theories of the pathogenesis of pruritus of renal failure related pruritus to secondary hyperparathyroidism. The thought was that parathyroid hormones might induce mast cell proliferation in the skin. Subtotal parathyroidectomy was occasionally associated with control of uremic pruritus. Current theories postulate the release of histamine and other mediators of inflammation or protease release by as yet undefined metabolites that accumulate in skin during chronic renal failure. These products might be inactivated by erythemogenic doses of ultraviolet light (see later discussion). Pruritus can be so intense and persistent that excoriations lead to cutaneous nodules (prurigo nodularis) or to damage of dermal connective tissue with subsequent transepidermal elimination (e.g., Kyrle's disease, reactive perforating collagenosis, or perforating folliculitis).

Obstructive Biliary Disease. Although pruritus does not accompany the hyperbilirubinemia associated with hemolysis, it is a common feature of obstructive biliary disease. The association with pruritus is a common feature of both intra- and extrahepatic cholestasis as well as of drug-induced cholestasis. Clinicians are familiar with the causes of cholestasis, including intrahepatic (e.g., hepatitis of all causes), extrahepatic (e.g., bile duct stricture, cholelithiasis, malignant bile duct or pancreatic tumors), and drug-induced (e.g., chlorpromazine, testosterone, norethindrone, phenothiazines, tolbutamide, erythromycin estolate, and estrogens). Bile salts possibly cause pruritus directly or through release of proteases from epidermal cells or tissue macrophages. Therapy with cholestyramine may be beneficial (see later discussion). Although pruritus may be the presenting symtom in up to 50% of cases of primary biliary cirrhosis, spontaneous disappearance of pruritus in patients with hepatitis may be a poor prognostic factor signifying severe deterioration in liver function.

Pregnancy. Pregnant patients may experience generalized pruritus as a result of all the dermatoses that affect non-pregnant patients. In addition, several dermatoses of pregnancy have been described. As with generalized pruritus in any patient, underlying primary cutaneous disease must be excluded. Generalized pruritus without a primary eruption may occur in up to 20% of pregnancies, usually beginning late in the first trimester. Generalized pruritus of the final trimester is often associated with mild elevations of serum alkaline phosphatase and bilirubin levels. This pruritus may be due to intrahepatic cholestasis related to increased estrogen levels, and it remits after delivery but may recur with use of oral contraceptives. This is discussed further in Chapter 43, Pregnancy and the Skin.

Lymphomas, Leukemia, and Hematologic Disease. Pruritus is an important sign that may have prognostic significance in several of the malignant lymphomas. Although plaques of cutaneous T cell lymphoma are usually pruritic, generalized pruritus may occasionally precede the primary eruption. Up to one fourth of patients with Hodgkin's lymphoma experience generalized nocturnal pruritus at some time during the course of their disease. The pruritus of Hodgkin's lymphoma is usually related to disease activity. Although most reference sources specify nocturnal pruritus, the reader should realize that pruritus from any cause is often experienced more intensely at night. This is due to a reduction in distracting stimuli with persistence of pruritic stimuli during the calm and quiet evening hours. Pruritus is less frequent in non-Hodgkin's lymphoma and in leukemias, with the exception of chronic lymphocytic leukemia, in which the frequency of pruritus approaches that seen in Hodgkin's lymphoma. Pruritus is an infrequent accompanying symptom of multiple myeloma. The mechanism of pruritus in these conditions remains unknown.

Iron deficiency is associated with pruritus. This is reversible with iron supplementation. The mechanism of pruritus in iron deficiency is unknown.

From 20 to 50% of patients with polycythemia rubra vera develop pruritus after a hot shower or bath. This short lasting pruritus is most probably mediated by histamine.

Carcinoid Syndrome and Other Malignant Disease. Pruritus is a feature of carcinoid syndrome. It may be related to histamine release in some tumors and to precursors of bradykinin in others.

It is sometimes difficult to unequivocally attribute pruritus to underlying solid tumors, as a temporal association must be established and chance association, particularly in the elderly, must be excluded. The association of pruritus with underlying solid tumors appears to be infrequent but is well documented in numerous reports.

Endocrine Disease. Pruritus is an important symptom of both hyper- and hypothyroidism. Whereas in hypothyroidism the mechanism may simply be related to the associated asteatosis (dry skin), there is a direct association with hyperthyroidism, albeit by an unknown mechanism. Hypoparathyroid-associated pruritus is most probably related to asteatosis. Secondary hyperparathyroidism is often associated with generalized pruritus. Diabetes mellitus is now believed to be a cause of localized, not generalized, pruritus.

Infestations. Various parasitoses may be associated with generalized pruritus in the absence of a primary cutaneous eruption. Examples of these may include trichinosis, schistosomiasis, onchocerciasis, and ruptured echinococcal cyst. Hookworm, tapeworm, and other roundworm infestations must also be excluded in evaluating the patient with generalized pruritus.

Drug Reaction. Most drug allergy is associated with a pruritic cutaneous eruption. Generalized pruritus may be associated with drug allergy in the absence of a primary eruption.

Psychiatric Disease. Psychologic causes of generalized pruritus should remain diagnoses of exclusion. Psychogenic pruritus should only be diagnosed in a patient whose condition exhibits positive psychiatric features.

Other Systemic Disease. Multiple sclerosis may be associated with paroxysmal pruritus. We have coined the diagnosis *unilateral neurogenic pruritus* for patients with contralateral pruritus associated with focal central nervous system lesions. Sjögren's syndrome has been rarely associated with generalized pruritus.

Idiopathic. Despite careful evaluation, a specific cause to explain generalized pruritus is not found in a majority (50–85%) of patients. These patients with idiopathic, or essential, pruritus should be monitored at intervals for systemic disease.

EVALUATION OF PATIENTS

A complete history and physical examination are obvious prerequisites to the laboratory evaluation of the patient with generalized pruritus. Exclusion of subtle primary cutaneous disease is critical, as is reversal of contributory factors such as asteatosis. Rectal and pelvic examinations are too often omitted as part of a complete patient evaluation for underlying systemic disease. Laboratory evaluation could include the following: complete blood count; chest roentgenogram; thyroid, liver, and renal function profiles; erythrocyte sedimentation rate; and stool guaiac and ova and parasite tests. A cost effective approach to the patient with generalized pruritus is critical. A "shotgun" complete laboratory evaluation on the first visit is not only wasteful but also may be counterproductive, as it may make the patient unduly anxious. Many patients, especially the elderly, have generalized pruritus induced by asteatosis. Reversing this skin dryness with emollients alone accompanied by reassurances from the physician may completely alleviate the pruritus.

Remembering that diagnosable systemic disease may be present in 10–50% of patients with generalized pruritus, the clinician must not lightly dismiss such a patient. If simple measures do not control the pruritus over a 1–2 week period, a more thorough history and complete physical examination are required. The laboratory tests mentioned compose the required screening evaluation; however, they may be performed in stages guided by the history and physical examination. The elderly adult with weight loss should have early stool guaiac evaluation and tests aimed at diagnosing occult malignancy; the patient with a rapid pulse and lid lag requires early thyroid function tests; and the recent immigrant from an underdeveloped tropical country with diarrhea should have early stool examination for ova and parasites. More complex evaluation can be guided by findings on history, physical examination, and laboratory screening tests.

TREATMENT

Control of the underlying systemic disease is often critical to treatment of generalized pruritus. Symptomatic treatment should accompany clinical and laboratory evaluation. Oral antihistamines are a key component to treatment. Antihistamine therapy is reviewed in more detail in the chapter on urticaria (Chapter 7). Hydroxyzine 10–30 mg at bedtime is sufficient for many patients. Other patients require higher dose, around the clock therapy. Emollients may reverse the asteatosis that exacerbates pruritus. Mild counterirritants such as 0.25% menthol may be compounded with the emollient. Topical therapy with non-sensitizing anesthetics (i.e., pramoxine hydrochloride) is useful for some patients. Sensitizers such as benzocaine should be avoided. Fluorinated topical corticosteriods should only be used on areas

of eczematized skin. Potent tranquilizers are only occasionally needed, but they may be very helpful in carefully selected cases.

The pruritus of renal failure is best treated with erythemogenic doses of ultraviolet B light (UVB: 290–300 nm). As few as 4–8 UV light treatments over a 1-month period have been associated with remissions of pruritus that last from weeks to months. The treatment is safe and can be repeated as necessary. Other reported treatments such as oral cholestyramine, oral activated charcoal, subtotal parathyroidectomy, and intravenous lidocaine are all less effective and are either more tedious to administer or are associated with more side-effects than UV light therapy.

The pruritus of liver disease may be benefited by oral cholestyramine treatment. Surgical drainage of the biliary tree relieves symptoms and is performed when surgically indicated.

In summary, the patient with generalized pruritus should be approached in a thorough, compassionate way, combining symptomatic treatment and gradually increasing diagnostic evaluation. Vigilant exclusion of subtle primary dermatological disease is important. Careful complete history, physical examination, and judicious use of laboratory testing accompanied by therapy aimed at reversible factors such as asteatosis, rather than a simple "shotgun" laboratory assessment, constitute the most cost effective approach to the patient with generalized pruritus.

Suggested Readings

Botero F: Pruritus as a manifestation of systemic disorders. Cutis 21:873–880, 1978.

Cormia FE: Pruritus: An uncommon but important symptom of systemic carcinoma. Arch Dermatol 92:36–39, 1965.

Gilchrest PA: Pruritus: Pathogenesis, therapy, and significance in systemic disease states. Arch Intern Med 142:101–105, 1982.

Jorizzo JL: The itchy patient: A practical approach. Primary Care 10:141–150, 1983.

Jorizzo JL, Gatti S, Smith EB: Prurigo: A clinical review. J Am Acad Dermatol 4:723–728, 1981.

Kantor GR, Lookingbill DR: Generalized pruritus and systemic disease. J Am Acad Dermatol 9:373–382, 1983.

11

Erythroderma

JOSEPH L. JORIZZO

Erythroderma, also called exfoliative dermatitis, is a clinical final common pathway for a number of underlying cutaneous diseases. Erythroderma should properly be viewed as representing "chronic cutaneous failure" analogous to chronic renal failure. Dermatoses as varied as eczemas, psoriasis, drug eruptions, and cutaneous T cell lymphoma (mycosis fungoides) can all eventuate in the clinicopathologic picture of erythroderma. The entire cutaneous organ is inflamed. Dermal inflammation, viewed as erythema and mild edema, is accompanied by a psoriasiform thickening of the epidermis. This combination of dermal and epidermal change is non-specific histopathologically, and is often termed "psoriasiform dermatitis." This "final common pathway" histopathologically is reminiscent of the non-specific glomerulonephritis often seen in chronic renal failure.

ETIOLOGY AND PATHOGENESIS

Although up to 30–40% of cases of erythroderma remain idiopathic after extensive evaluation, the list of underlying dermatological and internal medical conditions is varied (Table 11–1). In most series, about one third to one half of patients with erythroderma have had a pre-existing dermatosis that was thought to have generalized. The most common underlying dermatoses are psoriasis and atopic dermatitis. It should be emphasized that these two diseases are quite distinct clinicopathologic entities. Atopic dermatitis is an eczematous disease characterized histopathologically by exocytosis (entry into the epidermis) of mononuclear cells with resultant spongiosis (edema within and around epidermal cells). Psoriasis is a papulosquamous disease characterized by rapid epidermal turnover and exocytosis of neutrophils into epidermal microabscesses.

Other eczematous diseases can also eventuate in erythroderma. Allergic contact dermatitis is a delayed hypersensitivity reaction with the epidermis as a target organ. Seborrheic dermatitis, nummular dermatitis, and photoallergic reactions are examples of other eczematous diseases that can underlie erythroderma.

Other papulosquamous diseases that sometimes resemble psoriasis and can precede erythroderma are pityriasis rubra pilaris and Reiter's syndrome. Other, more rare dermatoses, such as pemphigus foliaceus (an autoimmune bullous disease that occurs spontaneously or is sometimes induced by D-penicillamine or captopril therapy) and various ichthyoses (genodermatoses characterized by fish-like scaling), can also produce erythroderma. The differential diagnosis of childhood erythroderma includes ichthyosis and a number of pediatric dermatological conditions, a review of which is beyond the scope of this chapter.

Drug eruption from many varied oral medications can eventuate in erythroderma. Probably about 10% of all erythrodermas are due to drug hypersensitivity. Common medications associated with this reaction pattern include sulfa drugs (and trimethoprim-sulfamethoxazole), allopurinol, chlorpromazine, gold salts, penicillin, barbiturates, and phenytoin.

Table 11–1. SOME CAUSES OF ERYTHRODERMA

I. Pre-existing dermatosis
   A. Eczema/dermatitis
      1. Atopic dermatitis
      2. Contact dermatitis
      3. Stasis dermatitis
      4. Seborrheic dermatitis
   B. Psoriasis
   C. Pityriasis rubra pilaris
   D. Ichthyosis
   E. Pemphigus foliaceus
II. Drug reaction
III. Malignancy
   A. Cutaneous T cell lymphoma
   B. Other lymphomas and leukemias
   C. Other malignancy
IV. Idiopathic

The 10–15% incidence of underlying malignancy seen in erythroderma patients should be of great concern to the evaluating physician. Sézary's syndrome is a form of cutaneous T cell lymphoma characterized by circulating malignant helper T cells (Sézary's cells) and erythroderma. Patients with other lymphoreticular malignancies such as Hodgkin's disease or B cell lymphomas as well as solid tumors from the lung or gastrointestinal tract have been repeatedly associated with erythroderma.

As is apparent from the varied list of underlying diseases, there is most likely not a single pathogenesis for erythroderma. Using the Gell and Coombs classification of diseases, erythroderma may be caused by diseases of presumed type II (circulating antibody directed against a peripheral target—pemphigus foliaceus), type III (circulating immune complexes—phenytoin syndrome), and type IV (delayed hypersensitivity—allergic contact dermatitis) mechanisms, as well as by diseases of unknown cause (psoriasis) and malignant diseases (e.g., cutaneous T cell lymphoma). Factors within each disease that trigger the entire cutaneous surface to become inflamed and to develop a non-specific "chronic cutaneous failure" pattern clinicopathologically remain speculative.

CLINICAL FEATURES

The entire cutaneous surface is generally hot, red, scaly, and indurated. Qualities that separate eczematous eruptions (vesiculation and distribution of lesions) from psoriasis (well-marginated plaques with silvery scale) are lost. Peripheral edema may be marked. The patient is usually shivering, owing to the loss of heat associated with the massive diversion of blood flow through the skin.

Pruritus leads to scratching, which often produces the secondary changes of excoriation, crusting, and lichenification (accentuation of skin markings as a result of rubbing). A diffuse, non-scarring alopecia may be present. Longstanding erythroderma is associated with the ridging and pitting of nails seen in proximal (i.e., nail matrix–related) nail dystrophies. Post-inflammatory hyperpigmentation may be generalized.

Almost all patients with erythroderma have associated generalized lymphadenopathy. This is believed to be a reactive process that, unless the patient is proved to have a lymphoma, resolves with resolution of the dermatosis. Hepatosplenomegaly may also be seen and is not necessarily a bad prognostic sign. Signs of high output cardiac failure must be sought in these patients, who are at risk as a result of large arteriovenous shunting that occurs in the inflamed skin.

HISTOPATHOLOGY

As discussed, the histopathologic appearance of the skin in erythroderma is non-specific. If the process is subacute, the stratum corneum often shows parakeratosis (retention of nuclei in corneocytes) and the epidermis shows eczema-like spongiosis. Mononuclear cells migrate into the epidermis (exocytosis). A psoriasis-like thickening of the entire epidermis is seen. Dermal changes include edema, vasodilation, and a primarily mononuclear cell infiltrate. Eosinophils may also be seen. In patients with Sézary's syndrome, the mononuclear cells may have primarily cerebriform nuclei (Sézary's cells).

The lymph node changes seen in the lymphadenopathy of erythroderma are called dermatopathic lymphadenopathy. Lymph node architecture is well preserved. Lymph follicles are enlarged, with large, germinal centers. The paracortical areas are dramatically enlarged. It should be emphasized that even in patients with cutaneous T cell lymphoma (Sézary's syndrome, mycosis fungoides), biopsy of lymph nodes early in the course of the disease may show only dermatopathic lymphadenopathy.

PATIENT EVALUATION

An overview of the evaluation of the patient with erythroderma is provided in Table 11–2. A thorough cutaneous examination of all patients with erythroderma must be undertaken. It is possible that a given patient does not in fact have involvement of the entire cutaneous surface. These patients do not technically have erythroderma (although management of the patient with "almost erythroderma" is similar), and residual areas diagnostic of an underlying dermatosis (e.g., psoriasis, an eczematous process) might be identifiable at the interface between normal and abnormal skin. A positive Nikolsky sign (creation of a superficial blister by rubbing the skin) may be obtained in the rare patient with erythroderma who has pemphigus foliaceus. Infiltrated plaques suggestive of cutaneous T cell lymphoma may be identified. It is particularly important to follow the cutaneous examination daily during treatment, as clues to a visible underlying cutaneous condition may be unmasked with healing.

The patient should be thoroughly assessed for lymphadenopathy. Unless the diagnosis is 100% clear (e.g., a patient with longstanding atopic dermatitis that gradually evolved into erythroderma or a patient with longstanding psoriasis showing a similar evolution), a lymph node biopsy searching for lymphoma should be performed.

The patient with erythroderma also warrants a careful complete history and physical examination and usually monitoring in the hospital. These patients lose their capacity for thermoregulation. They lose heat to the environment and usually present with shivering. A fever can be masked in this setting. In order to maintain a normal body temperature, these patients experience an increase in metabolism that may result in progressive debilitation.

Patients with erythroderma have increased cutaneous blood flow, raised venous pressure with hypervolemia, and increased cardiac output. Although those patients with normal cardiac reserve may not be affected, patients with cardiac disease or the elderly could suffer serious, even fatal, effects.

Individuals with erythroderma that is not acute are usually anemic, although hemodilution may be a factor acutely. The chronic anemia may be associated with iron and/or folate deficiency. Iron and folate may be lost from rapidly dividing epidermal cells from scale, although malabsorption is the currently accepted theory.

Patients with erythroderma experience increased thirst and oliguria acutely. These changes are attributed to water retention as edema and to mild increases in water loss through the skin.

Patients with erythroderma have been shown to have an associated protein-losing enteropathy with steatorrhea that responds to treatment of the skin alone. Patients also have a low serum albumin level. Although this may be in part dilutional, protein loss in the bowel and scale probably play a significant role. Hepatic synthesis of albumin may be normal to increased.

Obviously, the companion to a meticulous complete physical examination is a careful and complete history. The history should address personal and family history suggestive of underlying dermatoses, a complete medication history, and a list of exposures

---

Table 11–2. EVALUATION OF THE PATIENT WITH ERYTHRODERMA

1. *Complete history:* Particular attention should be paid to history of pre-existing dermatoses; family history of skin diseases; medication history; history of possible contactants, including work and hobby exposures; review of systems for clues of possible occult malignancy and for symptoms of high output cardiac failure, anemia, and hypothermia.
2. *Complete physical examination:* Particular attention should be paid to possible areas of normal skin (does border suggest a possible underlying disease?), lymphadenopathy, signs of anemia or high output cardiac failure, signs of underlying disease during resolution of erythroderma (e.g., plaques of cutaneous T cell lymphoma or of psoriasis), signs of underlying malignancy.
3. *Skin biopsy:* Non-specific changes of erythroderma or specific findings of cutaneous T cell lymphoma or pemphigus foliaceus.
4. *Lymph node biopsy:* Dermatopathic lymphadenopathy (reactive) versus lymphoma.
5. *Laboratory examination:* General tests such as complete blood count (e.g., eosinophilia possibly more suggestive of drug etiology, anemia secondary to malabsorption of iron or malignancy, etc.), sedimentation rate, chemistry screen, chest roentgenogram, stool guaiacs, urinalysis, electrocardiogram owing to increased cardiac demand, Sézary cell preparation.

thinking of possible contact dermatitis. A review of systems oriented toward detecting clues of possible underlying malignancy is also crucial.

Elderly patients or those with a history suggestive of possible underlying malignancy should be investigated for occult carcinoma and particularly for lymphoma. This evaluation should be guided by findings on the complete history, physical examination, and screening laboratory tests. A chest roentgenogram should be performed. A series of guaiac tests should be performed on stool samples. Lymph node biopsy to exclude lymphoma should be performed unless the cause of the erythroderma is clearly known.

Cutaneous biopsy, although usually nonspecific, must be performed, especially looking for a diagnostic feature of cutaneous T cell lymphoma, psoriasis, or rarely pemphigus foliaceus.

Routine laboratory abnormalities are not specific for erythroderma. Patients with Sézary's syndrome may have a high percentage of Sézary's cells in their circulation. Caution must be exercised because patients with erythroderma not associated with reticulosis may have activated T cells in their circulation, which are virtually indistinguishable from Sézary's cells. Laboratory monitoring of anemia, albumin, and electrolytes is a component of following the patients' systemic response to their cutaneous disease.

COURSE AND TREATMENT

Erythroderma should be considered a serious disease that usually requires management in a hospital. It may occasionally be fatal. The drug-induced form of erythroderma usually resolves completely within several weeks after discontinuation of the offending medication. Erythroderma induced by allergic contact dermatitis also has an excellent prognosis if the offending antigen is identified and eliminated. Obviously, patch testing cannot be performed during the acute stage of the illness.

Erythroderma associated with psoriasis or endogenous eczema (e.g., atopic dermatitis) may convert from erythroderma back to simply extensive involvement with those diseases. Erythroderma associated with occult malignancy often responds to treatment of the malignancy; however, the prognosis is related to that of the malignancy. In general, patients with malignancy and erythroderma do poorly. Finally, patients with idiopathic erythroderma often seem to experience a chronic course.

Deaths in patients with erythroderma may be due to malignancy, cardiovascular compromise, or infection (e.g., septicemia, pneumonitis, etc.). If patients are treated with systemic corticosteroid therapy or antitumor therapy, death may also be associated with complications of therapy.

Supportive care, in a hospital acutely, requires careful attention to dehydration, protein loss, electrolyte balance, circulatory status, and temperature regulation. The patient's room should be kept comfortably warm.

Whirlpool treatments once daily are invaluable in débriding excess scale and reducing bacterial colonization on the inflamed cutaneous surface. Wet compresses can also be used for this purpose. In this author's opinion, occlusive plastic (i.e., "sauna") suits should be avoided because their mechanism of enhancing topical corticosteroid penetration into the skin is via hydration as a result of sweating. Perspiration can be quite irritating to the inflamed skin, and the suit promotes bacterial overgrowth.

Systemic antibiotics are only required in patients with true cutaneous or systemic infection. Systemic corticosteroid therapy is often initiated to treat erythroderma; however, several words of caution are required. Short-term tapering courses of prednisone or other systemic corticosteroids may be associated with severe rebound flare-ups of the disease after tapering. Patients with psoriatic erythroderma should not be given systemic corticosteroid therapy, owing to the risk of rebound, life-threatening, pustular psoriasis on tapering. Patients with idiopathic erythroderma may have the condition for years, which would lead to unacceptable side-effects if high dose systemic corticosteroid therapy is continued long-term.

Topical corticosteroid therapy should be a mainstay of treatment. Middle strength corticosteroid should be applied frequently to a clean, dry, cutaneous surface. Wet wrap occlusion may be used; however, this author prefers to avoid "sauna suit" occlusion. Stubborn chronic cases of erythroderma may benefit from combined tar ointment and ultraviolet light treatments similar to the Goeckerman regimen used to treat psoriasis.

Underlying diseases such as malignancy must, of course, be diagnosed and treated appropriately.

Suggested Readings

Abrahams I, McCarthy JT, Sanders SL: One hundred and one cases of exfoliative dermatitis. Arch Dermatol 87:96–101, 1963.

Adam JE: Exfoliative dermatitis (erythroderma). Cur Prob Dermatol 4:1–23, 1972.

Hasan T, Jansen CT: Erythroderma: A followup of fifty cases. J Am Acad Dermatol 8:836–840, 1983.

Hurwitt E: Dermatopathic lymphadenitis. J Invest Dermatol 5:197–204, 1942.

Nicolis GD, Helwig EB: Exfoliative dermatitis. Arch Dermatol 108:788–797, 1973.

Winkelmann RK, Buechner SA, Diaz-Perez JL, et al: Sézary syndrome. J Am Acad Dermatol 10:992–999, 1984.

12

Purpura

WARREN W. PIETTE

The clinical finding of purpura is associated not only with some of the most rapidly life threatening illnesses known, but also with some of the most common and benign conditions of daily life. Although the evaluation of a patient with purpura can occasionally be quite complicated, a good history and physical examination used in conjunction with some very simple tests may be all that is required for the evaluation of many patients with this problem.

Purpura is a generic term for visible hemorrhage in the skin and mucous membranes. More specific terms exist to describe particular types of purpura, and the value of sub-typing purpura becomes important when approaching pathogenesis. The term *petechia* (pl. petechiae) generally implies an area of hemorrhage 3 mm or less in diameter (Fig. 12–1). Petechiae may become confluent, but the presence of discrete, non-palpable petechiae implies a problem with either platelet number or function. An *ecchymosis* (pl. ecchymoses) is a blue-black or purplish macule usually at least 2.0–2.5 cm in its greatest dimension, and is often due to minor trauma. Finally, a *contusion* is a major trauma–induced hemorrhage; as such, it is usually associated with significant soft tissue swelling or tenderness.

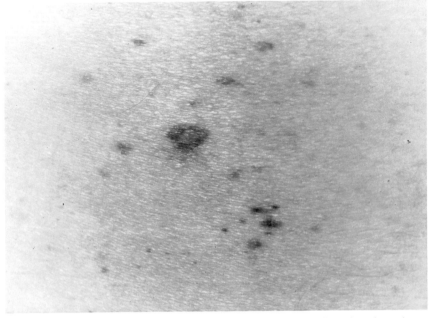

Figure 12–1. Small petechiae are present in this individual with thrombocytopenia.

PATHOGENESIS

Cutaneous hemorrhage may result from intravascular, vascular, and extravascular causes. These major divisions provide a useful framework for an organized approach to the pathogenesis of hemorrhage for a single patient (Table 12–1).

Intravascular Causes

Cutaneous hemorrhage can occur with decreased, normal, or elevated platelet counts.

Low Platelet Counts. Platelet counts above 50,000/mm³ are usually not accompanied by purpura unless a platelet function abnormality exists or unless there is a separate

Table 12–1. PARTIAL DIFFERENTIAL DIAGNOSIS FOR PURPURA

Intravascular Causes
Low platelet counts (<50,000/mm³)
  Idiopathic thrombocytopenic purpura
  Thrombotic thrombocytopenic purpura (hemolytic-uremic syndrome)
  Disseminated intravascular coagulation
  Drug-related thrombocytopenia
    Peripheral: quinidine, quinine
    Marrow: idiosyncratic or dose-related
  Marrow infiltration, inflammation, fibrosis, or failure
Normal platelet counts
  Congenital or hereditary platelet function defects
  Acquired platelet function defects
  Hemophilias
  Anticoagulants
  Intravascular pressure (Valsalva-like maneuvers)
Elevated platelet counts (≥1,000,000/mm³)
  Myeloproliferative diseases

Vascular Causes
Inflammatory
  Leukocytoclastic vasculitis
  Lymphocyte-predominant vasculitis
Non-inflammatory (or mildly inflammatory)
  Chronic pigmented purpura
  Benign hypergammaglobulinemic purpura of Waldenström
  Hereditary hemorrhagic telangiectasia
  Ehlers-Danlos syndrome
  Pseudoxanthoma elasticum
  Systemic amyloidosis (AL-fibril type)

Extravascular Causes
Major trauma
Minor trauma
  Actinic purpura, senile purpura
  Corticosteroid-induced purpura
  Scurvy
  Systemic amyloidosis (AL-fibril type)
  Ehlers-Danlos syndrome
  Pseudoxanthoma elasticum

injury. Therefore, the critical level of thrombocytopenia that might result in hemorrhage is 50,000/mm³ or less. Disorders in the intravascular thrombocytopenia category include idiopathic thrombocytopenic purpura; thrombotic thrombocytopenic purpura; hemolytic-uremic syndrome; disseminated intravascular coagulation (Fig. 12–2; Plate II*H*); purpura fulminans (Fig. 12–3); drug-related thrombocytopenia (whether a result of peripheral or marrow effects); and marrow infiltration, inflammation, fibrosis, or failure.

Normal Platelet Counts. Intravascular hemorrhage associated with normal platelet counts may result from congenital or hereditary platelet function defects or from acquired platelet function defects that are due to drugs or to metabolic abnormalities such as severe renal or hepatic impairment. Another type of acquired platelet function defect is seen in patients with plasma cell dyscrasias with monoclonal gammopathies. Here there may be interference with normal platelet function by the protein. Monoclonal proteins may also cause hemorrhage through another mechanism in which the protein forms gels in the vessel resulting in occlusion of the vessel with distal necrosis and hemorrhage. Such changes are characteristically seen in monoclonal cryoglobulinemia.

Because platelets are the most important factor for normal hemostasis in the small vessels that supply the skin, patients with hemophilia usually do not present with purpura unless it is trauma related. Injury of large vessels in fat or muscle with hematoma formation and the development of an overlying ecchymosis may result in these patients.

Petechiae may develop in non-dependent areas from abrupt increases in capillary and post-capillary venule pressure. Forceful and repetitive Valsalva-like maneuvers such as paroxysmal vomiting, violent coughing, or straining during childbirth can cause petechial hemorrhage in the head and upper trunk areas even in patients whose platelet number and function are normal.

The use of anticoagulants may result in functional changes of the coagulation cascade system, but this system is not nearly as important in the small vessels in the skin as it is in the larger vessels of the subcutaneous fat and elsewhere. The hemorrhage that occurs in patients on coumarin or heparin therapy is usually due to extravasation from

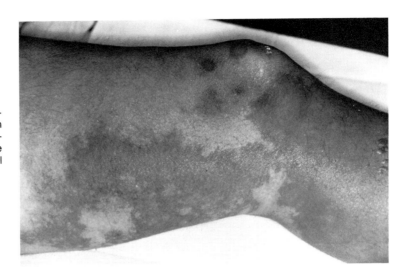

Figure 12–2. Large areas of purpura with necrosis in a patient with diffuse intravascular coagulopathy and gram-negative sepsis (see also Plate II*H*). (Courtesy of Dr. Neil A. Fenske, Tampa, FL.)

larger vessels following phlebotomy or significant trauma to the skin. A paradoxical state of intravascular thrombosis can develop in some patients while on either of these agents. The mechanism is not completely known, but it appears to be different for each drug and includes the formation of thrombi with distal necrosis and hemorrhage. The risk of coumarin necrosis is higher in women and is most likely to occur during initiation and termination of therapy. It is most likely to occur in sites with significant subcutaneous fat, such as the breast or buttock area. An important risk factor for the development of coumarin necrosis is protein C deficiency. This vitamin K–dependent anticoagulant factor is one of the first to be reduced by the administration of coumarin. Deficiency of this factor is an inherited trait. The mechanism of coumarin necrosis remains poorly understood because some patients without detectable protein C deficiency have also developed such necrosis. Heparin necrosis may develop either at the site of subcutaneous heparin injection or in areas distant from such a site.

The Gardner-Diamond syndrome, or psychogenic purpura, is sometimes included in discussions of intravascular causes of hemorrhage. Whether this syndrome results from an as yet unknown mechanism of hemorrhage or represents solely factitial disease remains a controversial issue.

Elevated Platelet Counts. Minor platelet count elevations are not important in altering hemostasis, but platelet counts in excess of a million can be associated with both bleeding and thrombotic problems in the same patient. Such counts usually occur in myeloproliferative disorders, but they may rarely occur in the immediate post-splenectomy period.

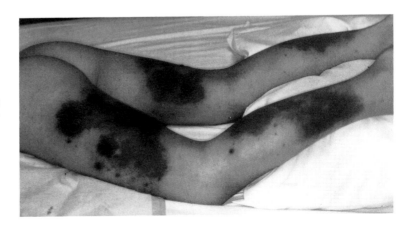

Figure 12–3. Purpura fulminans secondary to a varicella infection.

Vascular Causes

Vascular causes of hemorrhage include those disorders in which the vessel wall itself is the primary site of injury or abnormality.

Inflammatory hemorrhage should properly include only those disorders in which vessel-directed inflammation is evident, and includes both leukocytoclastic and true lymphocytic forms of vasculitis. Perivascular inflammation that is not vessel-directed should not be considered vasculitis, and it does not result in the hallmark lesion of inflammatory hemorrhage, palpable purpura. Although not all inflammatory hemorrhage presents as palpable purpura, palpable purpura is almost always due to a vasculitic process (Fig. 12–4). Lesions of palpable purpura are characterized by a port-wine color, incomplete blanching on pressure or diascopy, and palpability. Such lesions usually develop first in dependent areas (which may be the back and buttocks in a bedridden patient). An important cause of palpable purpura is small vessel leuko-cytoclastic vasculitis, which has a variety of etiologies, including cutaneous-systemic vasculitis; Henoch-Schönlein purpura; connective tissue disease, such as systemic lupus erythematosus and rheumatoid arthritis; and Wegener's granulomatosis or allergic granulomatosis of Churg-Strauss, with or without granulomatous changes. However, the physical findings of palpable purpura may occasionally result from disorders such as urticarial vasculitis, the "lymphocyte-predominant vasculitis" seen occasionally with Sjögren's syndrome, hypocomplementemic vasculitis, erythema multiforme, and the pityriasis lichenoides group. It is important to emphasize that the finding of palpable purpura indicates only inflammatory hemorrhage, and that a biopsy of an early lesion (less than 24–48 hours old) is necessary to demonstrate the type of vessel injury. This has important clinical implications, since a patient with cutaneous small vessel vasculitis may have associated visceral or renal involvement, whereas a patient with palpable purpura that is due to erythema multiforme would instead be at risk for the development of severe mucosal injury, as occurs in Stevens-Johnson syndrome.

Mild inflammatory conditions that may result in purpura and occasionally in palpable purpura include the syndromes of chronic pigmented purpura and benign hypergammaglobulinemic purpura of Waldenström. Chronic pigmented purpura includes several subsets, but usually patients with this problem have areas of recurring hemorrhage, often petechial, with surrounding erythema and brown hyperpigmentation as a result of hemosiderin deposition in the dermis (Fig. 12–5). Because petechial hemorrhage is common in this syndrome, often the patient or the physician is concerned that there is a serious underlying disorder such as leukemia. Chronic pigmented purpura is not associated with internal disease. Waldenström's hypergammaglobulinemic purpura is usually characterized by macular hemorrhage in either dependent areas or areas covered by restrictive clothing. This condition may be idiopathic or may occur in association with Sjögren's syndrome, sarcoidosis, or other diseases having a polyclonal gammopathy. These lesions may be associated with a burning sensation and may have little or no inflammation on biopsy. This disorder is characterized by the presence of an IgG–anti-IgG rheumatoid fac-

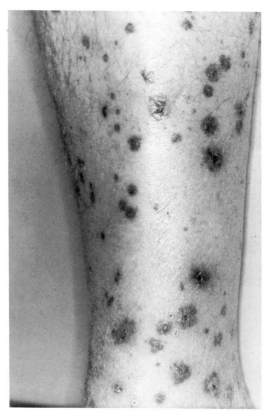

Figure 12–4. Typical, palpable purpura in a patient with leukocytoclastic vasculitis.

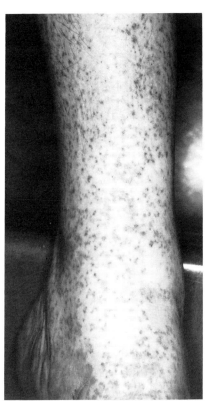

Figure 12–5. Pigmented purpuric eruption secondary to capillaritis. These lesions were non-palpable.

tor, which is demonstrable using analytic ultracentrifugation of serum or plasma.

Non-inflammatory vascular hemorrhage can occur in Osler-Weber-Rendu syndrome (hereditary hemorrhagic telangiectasia), Ehlers-Danlos syndrome, pseudoxanthoma elasticum, and light chain–related systemic amyloidosis. Because the collagen and elastin content of very small blood vessels is minimal, cutaneous hemorrhage in association with the Ehlers-Danlos syndrome or pseudoxanthoma elasticum is usually not due to a vessel wall abnormality but rather to poor vessel wall support by the surrounding connective tissue. The Kasabach-Merritt syndrome, usually seen in infants, occurs when the abnormal vasculature of a giant cutaneous or visceral hemangioma induces platelet consumption and thrombosis; a clinical picture mimicking disseminated intravascular coagulation may result.

Extravascular Causes

Extravascular causes of hemorrhage may include either major trauma or minor trauma to the skin. Major trauma is that which would result in hemorrhage even in normal skin; is associated with significant tissue swelling, tenderness, or obvious abrasions; and is seldom a diagnostic problem. Purpura related to minor trauma may occur in the absence of obvious tissue swelling and often without patient recollection of trauma. Such hemorrhage is usually due to poor support of the small blood vessels by surrounding abnormal connective tissue. The areas of skin most likely to be traumatized include the extensor surface of forearms, the anterior lower legs, and the dorsum of the hands. Purpura that is due in part to external trauma tends to be distributed in a geometric pattern: for example, linearly on the forearm in a scraping type injury, or linearly across a periarticular flexural crease. Perhaps the most common type of minor trauma–related purpura is senile purpura. Most senile purpura in reality should be classified as actinic or solar purpura, since it occurs only in chronically sun-exposed areas with actinic degeneration of the connective tissue. Corticosteroid excess (endogenous or iatrogenic) is another common cause of poor connective tissue support (Fig. 12–6).

The presence of perifollicular hemorrhage should suggest the diagnosis of scurvy, and requires a nutrition-directed history to exclude it as a cause. The reason for the initial perifollicular localization of vitamin C deficiency is not known. The hemorrhage is probably due to a collagen defect, since ascorbic acid is a necessary factor for the formation of normal collagen. Light chain–related systemic amyloidosis is a rare but important cause of dramatic minor trauma–related hemorrhage, owing to infiltration of vessel walls and to replacement of normal connective tissue by infiltration. Waxy appearing papules and plaques, or purpura easily induced by light stroking or pinching of skin, strongly suggests the diagnosis of light chain (AL)–related systemic amyloidosis. Cutaneous hemorrhage as a result of Ehlers-Danlos syndrome and pseudoxanthoma elasticum is usually due to the poor tissue support vessels receive in involved areas.

CLINICAL FEATURES

Any cutaneous eruption may become hemorrhagic when sufficiently traumatized:

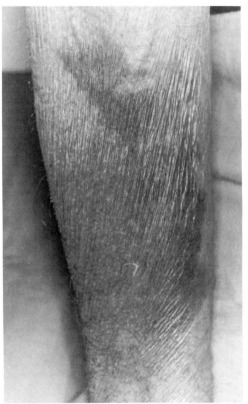

Figure 12–6. Ecchymosis as a result of steroid application. Also, note the cutaneous atrophy produced by topical steroids. (Courtesy of Dr. Neil A. Fenske, Tampa, FL.)

for example, by scratching. In contrast, the presence of symmetrical hemorrhage, especially in dependent areas, or hemorrhage in lesions that the patient cannot easily scratch, as well as the absence of excoriations, suggests that hemorrhage is primary rather than secondary. Because purpura has many different causes, the associated history and physical findings will vary greatly, depending on the etiology. For instance, arthralgias, arthritis, fever, and visceral lesions may accompany cutaneous small vessel leukocytoclastic vasculitis. Monoclonal cryoglobulinemia results from clonal plasma cell population expansion, which may be malignant. Widespread petechial hemorrhage developing into a disseminated intravascular coagulation–like state in an ill patient might result from the diffuse endothelial cell inflammation associated with Rocky Mountain spotted fever. Larger lesions of palpable purpura, often with central necrosis or pustule formation, may develop with other forms of sepsis from meningococcal, gonococcal, or staphylococcal infections.

DIFFERENTIAL DIAGNOSIS

The differential diagnosis has already been discussed in the section on pathogenesis. A complete differential diagnosis of purpura is beyond the scope of this chapter. However, by organizing the history and physical findings within the framework of intravascular, vascular, and extravascular causes of purpura, it may be possible to reach the correct diagnosis more rapidly and efficiently than simply through the indiscriminate use of laboratory studies.

HISTOPATHOLOGY

Histologically, purpura presents as the extravasation of red blood cells in the dermis. Both petechiae and ecchymoses show simple extravasation on biopsy examination, the difference being the extent of involvement. Patients with inflammatory hemorrhage may show leukocytoclastic vasculitis changes, characterized primarily by the presence of at least some neutrophils in and around vessel walls, the presence of perivascular nuclear dust representing degenerated neutrophil nuclei, and fibrinoid necrosis of the vessel wall. This is the histologic correlate of most forms of necrotizing vasculitis.

PATIENT EVALUATION

The value of a careful history, physical examination with detailed skin inspection, and examination of the peripheral blood smear cannot be overemphasized. They are essential ingredients to the proper evaluation of any patient with purpuric lesions. Purpura can be diagnosed visually on physical examination. In rare instances, evidence of hemorrhage may be detectable on biopsy alone, but the role of biopsy in the evaluation is usually most helpful in patients with palpable purpura or in diseases such as cryoglobulinemia, disseminated intravascular coagulation, thrombotic thrombocytopenic purpura, or vessel wall or connective tissue infiltration. A confirmatory biopsy is best performed on new lesions in order to observe the most typical histopathologic and immunofluorescent findings.

The complete blood cell count and peripheral blood smear are of vital importance in the evaluation of patients with purpura. Because platelets are the most important factor in maintaining hemostasis in small blood vessels, a platelet count and a bleeding time are usually much more important than a prothrombin time or partial thromboplastin time in evaluating causes of cutaneous hemorrhage. The blood smear should always be used as confirmatory test, especially when the complete blood cell count is performed by automation. For example, significant thrombocytosis can be missed by automated counters when the platelets have agglutinated, a common finding in the thrombocytosis of myeloproliferative disorders. Also, the presence of red cell spherocytosis on a peripheral smear may be due to an antibody-mediated hemolytic anemia, and might imply a distinct but concurrent autoimmune-mediated destruction of platelets, as in systemic lupus erythematosus.

TREATMENT

Almost all treatment for purpura is directed at the specific cause of hemorrhage, making the correct diagnosis absolutely critical to proper care. The treatment of cutaneous vasculitis is discussed in Chapter 4. The treatment of other forms of purpura depends on the underlying cause.

Suggested Readings

Braverman IM: The angiitides. *In* Braverman IM: Skin Signs of Systemic Disease, 2nd ed. Philadelphia, WB Saunders Co., 1981, pp. 378–452.

Gottlieb AJ: Nonallergic purpura. *In* Williams WJ, et al: Hematology, 3rd ed. New York, McGraw-Hill Book Co., 1983, pp. 1363–1368.

Marder VJ: Consumptive thrombohemorrhagic disorders. *In* Williams WJ, et al: Hematology, 3rd ed. New York, McGraw-Hill Book Co., 1983, pp. 1433–1461.

Moake JL, Funicella T: Common Bleeding Problems. Clinical Symposia 35. West Caldwell, NJ, Ciba Pharmaceutical Co., 1983, pp. 1–32.

Robboy SJ, Mihm ML, Colman RW, Minna JD: The skin in disseminated intravascular coagulation: Prospective analysis of thirty-six cases. Br J Dermatol 99:221–229, 1973.

Spicer TE: Purpura fulminans. Am J Med *61*:566, 1976.

Stone MS, Rosen T: Acral purpura: An unusual sign of coumarin necrosis. J Am Acad Dermatol *14*:797–802, 1986.

Williams WJ: Classification of disorders of hemostasis. *In* Williams WJ, et al: Hematology, 3rd ed. New York, McGraw-Hill Book Co., 1983, pp. 1288–1289.

III

CUTANEOUS HEMATOLOGY AND ONCOLOGY

13

Skin Signs of Internal Malignancy

JEFFREY P. CALLEN

The skin often reflects internal processes, and this awareness in our patients leads them to consider malignancy as a potential cause for many ailments of the cutaneous surface. In addition, there are many conditions that at one time or another have been linked to internal malignancy in both a specific and/or a non-specific manner. In this chapter, we consider those cutaneous disorders that have been linked to internal malignancies, and specifically attempt to answer the questions regarding whether or not a condition should be considered as a potential reflection of malignancy, the precise manner in which the skin disease and the neoplasm are related, and the evaluation necessary for the patient with the cutaneous disease.

Curth has previously suggested criteria by which we can gauge the potential relationship of two disorders, in this case a skin change and neoplasia (Table 13–1). The malignancy and the skin disorder should occur *concurrently*, the two disorders should follow a *parallel* course, there should be a *specific tumor site or cell type* associated with the skin disease, there should be a *statistical association* between the two processes, and there should be a *genetic association* between the two disorders. In each potential association, we will examine these factors in order to determine if a "true" association exists. There is no adequate method for ordering the entities that we will be examining, and thus we will attempt to deal with them alphabetically within three categories: (1) proliferative and inflammatory dermatoses, (2) hormone-secreting tumors, and (3) inherited syndromes.

PROLIFERATIVE AND INFLAMMATORY DERMATOSES

Acanthosis Nigricans

The characteristic feature of acanthosis nigricans (AN) is the presence of hyperpigmented, velvety thickening of the skin on intertriginous surfaces. The eruption usually involves the axillary vault (Fig. 13–1; Plate IIIA), the neck, the inguinal crease, the nipples, and the umbilicus, but may also involve areas of trauma such as the elbows, knees, and knuckles. Occasionally the oral mucosa can have a papillomatous change (Fig. 13–2). In rare instances, the eruption can become generalized. Verrucous or papillary lesions may also accompany the typical lesions of AN. Patients may also develop multiple seborrheic keratoses.

AN can occur in multiple clinical circumstances, including internal neoplasia, various endocrinopathies, a familial form, and a form associated with obesity (pseudo-AN).

Table 13–1. CRITERIA USED TO ASSOCIATE DERMATOSES AND NEOPLASIA

Concurrent onset
Parallel course
Uniform neoplasm (site of cell type)
Statistical association
Genetic association

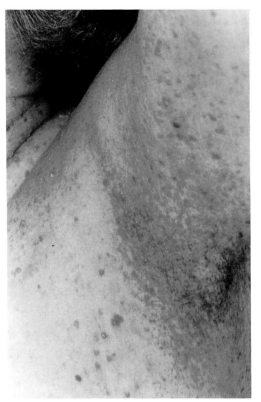

Figure 13–1. Acanthosis nigricans and multiple seborrheic keratoses and skin tags in an individual with adenocarcinoma of the stomach (see also Plate IIIA). (Courtesy of Dr. Neil A. Fenske, Tampa, FL.)

When other associations are ruled out, the possibility of an underlying neoplasm must be strongly considered. In general, the patients with malignant AN are older adults.

AN most often occurs simultaneously with the underlying malignancy; however, cases in which the dermatosis preceded or followed the malignancy have also been reported. Approximately 90% of the tumors associated with AN are within the abdominal cavity, including the gastrointestinal and genitourinary tracts. Furthermore, most of the tumors are adenocarcinomas. The most frequent single occurrence is the association of malignant AN with adenocarcinoma of the stomach. Malignancies outside the abdomen and non-adenocarcinomas have been reported. The course of AN in the presence of cancer seems to parallel the course of the tumor. The prognosis of malignant AN is poor, owing to the nature of the tumors with which it is associated. Thus, malignant AN is a prototype of dermatological conditions associated with malignancy in that it fits all

of Curth's "postulates" except the genetic association.

Acrochordons (Skin Tags)

Skin tags are extremely common skin lesions that have been believed to be of little or no significance. Recently, this long held belief has been questioned by the finding of colonic adenomatous polyps in patients with multiple acrochordons. A methodologic problem has been present in all the studies thus far reported. The patients selected for study have had symptoms that warranted an evaluation for polyps. The studies then assessed the frequency of skin tags in those patients with or without polyps. Until an appropriate study prospectively demonstrates that patients with skin tags have more frequent polyps regardless of the presence or absence of bowel symptoms, we should remain skeptical of this association.

Bazex's Syndrome

Acrokeratosis paraneoplastica, or Bazex's syndrome, is by definition always associated with an underlying malignancy. Acrokeratosis paraneoplastica develops progressively

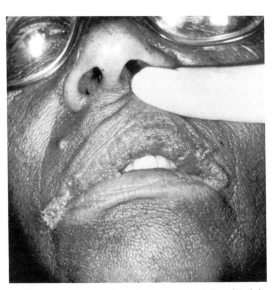

Figure 13–2. Mucosal surfaces may be involved in acanthosis nigricans, as demonstrated by this woman with adenocarcinoma of the stomach. (Courtesy of Dr. Mark Holzberg, Atlanta, GA.)

through three stages. The initial cutaneous signs consist of erythematous, violaceous, poorly defined macules with a fine, adherent scale that occur over the acral areas of the body, such as the fingers, toes, ears, and nose. Paronychial reaction is also said to be quite common. The second stage involves the development of a keratoderma, and the initial lesions become more generalized. In the third stage, the eruption generalizes but still maintains this violaceous nature, the keratoderma, and the predilection for acral involvement (Fig. 13–3; Plate IIIB). The three stages of the cutaneous disease parallel the growth and spread of the underlying tumor. Tumors associated with this process are generally found in the upper "aerodigestive" tract and are most often squamous cell carcinomas. The course of the cutaneous involvement has been found to often parallel the course of the tumor. Thus, this condition seems to fulfill the criteria necessary to consider it a marker of internal malignancy.

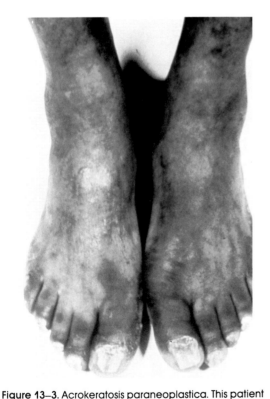

Figure 13–3. Acrokeratosis paraneoplastica. This patient demonstrates violaceous plaques in the acral areas. He also had squamous cell carcinoma of the larynx (see also Plate IIIB). (Courtesy of Dr. Charles Camisa, Columbus, OH.)

Bowen's Disease

Bowen's disease is a form of intraepidermal squamous cell carcinoma of the skin. Invasion of this neoplastic process can occur late in the course of the disease. Sun exposure and arsenic ingestion have been implicated in the etiology of Bowen's disease. The lesion of Bowen's disease is an erythematous plaque with scale and occasionally erosion. The lesion is often treated as an eczema or as psoriasis prior to biopsy, which reveals the true nature of the pathologic process.

The relationship of Bowen's disease and malignancy was reported by Graham and Helwig in 1959 to be as high as 80%; however, subsequently these same authors revised their figures downward. Later it was suggested that those patients with lesions on "non-exposed" surfaces had a much greater propensity for the presence of an underlying malignancy. Our data did not support this latter theory, but it did seem that our patients had a greater risk of having or developing a cancer than would be expected in the general population. Data from Denmark have failed to show any cancer risk for patients with Bowen's disease or other types of cutaneous malignancies. Recently, all these data have been called into question by epidemiologists. In addition, there is no type or site of neoplasm that has been associated with Bowen's disease, and there is no parallel course. Thus, at the current time this entity should not be considered to be a marker of internal malignancy, and patients should not have evaluations beyond the standard history, physical examination, and appropriate age-related testing.

Bullous Dermatosis

Several of the bullous dermatoses have been associated with malignancies. Traditionally, the most often mentioned disorder has been bullous pemphigoid, a blistering disorder that frequently occurs in older adults (see Chapter 45). The association of malignancy with this bullous disorder seems to be coincidental, and may be only related to the fact that both bullous pemphigoid and malignancy tend to occur in the elderly. Several authors have suggested that certain pemphigoid subsets may be associated with an increased risk of malignancy; in particular, those patients with negative immuno-fluorescence, those who have linear IgA disease, and those who have prominent mucosal lesions. There are a wide variety of neoplasms associated with pemphigoid, and there does not appear to be a specific course relating the pemphigoid to the malignancy. Epidermolysis bullosa acquisita, a related disorder, has only rarely been associated with malignancy. Thus at the current time, the data are not supportive of a relationship for pemphigoid or related disorders and malignancy.

The pemphigus group of disorders has been associated with thymomas, both benign and malignant. Those patients with this association tend also to have myasthenia gravis. The course of the pemphigus has not been found to coincide with that of the neoplasm. However, it seems wise to review the routine chest x-ray carefully to be certain not to miss the possible association with thymoma.

Dermatitis herpetiformis (DH) has been reported in association with intestinal lymphoma. This relationship appears to be due to the presence of gluten-sensitive enteropathy in patients with DH. In those patients whose DH is complicated by the appearance of an intestinal lymphoma, the removal of the tumor does not seem to have an effect on the course of the DH.

Porphyria cutanea tarda (PCT) has been associated with hepatic tumors, in particular primary hepatoma. The exact frequency of hepatic tumors in patients with PCT is not known; however, there are cases that have a concurrent onset and follow a parallel course. Thus, careful evaluation of the liver is necessary in all patients with PCT.

Dermatomyositis and Other Collagen-Vascular Disorders

The issue of dermatomyositis and its potential relationship to malignancy has been discussed elsewhere (see Chapter 2). This entity, although possibly statistically associated with malignancy, only rarely fulfills the other criteria suggestive of a relationship. Thus, at the current time the physician should be aware of a potential neoplasm and be certain that no unexplained symptoms or signs are overlooked.

Malignancies appear to be a coincidental occurrence in patients with lupus erythe-matosus (LE). Several reports of lymphoreticular malignancies in patients with systemic LE seem to be due to the therapy of the LE with immunosuppressive agents rather than to the presence of the LE. Myeloma and paraproteinemias have been reported in patients with chronic cutaneous LE, but the frequency and significance of this finding are elusive.

Scleroderma may be linked to malignancy of the lung and/or esophagus. The frequency of these complications is unknown, but they do appear to occur only in those patients with long-standing scleroderma involving the site affected by the neoplasm. Special evaluation of the patient with scleroderma for occult malignancy does not seem warranted.

The coexistence of necrotizing vasculitis and malignant neoplasms has been occasionally noted. Most of the tumors reported with vasculitis have been of the lymphoreticular system, but an occasional patient with a solid tumor has been seen. We reported a man with a carcinoma of the colon whose course seemed to be concurrent and parallel with his vasculitis. One additional neoplasm is worthy of notation: the association of hairy cell leukemia with various vasculitic syndromes. Despite these associations, the vasculitis patient does not need a special malignancy evaluation.

Eruptive Angiomas, Telangiectasias, and Seborrheic Keratoses

Reports linking the sudden appearance of angiomas or telangiectasias with internal malignancies have been published in the dermatological literature. The angiomatous lesions are quite common in an adult population and are seen as small, cherry-colored papules. However, possibly when there is a rapid onset of the lesions, we might be concerned with potential malignancy. The situation with telangiectasias is similar to that with angiomas.

The sudden appearance or growth of multiple seborrheic keratoses is known as the "sign of Leser-Trélat" (see Fig. 13–1). Numerous reports have linked this condition to various malignancies. In addition, many of the patients with this problem also have AN. The sign of Leser-Trélat is associated with intra-abdominal adenocarcinomas but to a lesser extent than is malignant AN. Although all of the criteria are not fulfilled, it seems reasonable to evaluate a patient with this sign carefully with a history, physical examination, and roentgenographic studies of the gastrointestinal and genitourinary systems.

Exfoliative Erythroderma

Exfoliative dermatitis (erythroderma) is a cutaneous reaction characterized by a generalized erythema, edema, and scaling. The reaction may be accompanied by fever, lymphadenopathy, organomegaly, and/or leukocytosis. Malignancy has been reported to be present in roughly 10–15% of patients. In most instances the malignancy is of the lymphoreticular system, but several reports of solid tumors have also appeared. The course of the skin disease often follows that of the tumor, and the discovery of the malignant process has often been linked to the diagnosis of the cutaneous disorder. Therefore, in all patients with erythroderma, the possibility of an underlying neoplasm must be considered.

Figurate Erythemas

There are multiple figurate erythemas, but the only one that truly appears to be related to malignancy is *erythema gyratum repens*. In this eruption, erythematous lesions form gyrate or serpiginous bands that rapidly spread across the cutaneous surface. The lesions produce a "grain of wood" appearance. Almost all cases have been associated with malignancy, which is often concurrently discovered. The course is also frequently parallel to that of the neoplasm. There is not a specific type or site of the malignant process. The presence of erythema gyratum repens should trigger an extensive search for cancer.

Herpes Zoster (Shingles)

Herpes zoster is an acute cutaneous eruption that represents a reoccurrence of a dormant varicella-zoster viral infection. The eruption is characterized by multiple crops of grouped vesicles on an erythematous base that follow a dermatomal distribution. Pain and/or fever may accompany the eruption,

but the patients are generally otherwise in good health. The notion that herpes zoster might be linked to occult malignancy was laid to rest by a study from the Mayo Clinic that demonstrated that there was no increased risk of malignancy regardless of the clinical characteristics of the eruption.

Hypertrichosis Lanuginosa (Malignant Down)

Hypertrichosis is the excessive growth of hair without signs of virilization (Fig. 13–4). The sudden development of fine, downy hair has been linked to the presence of an underlying neoplasm in all cases thus far reported. The malignancies reported have been of varied sites and cell types, but have often been discovered at the time of the diagnosis of hypertrichosis lanuginosa. Glossitis has also accompanied the malignancy-associated down, but it is felt to be a manifestation of a vitamin deficiency rather than a related finding. Patients with this type of hair growth who do not have an endocrinopathy that might cause their hair growth must be evaluated for the possibility of an occult malignancy.

Ichthyosis (Acquired)

Acquired ichthyosis is similar to ichthyosis vulgaris, which is characterized by rhomboidal scales with margins that are lifted off the surface of the skin. Acquired ichthyosis has been associated with malignancy, particularly lymphoreticular disorders. It has also been associated with other paraneoplastic conditions such as AN or the sign of Leser-Trélat. However, several other conditions have been associated with acquired ichthyosis, including hypothyroidism and sarcoidosis. Although there is a possible relationship to neoplastic diseases, it seems that the diagnosis of the malignancy is known at the time of the recognition of the ichthyosis.

Keratoacanthoma

The keratoacanthoma is a rapidly growing epidermal neoplasm that may be locally invasive but that otherwise exhibits a benign course. Multiple keratoacanthomas have been reported with malignancy, and in ad-

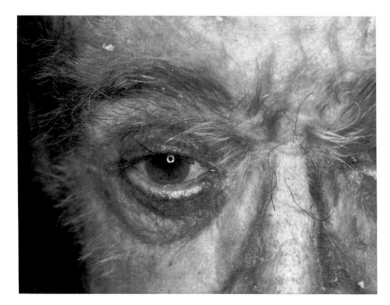

Figure 13–4. Hypertrichosis lanuginosa. This man developed fine lanugo hairs at the same time as he was discovered to have a squamous cell carcinoma of the lung.

dition the keratoacanthoma is one of the cardinal features of the Muir-Torre syndrome. Despite these sporadic reports of an association, we were unable to confirm a role for the keratoacanthoma as a marker of internal malignancy in our study of 78 patients. Patients with keratoacanthoma tend to be elderly, and thus the association appears to be age related.

Migratory Thrombophlebitis (Trousseau's Syndrome)

Although superficial thrombophlebitis is a common medical condition, the appearance of recurrent and migratory disease is potentially a manifestation of an underlying cancer, specifically within the pancreas. The disease is believed to be caused by a chronic, low grade, intravascular coagulopathy. The veins of the neck, chest, and abdomen, as well as those of the lower extremities, are involved sequentially or simultaneously. Patients with this finding should be evaluated thoroughly, including a CAT scan of the abdomen.

Multicentric Reticulohistiocytosis

Multicentric reticulohistiocytosis is a rare disorder characterized by polyarthritis and nodular skin lesions. The skin lesions are small, flesh-colored to violaceous nodules on the scalp, ears, face, extremities, trunk, and mucous membranes. The arthritis involves the joints of the hands and is destructive, eventually resulting in severe deformities of the fingers. Roughly one quarter of the patients have had an internal malignancy, usually a carcinoma. The exact relationship, specifically the manner in which the disorder is associated with cancer, is not clear.

Mycosis Fungoides (Cutaneous T Cell Lymphoma)

Cutaneous T cell lymphoma (CTCL) is often a chronic cutaneous disease characterized by poikiloderma or erythematous plaques. The disease is characterized histopathologically by epidermotrophic malignant T cells. Second primary malignancies have been reported to occur in patients with CTCL more frequently than would be predicted. The malignancies vary in their site and cell type and occur concurrently, prior to, or subsequent to the diagnosis of CTCL. The data do not suggest that an extensive search for malignancy be conducted, but they do suggest that new symptoms or signs must be carefully and thoroughly evaluated.

Necrobiotic Xanthogranuloma

The term necrobiotic xanthogranuloma with paraproteinemia was coined by Winkelmann to describe the destructive cutaneous lesions associated with the histopathologic finding of an inflammatory granuloma with xanthomatosis and panniculitis that was associated with a paraproteinemia. Clinically, the lesions are yellow to red papules, nodules, or plaques that enlarge and become ulcerative. The lesions have a predilection to occur on the periorbital skin. By definition, these lesions have been associated with paraproteinemia and infrequently with myeloma.

Paget's Disease of the Breast and Extramammary Paget's Disease

Paget's disease of the breast is characterized by an erythematous, eczematous plaque surrounding the nipple and areola (Fig. 13–5; Plate IIIC). This condition occurs in conjunction with a ductal adenocarcinoma of the breast, which has frequently metastasized to the axillary lymph nodes. Paget's disease is believed to be due to an upward migration of malignant cells, and as such it is not truly a paraneoplastic sign.

Extramammary Paget's disease is the same clinicopathologic lesion found in mammary Paget's, occurring on a non-mammary surface. The lesions most often occur on the genital, the axillary, or the perianal skin. Only 40–50% of the patients with this condition have an underlying neoplasm. The neoplasms generally occur in areas underlying the area of involvement, such as the genitourinary or gastrointestinal tract. In patients with extramammary Paget's disease, an evaluation of the areas contiguous to the disease should be undertaken.

Pityriasis Rotunda

Pityriasis rotunda is an unusual, round, non-inflammatory, circular lesion that occurs on the trunk and results in hyperpigmentation. Various malignancies have been reported to occur in conjunction with pityriasis rotunda, but in addition, this condition has been reported with numerous other potential etiologic agents. In a study from South Africa, pityriasis rotunda was reported in 10 patients, of whom 7 had hepatocellular carcinoma. The relationship of this skin condition to malignancy when present is not known; to date, there have not been patients whose pityriasis rotunda has followed the course of the neoplasm. Despite the lack of confirmatory data, it seems prudent to at least consider cancer in anyone with this rare cutaneous disease.

Punctate Keratoses of the Palms and Soles

Punctate keratoses are discrete, flesh-colored, hyperkeratotic papules that occur on the palms and soles. The lesions often have a central plug or a depressed, crater-like center (Fig. 13–6). The lesions are often numerous but remain distinct from one another. Symptoms are rarely experienced by the patient. Arsenical keratoses, although histopathologically different, are clinically indistinguishable from punctate keratoses. Occasionally, this type of lesion is seen in the familial syndrome of tylosis palmaris et plantaris.

With the exception of the familial syndrome that is associated with esophageal carcinoma, the relationship of punctate keratoses or arsenical keratoses to malignancy is controversial at best. Some studies have suggested that there is a relationship, whereas other studies have failed to find an increased incidence of neoplasia in patients with palmar keratoses. Furthermore, there is not a uniform type of malignancy, nor is there any distinctive relationship. Thus, at the current time it does not seem to be necessary to evaluate these patients in any specific manner.

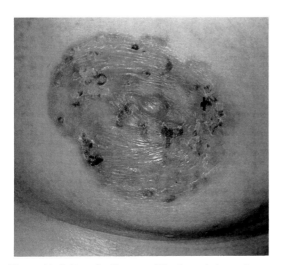

Figure 13–5. Paget's disease of the breast. An erythematous plaque surrounds the nipple in this female with ductal adenocarcinoma of the breast (see also Plate IIIC).

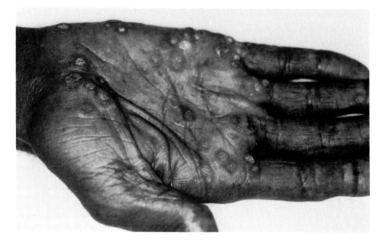

Figure 13–6. Arsenical keratoses. Multiple keratotic lesions exist in this individual. No other tumors were found.

Pyoderma Gangrenosum and Other "Neutrophilic" Dermatoses

Cases of various malignancies have been reported infrequently in patients with classic pyoderma gangrenosum. However, those patients with atypical bullous pyoderma gangrenosum have been frequently found to have myeloid leukemia or a pre-leukemic state (Fig. 13–7). Similarly, multiple patients with Sweet's syndrome (acute febrile neutrophilic dermatosis) have been reported to have myeloid leukemia. In these patients, the discovery of the leukemia often occurs with the recognition of the cutaneous abnormality. The skin lesions also disappear when the leukemia is in remission, and the skin disease recurs when the leukemia relapses. It seems reasonable to evaluate all patients with atypical pyoderma gangrenosum or Sweet's syndrome with careful hematologic studies, including a bone marrow examination.

Pachydermoperiostosis Acquisita

Acquired pachydermoperiostosis is represented by the combination of thickening of the skin, a hypertrophic osteoarthropathy, and clubbing of the nails. Facial skin can be affected and give the facies a coarse appearance similar to that seen with acromegaly. In addition, the skin of the distal extremities is also frequently involved. The palms and soles may also become hyperkeratotic. Clubbing, which is part of this "syndrome," can also occur without the other features of the disease, and essentially has the same implications regarding malignancy.

These disorders have been most frequently associated with cancers in the lungs. However, they occur in many benign pulmonary and cardiac disorders as well. The incidence of malignancy is unknown, as are the results of tumor therapy on the course of the skin and the nails. Thus, we should consider clubbing with or without pachydermoperiostosis to be a sign of cardiopulmonary disease, possibly of lung cancer.

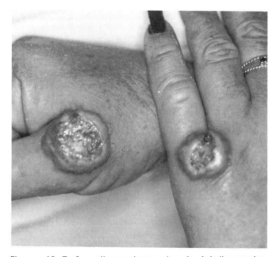

Figure 13–7. Sweet's syndrome (acute febrile neutrophilic dermatosis) in a patient with carcinoma of the thyroid.

Vitiligo

Vitiligo or a vitiligo-like leukoderma has been reported in conjunction with malignant melanomas. Furthermore, a report has linked vitiligo in older individuals (over age 40) with various malignant neoplasms. This association has not been confirmed. In our view, the onset of vitiligo in an adult does warrant a careful examination of the entire cutaneous surface. In addition, if in the future serologic testing for melanoma becomes available and is reliable, it would also be indicated.

HORMONE-SECRETING SYNDROMES

Carcinoid Syndrome

The carcinoid syndrome is produced by tumors that secrete 5-hydroxytryptamine and other vasoactive amines. The tumors are most common in the gastrointestinal tract, but also occur in the lungs or ovaries. Clinically, there is flushing, diarrhea, abdominal pain, wheezing, and occasionally shortness of breath. Tumors from the gastrointestinal tract do not produce symptoms until they metastasize to the liver, because the liver under normal circumstances is able to detoxify the amines responsible for the production of symptoms. Tumors in other locations are capable of producing the symptoms prior to metastasis. The diagnosis of carcinoid syndrome is made by finding elevated levels of 5-hydroxyindole acetic acid (or other metabolites or other vasoactive amines) in the urine. Removal of the tumor results in a cessation of the symptoms.

Ectopic ACTH Syndrome

Certain tumors are capable of amine precursor uptake and decarboxylation and are thus known as APUDomas. These tumors usually originate in the lungs (bronchial adenoma or oat cell carcinoma), gastrointestinal tract (carcinoid—see previous discussion), or in glands. Ectopic ACTH producing tumors result in many of the typical signs and symptoms of Cushing's syndrome, with the exception of obesity. Intense hyperpigmentation is rare in Cushing's disease but is common in the patients with ectopic production of ACTH. The most common tumor producing this syndrome is the oat cell carcinoma of the lung.

Glucagonoma Syndrome
(see Chapter 22)

Necrolytic migratory erythema is the term used to describe the rash associated with glucagon producing tumors. These tumors are APUDomas that involve the alpha-cell of the pancreas. The characteristic cutaneous eruption is widespread, beginning with irregular patches of erythema studded with superficial flaccid erosion, vesicles, and bullae. The erythema and bullae may coalesce into circinate and/or polycyclic lesions. The eruption may be widespread but tends to concentrate on the central areas of the body, in particular the groin. Erythematous lesions at the corners of the mouth (angular cheilitis) and glossitis are commonly seen. Other findings include the recent onset of diabetes mellitus, anemia, weight loss, and diarrhea. The eruption is often confused with seborrheic dermatitis, intertrigo, or candidiasis. It closely resembles the rash seen in acrodermatitis enteropathica or acquired zinc deficiency. The mechanism by which the rash is produced is not completely understood, but removal of the tumor results in a disappearance of the rash. About one half to two thirds of the patients with the glucagonoma syndrome have liver metastases at the time of diagnosis; thus, the prognosis is generally guarded.

INHERITED SYNDROMES ASSOCIATED WITH INTERNAL CANCER

Cowden's Disease

Cowden's disease (multiple hamartoma syndrome—MHS) is a multisystem disease complex with an autosomal dominant inheritance pattern. The mucocutaneous findings are the most characteristic features of this disorder and include multiple facial trichilemmomas located around the nose and central face (Fig. 13–8); multiple keratotic papules on the face, neck, ears, and hands; and multiple papules on the oral mucosa that

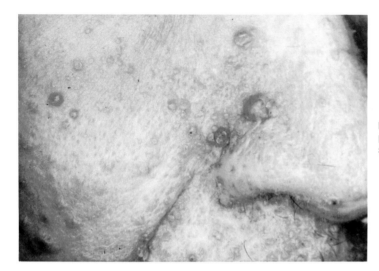

Figure 13–8. Cowden's disease. Multiple keratotic papules exist in the nasolabial fold and on the nose.

coalesce to form a cobblestone appearance. The systemic manifestations include multiple hamartomatous polyps in the gastrointestinal tract, tumors of the thyroid gland, ovarian cysts, and fibrocystic disease of the breast. The most important feature of Cowden's disease is an increased prevalence of malignant tumors of the breast, often bilateral. In addition, malignancy of the thyroid gland may occur. The percentage of malignant tumors may be as high as 40–50%, including adenocarcinoma of the breast (20%); adenocarcinoma of the thyroid (7%); squamous cell carcinoma of the skin (4%); and cancers of the colon, prostate, uterus, cervix, bladder, or blood (less than 1% each). Careful evaluation of patients with this syndrome for underlying malignancies is necessary in all individuals and all family members. Some authorities have even gone so far as to suggest prophylactic mastectomy in the female patients with this disease.

Gardner's Syndrome

Gardner's syndrome is an autosomal dominant disorder characterized by polyposis coli, cutaneous cysts, and multiple osteomas. The cysts are epidermoid cysts that appear in early childhood on the face, trunk, and scalp and that can precede the recognition of the colonic polyps by many years. In addition, fibromas, desmoid tumors, and lipomas may also be present on the skin. The colonic polyps are adenomatous in their

nature, and thus have the potential to degenerate into adenocarcinomas. If the polyps are left in place long enough, all patients will develop cancer of the colon; thus, prophylactic total colectomy is usually recommended in early adulthood.

Peutz-Jeghers Syndrome

Mucocutaneous pigmented macules and hamartomatous polyps of the gastrointestinal tract are characteristic of the Peutz-Jeghers syndrome. The hyperpigmented macules tend to cluster around the lips, on the oral mucosa, and on acral areas of the body. This disorder is inherited in an autosomal dominant pattern, but spontaneous mutations seem to account for 50% of the cases. The polyps, which may involve the entire gastrointestinal tract, are hamartomatous in nature and are thus not pre-malignant. However, in a small percentage of the patients, malignant degeneration of the polyps is possible, and additionally tumors of the breast have been reported in some pedigrees. Close follow-up of these patients is necessary, but no prophylactic surgery is needed.

Torre's Syndrome (Muir-Torre Syndrome)

Torre initially described a man with multiple sebaceous adenomas and carcinoma of the ampulla of Vater. Subsequently, this syndrome was characterized as an autosomal dominant disorder. Clinically, the patients have multiple sebaceous tumors, including adenomas, adenocarcinomas, and epitheliomas, in association with multiple adenocarcinomas of the colon. Other internal tumors have been reported, as well as other cutaneous neoplasms such as squamous cell carcinoma and keratoacanthomas. It was believed that the recognition of the syndrome rested on the appearance of a sebaceous tumor; however, it has been found that many patients with sebaceous neoplasms do not have internal malignancies. Thus, the presence of this neoplasm should not result in an extensive evaluation unless a positive family history exists. Lastly, it has been of interest that the visceral tumors seem to behave in a more benign fashion than would be expected from their histopathologic appearance.

von Recklinghausen's Disease

Neurofibromatosis is an autosomal dominant disorder that is discussed elsewhere (see Chapter 41). Somewhere between 2 and 5% of the patients with this syndrome will develop a malignancy, many of which represent a malignant degeneration of the neurofibroma. However, these patients may also develop astrocytomas, glioblastomas, meningiomas, and bilateral pheochromocytomas. Thus, if the patient with neurofibromatosis develops symptoms of headache, backache, or hypertension, the potential of an internal malignancy must be considered and appropriate tests ordered.

CONCLUSIONS

The cutaneous disorders associated with malignancy are reviewed in Table 13–2. They are classified as (1) those that fit the criteria to warrant specific investigations, (2) those that are statistically related to internal malignancy but that do not require extensive

Table 13–2. PARANEOPLASTIC DISORDERS

Disorders that Fit Curth's Criteria
Acanthosis nigricans and possibly the sign of Leser-Trélat
Bazex's syndrome
Carcinoid syndrome
Erythema gyratum repens
Hypertrichosis lanuginosa
Ectopic ACTH syndrome
Glucagonoma syndrome
Neutrophilic dermatoses
Paget's disease

Disorders Associated Statistically with Cancer
Acrochordon
Bowen's disease
Dermatomyositis
Extramammary Paget's disease
Exfoliative dermatitis
Mycosis fungoides
Palmar keratoses
Pruritus
Porphyria cutanea tarda
Pityriasis rotunda

Dermatoses Possibly Associated with Cancer
Arsenical keratoses
Erythema annulare centrifugum
Acquired ichthyosis
Multicentric reticulohistiocytosis
Necrobiotic xanthogranuloma
Classic pyoderma gangrenosum
Polymyositis
Vasculitis
Vitiligo

malignancy searches, and (3) those with only a possible association with cancer. Further work is still needed to delineate the exact relationship of these skin disorders with their potentially associated internal neoplasms. Epidemiologic studies that involve statisticians in the experimental design are needed for many of the syndromes that may be related to malignancy.

Suggested Readings

Callen JP (ed): Skin signs of internal malignancy. Sem Dermatol 3:265–359, 1984.
Curth HO: Skin lesions and internal carcinoma. In Andrade R, Gumport SL, Popkin GL, Rees TD (ed): Cancer of the Skin. Philadelphia, WB Saunders Co., 1976, pp. 1308–1343.

14

Metastatic Disease to the Skin

WARREN W. PIETTE

Although malignancies such as leukemias and lymphomas are more likely to be associated with cutaneous involvement (see Chapters 15, 16, and 20), such malignancies are relatively rare compared with solid tumors, especially carcinomas. For this reason, despite a relatively low incidence of cutaneous metastases, carcinomas account for most instances of metastatic disease to the skin. The overall incidence of metastatic disease to the skin is low, ranging from 1.4 to 4.4% in three autopsy series and up to 20.4% in a large non-autopsy series; most authors consider the clinical incidence of cutaneous metastases to be 5–10% or less. The series by Brownstein and Helwig provides some important epidemiologic information. Cutaneous metastases were the initial manifestation of malignancy in 27% of men and 6% of women; these figures are much higher than expected because this series was based on biopsy material referred to the Armed Forces Institute of Pathology and represents primarily confusing or unusual cases. Most patients in this series were 40 years of age or older. In women, 69% of cutaneous metastases were due to breast carcinoma; 9% to colon carcinoma; and 4–5% each to melanoma, lung, and ovarian carcinoma. With the significantly increased incidence of lung carcinoma in women since this study was conducted (1972), lung carcinoma may now be a more important cause of cutaneous metastases in women. In men, lung carcinoma accounted for 24% of cutaneous metastases, colon carcinoma for 19%, malignant melanoma for 13%, oral cavity

tumors for 12%, renal tumors for 6%, and gastric carcinoma for 6%. Adults under 40 years old were most likely to have melanoma as the primary tumor.

Recognition of metastatic disease to the skin is important for two reasons. First, a cutaneous metastasis may present before there are clinical signs of an internal malignancy. Second, should a cutaneous metastasis be present, the skin lesion may be the best means of confirming a suspected diagnosis of cancer suggested by findings in other organs much more difficult to biopsy, or may lead the clinician to search for the primary tumor in the correct organ system.

PATHOGENESIS

The exact mechanisms leading to invasion and metastasis of tumors are not known, but a number of factors have some theoretical and experimental support. There is evidence that some metastases are produced from a specialized minor subpopulation of cells, that some metastases are clonal in origin, that different metastases can originate from different progenitor cells, and that metastatic tumor cells are usually less genetically stable than are non-metastatic tumor cells. This evidence would suggest that most cells in a tumor are not important in terms of tumor metastasis, since they lack the particular factors needed to establish distant metastases.

Mutations may change cancer cells so that they become more or less prone to metastasize, and that some organic specificity for metastases may result. There is also evidence that tumor cells may gain the ability to metastasize by gaining genetic material from either normal cells or other tumor cells. Finally, in certain tumor models the ability to metastasize depends on the failure of the cell to express a particular antigen such as a particular class 1 major histocompatibility complex antigen. If the cell line is induced to express this antigen, its ability to metastasize is considerably reduced, suggesting a possible role for host immunologic response in defense against tumor growth.

The relative role of tumor cell properties and host defense mechanisms in the metastatic process is unknown. Macrophages may also be important in host tumor defenses, whether by an immunologic or non-immunologic mechanism. Even the specific factors required for local invasion or distant metastases are not well known, and are an area of considerable debate. The traditional concept of tumor invasion and metastasis begins with tumor cell proliferation, resulting in mechanical growth pressure, active tumor cell locomotion, and degradation of host interstitial matrix, possibly by enzymatic means. However, experimental evidence suggests that there is a much more complicated process involved.

If distant metastases are to occur, a capacity for tumor cell binding to endothelium and crossing vessel walls would seem to be important. Cell surface markers, host endothelial cell reactions, fibrin, and other potential surface bonding materials might also be important in facilitating this process. However, despite intense interest and efforts directed toward understanding the mechanisms for metastasis, more questions than answers remain.

CLINICAL FEATURES

Site

Several possible routes of tumor spread to the skin exist: direct extension into skin from an underlying malignancy, propagation of a tumor through lymphatics connecting with the skin, metastatic spread (embolization) through lymphatic and blood vessels, and rarely implantation of tumor during surgery with proliferation in the wound or scar.

The site of cutaneous metastasis depends in part on the site of the primary tumor and in part on the mechanism of metastasis for that tumor. In the Brownstein and Helwig series, the anterior chest wall and abdomen of women, and the anterior chest wall, abdomen, head, and neck of men accounted for 75% of observed cutaneous metastases, despite the fact that these skin sites compose less than 25% of the body surface area. Conversely, the back, flanks, and extremities were seldom the site of metastatic disease.

Malignant neoplasms that invade the lymphatics, such as breast carcinoma, squamous cell carcinoma of the oral cavity, and most pelvic neoplasms, will tend to metastasize to the skin overlying the neoplasm. Tumors that spread hematogenously, such as renal cell carcinoma and some pulmonary tumors, will often metastasize to distant sites. Many tumors have the capacity to spread by either means. Therefore, the type of cutaneous metastases at specific sites depends on the relative incidence of primary tumor types, the usual route of invasion or metastasis for that tumor type, the pattern of lymphatic drainage or relative blood flow in a particular site, and the proximity of a tumor to the skin surface. For example, a relatively rich blood supply may explain the increased incidence of scalp metastasis for such hematogenously spread tumors as leukemia, lymphoma, renal cell carcinoma, and some pulmonary carcinomas. Brownstein and Helwig detailed the most frequent tumor metastases by anatomic sites: (1) for the scalp: lung and renal cell carcinoma in men, breast carcinoma in women; (2) for the face: oral cavity squamous cell carcinomas in both men and women; (3) for the anterior chest: lung carcinoma in men and breast carcinoma in women; (4) for the abdomen: lung and large bowel carcinoma in men, ovarian carcinoma in women; and (5) for the extremities: melanoma in both sexes.

Clinical Appearance

Cutaneous metastases most commonly present as flesh-colored or slightly erythematous nodules or tumors involving the dermis and often the subcutaneous tissue; ulceration of such nodules is unusual (Fig. 14–1). Metastatic lesions may also be violaceous, pink, brown, or black in color, de-

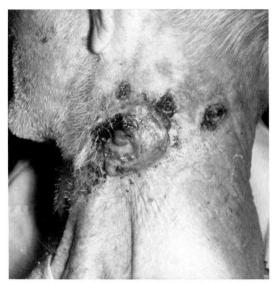

Figure 14–1. In this patient, a large, nodular lesion is present, representative of metastatic disease from the larynx.

pending on the type of tumor, its vascularity, and any associated pigment production. The consistency of lesions is characteristically firm or even rock hard. A rubbery consistency on palpation can be seen with any tumor type, but is more typical of hematopoietic malignancies or some sarcomas. Nodules may be freely movable or fixed to underlying tissue.

Other patterns of metastasis can be seen, particularly with certain tumor types. The *peau d'orange*, or orange peel, appearance of skin lesions in some patients is the result of lymphatic blockage by tumor, resulting in local lymphedema with "tethering" of the skin by skin appendages (Fig. 14–2; Plate IIID). This produces non-pitting edema with depressions at the site of hair follicle openings. Although this appearance is suggestive of cutaneous lymphatic invasion by breast carcinoma, particularly on the anterior chest wall, other tumors may also cause similar changes, and non-neoplastic diseases resulting in chronic lymphedema may also produce the same orange peel appearance. When such cutaneous changes are tumor related and extensive owing to involvement of the regional lymphatics, a condition known as *carcinoma en cuirasse* may develop. This condition is characterized by large sclerotic plaques that may be studded with nodules and, again, is most commonly seen with breast carcinoma. A variant known as carcinoma telangiectaticum consists of broad sclerotic plaques with multiple overlying telangiectases and telangiectatic papules. Inflammatory carcinoma (carcinoma erysipelatoides) mimics erysipelas or acute cellulitis, presenting as red, swollen, painful plaques; it results from lymphatic obstruction and associated acute inflammation (Fig. 14–3). Though rare, it typically is associated with breast carcinoma, especially in women with large, pendulous breasts, but can occur elsewhere and with other tumor types. A very sclerotic variant of metastasis (sometimes termed eburnean carcinoma) can present as morpheaform plaques. Tumor

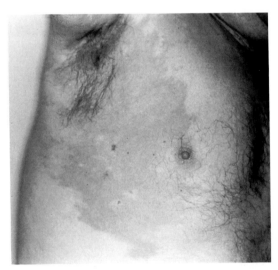

Figure 14–2. Metastatic carcinoma with a cellulitic appearance on the anterior chest wall as a result of carcinoma of the lung (see also Plate IIID).

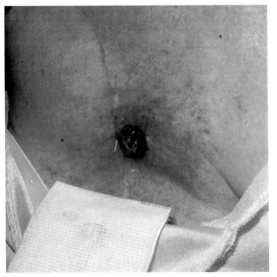

Figure 14–3. Metastatic nodule developing in a scar as a result of a local recurrence of breast carcinoma.

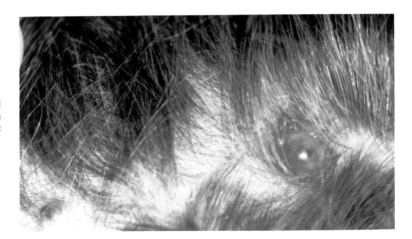

Figure 14–4. Metastatic renal cell carcinoma. This nodule in the scalp represents metastatic renal cell carcinoma.

cells may be very sparsely distributed within the lesion, and the fibrotic response of the skin may compress or distort the cancer cells, making their detection difficult.

Scalp metastases are often atypical in appearance, and may mimic cylindromas (turban tumors) or pilar cysts, or may present as patchy, usually scarring, alopecia (Fig. 14–4).

Metastases may sometimes cluster about the umbilicus, a phenomenon known by the eponym of Sister Mary Joseph's nodule (Fig. 14–5). Powell and colleagues reviewed 85 cases of tumor metastatic to the umbilicus. The lesions were usually firm, indurated nodules, often vascular in appearance and sometimes associated with fissuring or ulceration of the nodules. In 12 cases, this finding was the initial presentation of the internal malignancy. In 17 cases, despite review of the histologic material, the primary tumor site was never determined. In the remaining 68 cases, the tumors were primarily from the stomach, large bowel, ovary, and pancreas, in that order. Patients were 32–91 years of age (average age 61), men and women were roughly equal in number, and most patients died within months of the nodule's appearance. Most malignancies were intra-abdominal in origin, but 5 were female breast carcinoma. The tumors were overwhelmingly adenocarcinoma (79 cases), but 3 were undifferentiated tumors, 2 were squamous cell carcinomas, and one was a leiomyosarcoma.

Other unusual forms of cutaneous metastases include a zosteriform eruption with vesicle formation as a result of prostate or pulmonary adenocarcinoma, a chancriform metastasis to the penis caused by a transitional cell carcinoma or colonic adenocarcinoma, and verrucous nodules on the lower extremity in a patient with a chronically lymphedematous leg.

The characteristic pattern and appearance of metastatic lesions may be altered when such lesions arise in areas of previously damaged skin. For example, if metastases develop in an area of skin previously injured by radiation therapy directed at the primary tumor, the cutaneous metastases are much more likely to show early erosion or ulceration and may be associated with radiation therapy–related hyperpigmentation, telangiectases, or atrophy. Metastatic lesions in such a location may be difficult to differen-

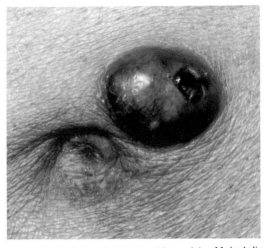

Figure 14–5. Sister Mary Joseph's nodule. Metastatic adenocarcinoma of the stomach to an area near the umbilicus.

tiate from a primary carcinoma because neoplasms such as basal cell and squamous cell carcinomas, sarcoma, and atypical fibroxanthoma may arise *de novo* in areas of radiation dermatitis, as well as occasionally from other types of chronic injury such as burn scars or chronic cutaneous ulcers.

Special Types

Cutaneous angiosarcomas usually present in elderly individuals as ill-defined, dark red to dark blue nodules and plaques, often located on the scalp or face. Though this type of angiosarcoma is thought to arise in the skin, it has often spread well beyond clinically apparent margins at the time of its diagnosis, both by direct invasion and by more distant cutaneous metastasis. Also, angiosarcoma or lymphangiosarcoma may arise in vessels of chronic cavernous hemangiomas (very rarely in port-wine stains), or in areas of chronic lymphedema such as those that may develop in upper extremities following mastectomy and axillary node dissection (Stewart-Treves syndrome). Though probably beginning at a single site, these types of tumors often remain undetected until multiple local metastases have developed.

Metastatic renal cell carcinoma accounts for some particularly interesting phenomena. Although renal cell carcinoma accounts for only about 2% of neoplasms, it may account for up to 10% of cutaneous metastases. As previously mentioned, it more frequently metastasizes to the scalp than most other tumors. Moreover, there is a high incidence of metastasis occurring late, often 3 or more years after apparent complete removal of the primary tumor. Renal cell carcinoma and thyroid carcinoma are the two types of internal malignancies most likely to have frankly vascular cutaneous metastases, which may be easily compressible, may rapidly refill on release of pressure, and may even pulsate spontaneously, especially if situated over bone surfaces such as on the scalp or forehead. At least one case of renal cell carcinoma mimicking Kaposi's sarcoma clinically and histologically has been described.

Neuroblastoma is the most common solid malignant tumor of childhood, and cutaneous metastases are very frequent in young infants with this disease, becoming much less frequent with increasing age (32% of neonatal patients, but only 3% of patients of all ages). The lesions are usually bluish nodules, sometimes termed "blueberry muffin" in appearance. In addition, a characteristic feature is blanching induced by palpation of the lesions. This blanching usually lasts 30–60 minutes and is followed by a 2-hour refractory period. Two other frequent manifestations of neuroblastoma include periorbital ecchymoses ("raccoon eyes"), and heterochromia iridis—a variation in the color of the iris.

Melanoma is usually cutaneous in origin, and it is a tumor that often develops multiple metastatic cutaneous or visceral lesions; it is discussed elsewhere. Kaposi's sarcoma is another tumor that is cutaneous in origin and that frequently has multiple cutaneous and occasionally visceral lesions. Evidence suggests that these multiple lesions represent a multifocal origin of tumor rather than multiple metastatic lesions, though definitive proof is lacking. Primary cutaneous tumors such as Merkel cell tumors, atypical fibroxanthomas, malignant fibrohistiocytomas of the skin, dermatofibrosarcoma protuberans, sebaceous carcinomas, melanomas, squamous cell carcinomas, and even basal cell carcinomas may occasionally develop non-cutaneous metastatic lesions. In this setting, it is important to recognize the cutaneous lesions as the primary malignancy rather than as a manifestation of a non-cutaneous primary tumor.

DIFFERENTIAL DIAGNOSIS

Because of the multiple clinical presentations of cutaneous metastases, the differential diagnosis can include a wide range of skin changes induced by inflammation, infection, benign neoplasias, and primary benign and malignant cutaneous tumors. Certainly, a biopsy should be obtained from any patient presenting with the recent finding of one or more growing nodules, particularly if inflammation is absent. In other settings, the physician must maintain a high index of suspicion that a localized eruption might be due to cutaneous metastases, particularly in a patient with unexplained systemic findings.

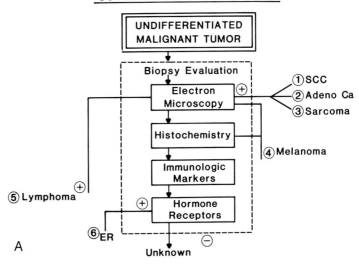

CUTANEOUS METASTASES

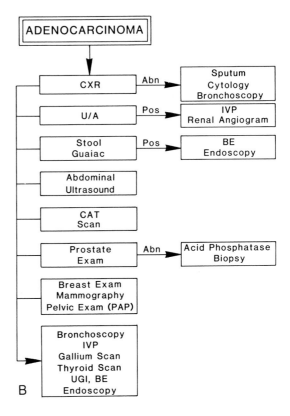

Figure 14–6. Evaluation of patient with cutaneous metastases. SCC = squamous cell carcinoma; Adeno Ca = adenocarcinoma; ER = estrogen receptors; ENT = ear, nose, and throat; CXR = chest x-ray; IVP = intravenous pyelogram; UGI = upper gastrointestinal x-rays; BE = barium enema.

Illustration continued on following page

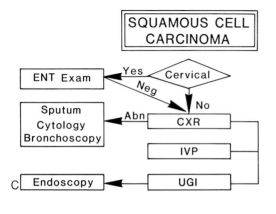

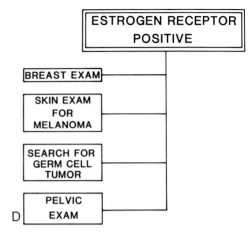

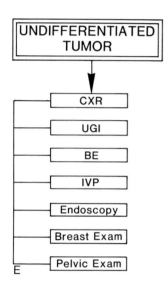

Figure 14–6 *Continued*

HISTOPATHOLOGY

The cutaneous pathology of hematopoietic tumors is discussed elsewhere (Chapters 15, 18, and 19). Most cutaneous metastases of solid tumors tend to show one of two histologic patterns. The first pattern is that of an "Indian file" appearance, with strands of malignant cells lining up in the spaces between the collagen bundles in the dermis. The second pattern is that of bulkier collections of cells in the dermis and subcutaneous fat, often with evidence of proliferation within the lymphatics. Most tumors metastatic to the skin are carcinomas, and most of these are adenocarcinomas. Even with cutaneous histologic examinations, it can be difficult to determine the primary site of the tumor. For example, renal cell carcinoma can be as difficult to diagnose on biopsy as it is clinically; in one series, there was nearly

a 50% misdiagnosis rate of renal cell carcinoma as a benign cutaneous lesion when the primary tumor site was unknown. Cases have been misdiagnosed as hemangioma, "pigmented papilloma," clear cell hidradenoma or other sweat gland tumor, angiosarcoma, or Kaposi's sarcoma. It is also important to remember that many inflammatory and benign neoplastic conditions can be mistaken for metastatic malignant lesions, so associated clinical findings are of considerable importance.

PATIENT EVALUATION

In a patient with a suspected malignancy, careful examination of the skin may reveal a cutaneous lesion that on biopsy might confirm the diagnosis. In a patient with a biopsy-proven cutaneous metastasis, further work-up should be directed by the usual behavior of the primary tumor when known, or by the most probable sites of the primary lesion when only a histologic type (e.g., adenocarcinoma) is known (Fig. 14–6). The cutaneous examination may also be helpful in directing a work-up if other signs of internal malignancy are present, such as acanthosis nigricans or digital clubbing.

TREATMENT

Cutaneous metastases usually indicate significant tumor burden, and as such are usually a poor prognostic sign. Some tumors may present with cutaneous metastases early in the course of disease, whereas others may be treatable even in the face of significant tumor burden. Metastatic carcinoma to the skin is almost always a poor prognostic sign,

however. For those tumors unlikely to respond to systemic therapy, local radiotherapy may be indicated if the lesion is symptomatic. On rare occasions, surgical excision of cutaneous metastases may be indicated.

Suggested Readings

Brownstein MH, Helwig EB: Patterns of cutaneous metastasis. Arch Dermatol *105*:862–868, 1972.

Brownstein MH, Helwig EB: Metastatic tumors of the skin. Cancer *29*:1298–1307, 1972.

Hagmar B, Ryd W, Erkell LJH: Why do tumors metastasize? An overview of current research. Tumor Biol *5*:141–149, 1984.

Lucky AW, McGuire J, Komp DM: Infantile neuroblastoma presenting with cutaneous blanching nodules. J Am Acad Dermatol *6*:389–391, 1982.

Powell FC, Cooper AJ, Massa MC, et al: Sister Mary Joseph's nodule: A clinical and histologic study. J Am Acad Dermatol *10*:610–615, 1984.

Rosen T: Cutaneous metastases. Med Clin North Am *64*:885–900, 1980.

15

Leukemia and Lymphoma

WARREN W. PIETTE

Specific or non-specific lesions of the skin may occur in many hematopoietic malignancies or destructive reactive processes. Specific lesions are those in which there are tumor cells in the skin; non-specific lesions, which are more common, do not have tumor cells but must be considered to be a cutaneous reaction to the malignancy.

PATHOGENESIS

Specific cutaneous lesions of leukemia or lymphoma result from direct infiltration of the epidermis, dermis, or subcutaneous fat by malignant cells. Depending on the degree and depth of infiltration, specific cutaneous lesions can present as papules, plaques, nodules, or ulcers. Early cutaneous involvement is usually related to specific tissue homing (or cell trafficking) patterns of the malignant cell. Late cutaneous involvement is usually due to a large tumor cell burden. Non-specific lesions do not contain obvious tumor cells, but may be due to tumor-related cytopenias resulting in infection or bleeding. In these cases, the pathogenesis of the lesions is easy to explain. However, when other paraneoplastic changes such as acquired ichthyosis, exfoliative dermatitis, or generalized pruritus occur, the causal relationship is unknown.

CLINICAL FEATURES

Specific Lesions

In general, specific cutaneous lesions occur much less frequently and develop much later in the course of non–T cell malignancies compared with T cell malignancies, especially mycosis fungoides (see Chapter 20 for a discussion of cutaneous T cell lymphoma). Specific cutaneous lesions in leukemias and lymphomas usually present as flesh-colored, erythematous, or more distinctively plum-colored papules or nodules that often have a rubbery consistency on palpation (Fig. 15–1; Plate IIIE). Specific lesions range in size from a few millimeters to several centimeters in diameter and tend to develop in a random distribution. Ulceration of primary cutaneous nodules is not common but can occur. Cutaneous ulceration may also result from necrosis of involved lymph nodes with secondary overlying cutaneous necrosis.

Early cutaneous involvement occurs more frequently in acute myelomonocytic and monocytic leukemia than in other non–T cell leukemias and lymphomas. Infiltrated, hyperplastic, friable gingival tissue strongly favors the diagnosis of acute myelomonocytic or monocytic leukemia, and biopsy of such tissue should confirm the diagnosis. Oral involvement can occur rarely with other types of acute leukemia, and even more rarely with chronic leukemias and lymphomas.

Non–T cell lymphoma can present with specific skin lesions and can be apparently limited to the skin for months to years before obvious extracutaneous involvement is noted. This is unusual, however, and most patients who appear to have skin-limited disease will be found to have visceral or nodal involvement on careful work-up.

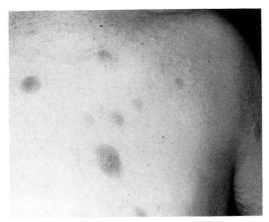

Figure 15–1. Multiple erythematous to violaceous nodules are present in this man with lymphoblastic lymphoma (see also Plate III *E*).

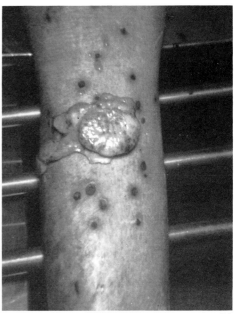

Figure 15–2. Late onset of lesion shown was present in a patient with Hodgkin's disease.

Those few patients who present with skin disease alone usually have lymphocytic lymphoma, and only rarely will patients with large cell (histiocytic) lymphoma present in such a fashion.

Although some reports do exist of Hodgkin's disease presenting as a skin-limited disorder, specific cutaneous lesions of Hodgkin's disease are very rare at any stage of the disease. Most commonly, when specific lymphomatous infiltrates of Hodgkin's disease do occur in the skin, they develop late in the course of the disease (Fig. 15–2), and they are thought to result from retrograde flow of lymphoma cells from obstructed, infiltrated lymph nodes. Another setting for specific cutaneous involvement of Hodgkin's disease occurs when massive nodal enlargement results in necrosis of overlying skin. Some reports do exist of both Hodgkin's disease and mycosis fungoides developing in the same patient, and the argument has been made that these diseases may be predisposing factors for each other. Some of these patients presenting with Hodgkin's disease have had prominent early cutaneous specific lesions. Because this is such a rare finding in most patients with Hodgkin's disease and an expected finding for mycosis fungoides, and since the histologic appearance of both diseases may at times mimic each other, it seems likely that at least some of these cases are simply a single lymphomatous process from the start. Such a conclusion does not reflect unfavorably on the skill of the hematopathologist, but merely points out the limitations of morphology in assessing polymorphous lymphomatous processes. The continuing improvements in cell marker studies should make such distinctions increasingly easier to demonstrate. Rarely, other leukemias and lymphomas may present as plaques, arciform papules, or ulcerated nodules that are indistinguishable clinically from lesions of mycosis fungoides.

Granulocytic sarcoma is another rare lesion that may precede the onset of acute granulocytic leukemia. Usually the lesions are flesh-colored or erythematous, but the solid mass of blast cells in the skin may also have a diagnostic yellowish-green coloration, in which case the term chloroma may be applied. The greenish coloration is thought to be due to the presence of high concentrations of myeloperoxidase. Granulocytic sarcoma is usually seen in children or young adults who have or will soon develop acute granulocytic leukemia.

Chronic granulocytic leukemia tends to spare the skin until an accelerated blast phase or blast crisis develops, at which time multiple flesh-colored or erythematous papules and nodules may rapidly develop (Fig. 15–3; Plate IIIF). An unusual manifestation of chronic granulocytic or myelogenous leukemia has been reported in a patient with a tender, edematous, purpuric area of induration on the lower leg that resembled stasis dermatitis but that was shown following biopsy to consist of a perivascular and peri-

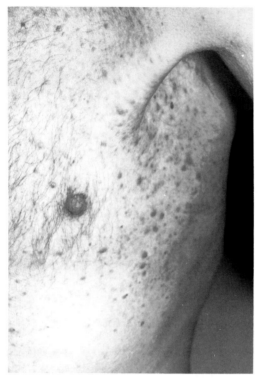

Figure 15–3. Multiple small violaceous papules and small nodules are present in this man with a blast cell crisis (see also Plate IIIF).

appendiceal myeloid infiltration of the dermis.

Hairy cell leukemia, or leukemic reticuloendotheliosis, is associated with mucocutaneous manifestations in roughly 20% of patients. It is presumably related to disease-associated thrombocytopenia, and patients have developed spontaneous purpura or epistaxis. Macular and papular lesions have also been described in patients with hairy cell leukemia, but the exact character of the infiltrate in such lesions is not well described. A patient with macrocheilitis mimicking the Melkersson-Rosenthal syndrome has been described, and the condition was due to specific infiltration of the lips by the hairy cell leukemia.

Leukemia or lymphoma, particularly chronic lymphocytic leukemia, rarely may infiltrate the facial tissues so extensively that a leonine facies results. The Mikulicz's syndrome may result from malignant lymphocytic infiltration of the lacrimal, orbital, and salivary glands and, although rare, is more frequently seen in leukemia and non-Hodgkin's lymphoma than in Hodgkin's disease.

Specific leukemic infiltrates may be localized by dermal inflammation resulting from processes as varied as surgical, thermal, or traumatic injury; intramuscular injections; and herpes simplex or herpes zoster lesions.

The type of cutaneous lesions and the phase of the disease during which it develops may be helpful in determining the cell type of the leukemia or lymphoma.

Non-specific Lesions

There are a number of non-specific cutaneous lesions that may occur in association with leukemia and lymphoma. Some non-specific cutaneous manifestations are so common that they are seldom helpful in diagnosis, but they can prove to be very difficult therapeutic problems. Other types of non-specific involvement may be so uncommon in other settings or so distinctive in appearance that not only is a specific diagnosis of leukemia or lymphoma suggested, but also sometimes even the exact type of lymphoma or leukemia can be inferred (Table 15–1).

Non-specific associations favoring the diagnosis of acute leukemia may result from marrow failure as a result of replacement of normal marrow by abnormal blasts. The resulting anemia will produce skin pallor; a marked thrombocytopenia may produce cutaneous hemorrhage (especially petechiae); and severe neutropenia may be suspected when certain opportunistic infections such as disseminated candidiasis, disseminated aspergillosis, or mucormycosis develop.

DIFFERENTIAL DIAGNOSIS

Clinical findings may suggest the presence of (and occasionally the specific type of) a leukemia or lymphoma, but the diagnosis of leukemia or lymphoma ultimately depends on firm histologic evidence, often in conjunction with specialized cell marker studies. Early cutaneous involvement by a leukemia or lymphoma suggests a T cell origin for the tumor (see Chapter 20). Because the prognosis and therapy of many T cell tumors may differ radically from those of non–T cell tumors, cell marker studies to determine the lineage of the malignant cell are especially important.

Table 15-1. NON-SPECIFIC MUCOCUTANEOUS LESIONS ASSOCIATED WITH LYMPHOMAS AND LEUKEMIA

Due to marrow failure:
  Pallor
  Petechiae
  Purpura
  Bleeding gums
  Infections
    Opportunistic infections
  Non-specific mucocutaneous syndrome
  (see Chapter 13)

Syndrome	Associated Neoplasia
Acute febrile neutrophilic dermatosis	Acute myelogenous leukemia
Atypical pyoderma gangrenosum	Acute myelogenous leukemia
Generalized pruritus	Hodgkin's disease
Vasculitis	Paraproteinemias
	Other leukemias or lymphomas
	Hairy cell leukemia
Exfoliative erythroderma	Mycosis fungoides
	Hodgkin's disease
	Sézary's syndrome
Acquired ichthyosis	Hodgkin's disease
	Lymphocytic lymphoma
	Kaposi's sarcoma

Cutaneous disease secondary to therapy
  Opportunistic infections
  Bleeding
  Kaposi's sarcoma
  Stomatitis (methotrexate, antibiotic therapy)
  Radiation recall

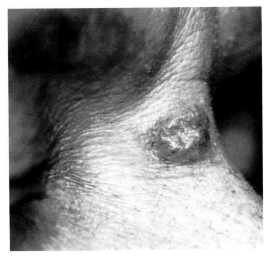

Figure 15-4. A small nodular lesion is present on this patient's nose and is representative of a benign lymphocytic infiltrate.

Pseudolymphoma of the skin is a term applied to a group of dermatoses that on the basis of clinical and histologic findings are difficult to distinguish from leukemia or lymphoma involving the skin (Fig. 15-4). Such dermatoses include lymphocytic infiltration of Jessner, reticular erythematous mucinosis, arthropod bite reactions, nodular scabies, actinic reticuloid, lymphomatoid papulosis, angioimmunoblastic lymphadenopathy syndrome, drug-induced pseudolymphoma syndrome, and lymphocytoma cutis.

The first 4 conditions are usually a diagnostic problem on histologic grounds only, and will be discussed in the next section. Actinic reticuloid and lymphomatoid papulosis are usually considered non-malignant conditions, but both have some risk of evolving into lymphoma, particularly a T cell type, and are discussed in Chapter 13.

Angioimmunoblastic lymphadenopathy with dysproteinemia, or immunoblastic lymphadenopathy, is a rare disease associated with polyclonal B cell activation. It usually starts with the rapid onset of generalized lymphadenopathy with fever, malaise, and weight loss in older individuals. Hepatosplenomegaly is frequently present. Polyclonal hypergammaglobulinemia, anemia, a positive direct Coombs test, leukocytosis, eosinophilia, thrombocytopenia, and hypoalbuminemia are frequent laboratory findings. Cutaneous manifestations are common in this syndrome. Generalized pruritus or excessive sweating occurs in up to one third of patients. Up to 40% of patients will have some type of cutaneous eruption. Generalized macular or papular erythema is most common, but purpura, urticaria or urticarial lesions, scleromyxedema-like lesions, and erythroderma have also been described. Patients may progress to definite lymphoma, usually with an immunoblastic sarcoma morphology. Despite the B cell nature of the most obvious immunologic abnormalities and lymphocyte proliferation, some researchers believe that angioimmunoblastic lymphadenopathy may actually result from an underlying T cell malignancy.

Drug-induced pseudolymphoma syndrome is usually due to phenytoin administration, but can occur with related compounds and with some barbiturates. Generalized lymphadenopathy, hepatosplenomegaly, fever, arthralgias, and eosinophilia are typical findings; generalized pruritic erythematous macules or papules are the most common cutaneous manifestations.

Rare instances of cutaneous nodule formation have been described. This syndrome is usually reversible following discontinuation of the offending drug, but progression to lymphoma has occurred.

Lymphocytoma cutis is known by a number of other names, including cutaneous lymphoid hyperplasia, cutaneous lymphoplasia, and Spiegler-Fendt sarcoid. The skin lesions are usually asymptomatic violaceous or flesh-colored papules or nodules. Lesions are most commonly located on the face, but can occur anywhere in either a grouped or a random pattern and may develop into large, confluent plaques. On rare occasions, spontaneous ulceration of these lesions may occur. Changes in the size and extent of established lesions are frequent, and spontaneous regression, which may take years to occur, is common. Lesional histologic examination is important in the differentiation from lymphoma, as is the absence of visceral lesions. Some patients originally diagnosed as having lymphocytoma cutis have later developed lymphoma, but it is unclear whether these instances indicate a true transformation, or merely reflect the impossibility of an absolutely accurate determination of malignancy by microscopic morphology alone.

Lymphomatoid granulomatosis is a condition classically considered a vasculitis with roughly a 30% incidence of cutaneous involvement, but has a definite risk of progression to lymphoma and may be a lymphoma from its inception (see Chapter 4). Cutaneous manifestations are frequent, and the biopsy of such lesions may be diagnostic. The morphologic and histologic appearance of cutaneous lesions is not that of lymphoma.

HISTOPATHOLOGY

Though the microscopic picture of the cutaneous lesions of non–T cell lymphoma or leukemia depends on the specific type of malignancy, certain generalizations can be made. Most leukemias and non-Hodgkin's lymphomas that involve the skin will histologically show a monomorphous infiltrate, which may be vasocentric or which may extensively infiltrate or efface portions of the dermis and subcutaneous fat. A thin upper dermal zone immediately below the epidermis is usually spared, even in extensively infiltrated lesions of non–T cell tumors. Nodular lymphomas are defined by nodular or follicular arrangements of lymphoma cells in involved lymph nodes, but despite this the cutaneous lesions resulting from the infiltration of nodular lymphoma will almost never show follicular or nodular patterns. Therefore, a skin biopsy is not reliable to distinguish nodular from diffuse lymphoma. Rare cases of true follicular cutaneous lymphoma, some with associated visceral disease, have been described, but the diagnosis is very hard to prove in the absence of extracutaneous lesions. Any condition that results in lymphocyte follicle development in the skin is unlikely to be lymphoma; this morphology usually suggests the diagnosis of an arthropod bite, nodular scabies, or lymphocytoma cutis.

Diffuse and confluent masses of lymphocytes in the dermis are typical of lymphocytoma cutis. Germinal centers may be seen, and are highly suggestive of this diagnosis. As noted, follicular centers are extremely rare in cutaneous lymphoma lesions but may surround a lymphomatous infiltrate. Because of this, the finding of germinal centers cannot be used to absolutely rule out malignancy, particularly if a biopsy is taken from the periphery of a large lesion.

The type of dense lymphocytic perivascular infiltrate typically seen in a cutaneous lesion of chronic lymphocytic leukemia and well-differentiated lymphocytic lymphoma can be seen in a number of non-malignant settings (e.g., cutaneous lupus erythematosus, lymphocytic infiltrate of Jessner, polymorphous light eruption, and drug-induced pseudolymphoma). Such histologic findings can only be properly interpreted in conjunction with the clinical setting, the lesional morphology, and occasionally additional special studies including cell marker surveys.

The histologic findings in cutaneous lesions of angioimmunoblastic lymphadenopathy are often similar to those found in lymph nodes, but they are much less specific in the skin. A perivascular lymphohistiocytic infiltrate is usually present, sometimes with evidence of vessel-directed injury as manifested by disruption of blood vessel walls, mild fibrinoid necrosis, swelling or necrosis of endothelial cells, intraluminal thrombi, or red cell extravasation. Eosinophils or neutrophils are occasionally present in this perivascular infiltrate. Unlike the more specific lymph node findings, immunoblasts, plasma cells, and amorphous eosinophilic background material are usually not prominent in the cutaneous infiltrate.

A variety of granulomatous reactions mimicking sarcoidosis or extravascular granulomas of granulomatous vasculitides have been reported in the settings of lymphoma and leukemia. Although not specific, such lesions may suggest the correct diagnosis when the clinical findings are not consistent with those of sarcoidosis or granulomatous vasculitis.

Although the skin biopsy findings may strongly suggest the diagnosis of leukemia or lymphoma, both the clinical findings and extracutaneous biopsy material are important in confirming the diagnosis.

PATIENT EVALUATION

The history and physical examination with special emphasis on skin and lymph nodes remain the keystone for proper diagnosis of leukemia, lymphoma, and pseudolymphoma involving the skin. The type of skin lesion (specific or non-specific), the histologic appearance of specific lesions, the pace of the disease, and the hematologic findings are all useful in establishing the need for further studies, including bone marrow examination or lymph node biopsy, routine and scanning radiography, or a diligent search for an associated underlying infection.

Improvements in cell identification by immunologic techniques have led to specific therapy tailored to the malignant cell types found in leukemias and lymphomas. The particular clinical findings, lesional morphology, lesional histologic examination, and associated disease processes are important in suggesting the proper diagnosis of a leukemic or lymphomatous process involving the skin.

TREATMENT

The best treatment for both specific and non-specific eruptions of leukemia or lymphoma is the cure or control of the underlying systemic disease. When such control cannot be achieved by currently available chemotherapy, immunotherapy, or radiation therapy, or where responses are slow or incomplete, local therapy may be more important. Local radiation therapy can often induce regression or remission of specific (tumor-containing) cutaneous lesions. If radiation therapy fails or is not acceptable to the patient, or if previous treatment precludes further local radiation, the intralesional injection of triamcinolone acetonide at a concentration between 5 and 20 mg/ml may occasionally be helpful. Cutaneous and subcutaneous atrophy may be severe following such injections, and the full effect of intralesional therapy may not be evident for 3–4 weeks following the injection.

Therapy for non-specific lesions, when treatment for systemic disease is inadequate, depends on the particular type of cutaneous involvement. Emollients, which might contain 0.25% menthol, and oral antihistamines can be helpful in relieving generalized pruritus. Prurigo nodules may require intralesional corticosteroid injections if potent topical corticosteroid therapy of lesions proves ineffective. Urticaria may be at least partially controlled through the use of oral antihistamines. Urticarial vasculitis or small vessel leukocytoclastic vasculitis may require daily or alternate day prednisone therapy when lesions are symptomatic and recurrent. Patients with erythroderma may require intensive topical therapy with wet-to-dry soaks if there is exudation, emollients for xerotic changes, and intermediate strength topical corticosteroid therapy. Occasionally, high dose systemic corticosteroid therapy may be required. Patients with an exfoliative erythroderma may require careful monitoring of body temperature, regulation of fluid and electrolyte balance, nutritional monitoring, and attention to the cardiac status (because of the risk of high output failure, which is very rare).

The possibility that there may be viral, fungal, or bacterial origin for the skin lesions must always be considered. Therefore, early biopsy of suspicious lesions for histology and culture should be considered, especially in patients who are leukopenic or immunocompromised.

Intralesional corticosteroid injections are often helpful in treating lesions of lymphocytoma cutis. Although reports cite the rapid response of lymphocytoma cutis to low dose radiation therapy, this should probably be used only for lesions that are symptomatic. The possibility of misdiagnosing leukemia or lymphoma as lymphocytoma cutis must always be considered, and the correct interpretation of clinical or histologic changes in a recurrent lesion treated initially with radiation therapy may be made much more difficult by such therapy.

Suggested Readings

Braverman IM: Lymphomas and allied disorders; and Leukemia and allied disorders. *In* Braverman IM: Skin Signs of Systemic Disease, 2nd ed. Philadelphia, WB Saunders Co., 1981, pp. 109–196.

Matloff RB, Neiman RS: Angioimmunoblastic lymphadenopathy: A generalized disorder with cutaneous manifestations. Arch Dermatol 114:92–94, 1978.

Weis JW, Winter MW, Phyliky RL, Banks PM: Peripheral T-cell lymphomas: Histologic, immunohistologic, and clinical characterization. Mayo Clinic Proc 61:411–506, 1986.

Wood GS, Burke JS, Horning S, Doggett RS, et al: The immunologic and clinicopathologic heterogeneity of cutaneous lymphomas other than mycosis fungoides. Blood 62:464–472, 1983.

16

Dysproteinemias, Plasma Cell Disorders, and the Skin

WARREN W. PIETTE

A wide variety of diseases associated with monoclonal immunoglobulin or light chain production may cause skin lesions. In some instances, the skin lesions are directly related to the monoclonal protein, as in many cases of cryoglobulinemia. In other instances, skin lesions result from abnormalities in the metabolism of monoclonal proteins, as in light chain–related systemic amyloidosis. In still others, skin lesions occur in diseases frequently associated with benign or malignant clonal plasma cell proliferation.

Any discussion of monoclonal proteins must include monoclonal gammopathy of unknown significance. Though uncommon in youth, the incidence of this disorder increases with age, reaching 3% in individuals 80 or more years old. Roughly 5–10% of patients with such a gammopathy will eventually develop a malignant disease.

This discussion of cutaneous disease associated with monoclonal protein disorders is divided into three parts: disorders directly related to monoclonal proteins (cryoglobulinemia, hyperviscosity syndrome, cold agglutinin disease), disorders directly related to amyloid deposition (see Chapter 17), and disorders associated with monoclonal protein production (such as POEMS syndrome, cutaneous plasmacytomas, and scleromyxedema).

DISORDERS DIRECTLY RELATED TO MONOCLONAL PROTEINS

Pathogenesis

Monoclonal proteins may cause disease directly by acting as cryoglobulins, by raising serum viscosity, or by acting as cold agglutinins. Cryoglobulins are immunoglobulins that precipitate on exposure to cold. Cryoglobulins may be unstable in other settings, such as in the hyperosmotic environment found in the kidneys or in microvascular areas with very slow blood flow. The most critical factor that determines cryoglobulin behavior *in vivo* is the temperature at which it begins to precipitate. If that temperature approaches those found in the cutaneous microvasculature on cold exposure, cold-induced disease is usually significant. If it precipitates only at well below room temperature, symptoms will not be cold related. Cryoglobulins are divided into three categories, depending on their composition. Type I cryoglobulins consist of a single, monoclonal protein; type II cryoglobulins are composed of a monoclonal immunoglobulin with anti-IgG activity that binds to polyclonal serum IgG (a rheumatoid factor with a monoclonal component); and type III cryoglobulins consist of polyclonal immunoglobulins, usually with anti-IgG activity, that bind to polyclonal serum IgG (a polyclonal rheumatoid factor). Roughly 5–10% of myeloma proteins and macroglobulins are cryoprecipitable. Types I and II cryoglobulinemia are often, but not always, associated with a lymphoproliferative disorder. Patients with type II cryoglobulinemia may have IgM, IgG, or IgA as their monoclonal rheumatoid factor. The possibility that rheumatoid factor may be an IgM or IgA is important; they may not be detected on routine serum protein electrophoresis when bound to polyclonal IgG.

The hyperviscosity syndrome results from a significant increase in whole blood viscosity. Such an increase may be related to an increase in the cellular elements in the blood, as in polycythemia rubra vera or primary thrombocythemia. It may also result from a change in serum viscosity as a result of the presence of large amounts of monoclonal protein in the blood. If immunoglobulin related, the hyperviscosity syndrome is usually due to a monoclonal IgM protein. Monoclonal IgG or IgA can cause the hyperviscosity syndrome, but must either be present in the serum in higher amount or have an increased tendency to aggregate in the serum.

Cold agglutinin disease is actually a cold antibody–induced autoimmune hemolytic anemia. The antibody, usually IgM, binds to the red cell in the cold and initiates complement activation, then elutes at body temperature while the complement activation proceeds to red cell lysis. The cold agglutinin also promotes the agglutination of red cells, leading to sludging or occlusion of blood flow in the microvasculature exposed to cold temperatures.

Clinical Features

Cryoglobulinemia. Type I cryoglobulins are usually IgM and therefore primarily intravascular. They are likely to precipitate at temperatures easily attained in the cutaneous microvasculature. Both of these factors contribute to clinically important cold-induced disease. Such disease may present as Raynaud's phenomenon; livedo reticularis; digital infarcts; peripheral gangrene; or purpura, which may be palpable (Fig. 16–1) or may have central necrosis.

Cold sensitivity is more variable with type

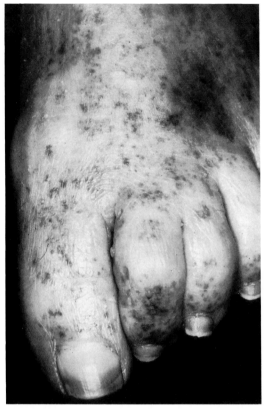

Figure 16–1. Small petechiae are present in this patient with cryoglobulinemia.

II and type III cryoglobulins, since these are usually bound to normal IgG. These mixed cryoglobulins may be detected as cryoproteins in the laboratory; in the patient, their rheumatoid factor activity usually results in immune complex formation and enhances the ability of these proteins to fix complement. For this reason, mixed cryoglobulinemias tend to present with features of leukocytoclastic (necrotizing) vasculitis affecting both small- and medium-sized vessels in the skin and elsewhere, and they are not usually responsible for cold-induced disease. Palpable purpura, digital infarcts, arthralgias and arthritis, and glomerulonephritis are the usual clinical features. Angioedema with urticaria may develop in some patients who have an antibody to C_1-esterase inhibitor; this antibody may also behave as a cryoglobulin in the test tube. Most patients with these features have an underlying malignant lymphoproliferative disease. Finally, some cases of cold-induced urticaria are due to a circulating cryoglobulin without evidence of any associated disease.

Hyperviscosity Syndrome. The hyperviscosity syndrome may present as mucous membrane bleeding, retinopathy, neurologic disturbances, hypervolemia, or cardiac failure, and if due to a cryoglobulin, as Raynaud's phenomenon. Symptoms require a 4–5 fold increase in blood viscosity, seldom seen with less than 2–3 gm/dl serum concentrations of IgM if a result of monoclonal proteins. Hyperviscosity alone may not fully explain the increased bleeding tendency in these patients. Additional factors in some patients are antibody activity against clotting factors, platelet dysfunction as a result of surface coating by immunoglobulin, or other poorly understood clotting defects.

Cold Agglutinin Disease. Cold agglutinin disease is characterized clinically by episodes of hemolytic anemia, hemoglobinuria, and cold-mediated vaso-occlusive phenomena. Patients may develop acrocyanosis, Raynaud-like phenomenon, or generalized livedo reticularis, but skin ulcerations or necrosis are unusual. Jaundice or pallor may follow a severe episode of hemolysis. Cold agglutinin disease occurs in two forms: primary (idiopathic) and secondary. Patients with primary cold agglutinin disease may develop features diagnostic of, or very similar to, Waldenström's macroglobulinemia, whereas secondary forms follow certain infections. Cold agglutinins can also be categorized by their red cell antigen affinity. The antibodies are usually directed against the I/i antigen system, and very rarely against Pr group antigens. Anti-I antibodies occur primarily in association with idiopathic disease, with mycoplasmal pneumonia, and with some lymphomas; anti-i specific antibodies are associated with infectious mononucleosis and with some lymphomas. The cold agglutinins are monoclonal in primary and lymphoma-associated disease, and polyclonal in post-infectious disease. Interestingly, the rare cases of cold agglutinin disease that are due to an IgA cold agglutinin are characterized by red cell agglutination in the microvasculature, but by an absence of hemolytic anemia because the cell-bound IgA does not fix complement.

Waldenström's Macroglobulinemia. This is a disease characterized by a serum monoclonal IgM spike and by malignant lymphoplasmacytoid proliferation, primarily in the bone marrow, liver, spleen, and lymph nodes. The IgM paraprotein may behave as a monoclonal (type I) cryoglobulin or as a cold agglutinin in some patients.

Differential Diagnosis

The differential diagnosis for cryoglobulinemia or cold agglutinin disease depends on the disease manifestations. In cases of mixed cryoglobulinemia presenting as leukocytoclastic vasculitis, the differential diagnosis primarily includes other necrotizing vasculitides. The hyperviscosity syndrome is usually due to a clonal lymphoproliferative disorder, but can result from other blood disorders such as polycythemia vera. Raynaud's phenomenon can be idiopathic (Raynaud's disease), but is usually secondary to a connective tissue disease. Other diseases may resemble Raynaud's phenomenon; in addition to those mentioned in this section, conditions such as ergotism, Buerger's disease, pernio, and acrocyanosis should be considered. In patients presenting with lesions of thrombosis (cold agglutinin disease) or protein precipitation (monoclonal cryoglobulinemia) in dermal vessels, disorders that must also be considered include disseminated intravascular coagulation, thrombotic thrombocytopenic purpura, coumarin necrosis, and heparin necrosis. Three rare disorders should also be considered: cryofibrinogenemia, paroxysmal cold hemoglobinuria, and paroxysmal nocturnal hemoglobinuria.

Histopathology

Cutaneous lesions of monoclonal cryoglobulinemia demonstrate intravascular amorphous eosinophilic material that is principally composed of precipitated cryoglobulin. Red blood cell extravasation in the dermis is often present. Inflammation is usually minimal, is located perivascularly, is lymphohistiocytic, and appears to be a response to, rather than a cause of, necrosis resulting from vessel occlusion. In contrast, on biopsy cutaneous lesions of mixed cryoglobulinemia show changes of leukocytoclastic (necrotizing) vasculitis, including neutrophil infiltration of the vessel wall, nuclear fragments of dead neutrophils (nuclear dust), and fibrinoid necrosis of the vessel walls. Immunoreactant deposition in vessel walls can be seen on direct immunofluorescence microscopy. The exact histologic picture depends on the age of the lesions biopsied. Positive immunofluorescence microscopy findings are not expected in lesions more than 24–48 hours old, and the neutrophil infiltrate may be largely replaced by a lymphohistiocytic infiltrate as the lesion evolves. These patients do not develop the intravascular occlusion so typical in lesions of monoclonal cryoglobulinemia.

Lesions that are due to cryofibrinogenemia, cold agglutinin disease, paroxysmal cold hemoglobinuria, and paroxysmal nocturnal hemoglobinuria should show cutaneous biopsy evidence of multiple dermal vessel thrombosis, usually in the absence of significant inflammatory infiltrate. The histologic findings are essentially identical to those seen in cutaneous lesions of disseminated intravascular coagulation or thrombotic thrombocytopenic purpura, but can usually be distinguished from the intravascular occlusion that is due to monoclonal cryoglobulinemia, which usually has a more amorphous and paler eosinophilic staining pattern.

Patient Evaluation

The detection and analysis of a serum or urine monoclonal immunoglobulin or Bence Jones protein are usually easily accomplished through serum or urine protein electrophoresis testing and immunoelectrophoresis or immunofixation techniques. If a patient is suspected of having a cryoprotein-related disease, a very simple screening procedure may be helpful. Blood is drawn for both serum and plasma sampling, and kept warm until the cellular elements have been removed. Following at least overnight refrigeration, each sample is then examined for evidence of a cryoprecipitate. A cryoglobulin should appear in both the serum and the plasma sample, whereas a cryofibrinogen will only appear in the plasma fraction. Immunoelectrophoresis of the precipitated cryoglobulin can then define its composition. Patients found to have type I or II cryoglobulins should be examined for an underlying malignant lymphoproliferative disorder. Patients with type II or III cryoglobulins should be evaluated for an underlying connective tissue or autoimmune disease, or for the presence of chronic infection or antigenemia such as that associated with hepatitis B virus.

Confirmation of a presumptive diagnosis of cold agglutinin disease, paroxysmal cold hemoglobinuria, or paroxysmal nocturnal hemoglobinuria usually requires consultation with hematologists and hematopathologists. If the hyperviscosity syndrome is suspected, serum viscosity measurements are usually easily obtained from routine laboratories, but whole blood viscosity measurements remain a specialized research procedure.

Treatment

Treatment of cryoglobulinemia depends on the clinical features. If clinically relevant cold sensitivity is present (almost exclusively associated with IgM type I cryoglobulin), adequate clothing and avoidance of cold exposure may be all that is required. In patients with type II or III cryoglobulinemia, in which necrotizing vasculitis is the usual presenting finding, therapy will depend on the manifestations. Cutaneous lesions may respond to oral dapsone therapy, whereas aggressive therapy with systemic steroids in combination with immunosuppressive agents may be required when there is significant systemic disease. Patients with specific underlying etiologic disorders may respond to effective treatment for that disorder. Patients with essential (idiopathic) mixed cryoglobulinemia may benefit from chemotherapy even in the absence of obvious lymphoproliferative disease. Plasmapheresis may provide temporary but rapid relief of symptoms in patients with high levels of circulating cryoglobulins, and may be synergistic when combined with chemotherapy in appropriate cases.

Cold agglutinin disease is best treated by keeping the patient (particularly the extremities) warm. Cytotoxic agents may be useful in some patients, but plasmapheresis is contraindicated because it may induce severe hemolytic anemia. Post-infectious cases of cold agglutinin disease are usually self-limiting.

DISORDERS ASSOCIATED WITH MONOCLONAL PROTEIN PRODUCTION

Pathogenesis

The group of disorders associated with monoclonal protein production does not occur by a single pathogenetic mechanism, but are united by the frequent finding of an associated monoclonal gammopathy. Some diseases are almost always associated with plasma cell neoplasia, often malignant (e.g., cutaneous plasmacytoma, POEMS syndrome); others are frequently associated with plasma cell proliferation or monoclonal gammopathy (e.g., necrobiotic xanthogranuloma with paraproteinemia). Many diseases have a greater than chance association with the presence of a monoclonal serum or urine protein, but this is nonetheless not required for typical disease expression (scleromyxedema, scleredema). The known relationship between these diseases and the expression of monoclonal protein will be mentioned in the context of the individual diseases.

Clinical Features

The POEMS Syndrome. This syndrome, recognized as a distinct entity in Japan in 1968, is also known as the PEP, Crow-Fukase, or Takatsuki syndrome. This disease is primarily reported from Japan, but a few cases have now been reported in the United States. The acronym stands for polyneuropathy, organomegaly, endocrinopathy, M protein, and skin disease or sclerosis. In the largest series (102 patients), men were affected twice as frequently as women, and patients were young to middle-aged adults, with a mean age of 46. All patients had a peripheral polyneuropathy, usually sensorimotor; 97% had elevated cerebrospinal fluid protein, and 62% had papilledema. Organomegaly was manifested by hepatomegaly in 82%, lymphadenopathy in 65%, and splenomegaly in 39% of the patients. The most common endocrine abnormalities were impotence (78%) and gynecomastia (68%) in men, and amenorrhea (68%) in women. Other endocrine findings in this and other series include glucose intolerance (28–48%); hyperthyroidism (10–24%); and hyperprolactinemia, adrenal insufficiency, and hypercalcemia (rare).

Most patients (75%) have had a serum or rarely a urine monoclonal spike. In 95% of the cases with a spike, the monoclonal protein has had a lambda light chain component. Though many of these patients may ultimately progress to multiple myeloma, this does not always occur. Slightly more than half the patients with POEMS syndrome have bone lesions, and 85% of pa-

tients with bone lesions had osteosclerotic lesions, with or without osteolytic lesions. This is in contrast to large series of myeloma patients in which osteosclerotic lesions make up only 0.5–3.0% of bone lesions. Also, unlike the findings in osteolytic multiple myeloma, anemia, hypercalcemia, and renal insufficiency are uncommon, and extensive bone marrow infiltration by plasma cells is rare.

Skin changes are very common in this disorder, and reported changes include diffuse hyperpigmentation (93–98%); peripheral edema (92%); and sometimes anasarca, hypertrichosis (78–81%), a poorly characterized skin thickening (77–85%), and digital clubbing (56%). Verrucous angiomas, "white fingernails," Raynaud's phenomenon, and sicca syndrome have also been described.

Variable findings include ascites, pleural effusions, fever, polycythemia, leukocytosis, thrombocytosis, and an elevated sedimentation rate. As awareness of this syndrome increases, it is likely that its recognition in the United States will increase, particularly in the group of patients with cryptogenic polyneuropathies or isolated osteosclerotic bone lesions.

Cutaneous Plasmacytomas. Cutaneous plasmacytomas are very rare, and may be solitary or multiple. Most of these skin lesions are smooth, non-tender, cutaneous or subcutaneous nodules, flesh colored to violaceous, 1–5 cm in diameter, and they may be crusted or ulcerated. They are usually located on the trunk, extremities, or face. Cutaneous plasmacytomas indicate a large tumor cell burden in multiple myeloma, and therefore usually occur late in the course of the disease. Lesions may develop either as an extension from underlying bone or as distinct cutaneous metastases. All immunoglobulin classes have been associated with cutaneous plasmacytomas, but most are IgG- or IgA-producing cells. IgD myeloma is very rare; patients with this disease are apt to be young men, to have a much more aggressive course, and to have a very high incidence of extramedullary lesions, including cutaneous plasmacytomas (up to 18%). In a very few instances, a solitary cutaneous plasmacytoma may be an isolated finding, even with long-term follow-up. Because the number of plasma cells in such a lesion is small and the amount of immunoglobulin synthesized is directly related to cell numbers, such patients are unlikely to have a serum M spike. The presence of an M spike should strongly suggest occult extracutaneous disease. Some authors have argued that patients with long-term isolated cutaneous plasmacytomas actually have an indolent follicular B cell lymphoma that develops primarily in the skin. Plasma cell–rich lesions have been described in plasma cell orificial mucositis and systemic plasmacytosis. Though rare disorders, these present with so extensive an infiltration of plasma cells that on biopsy they may mimic cutaneous plasmacytomas.

Necrobiotic Xanthogranuloma with Paraproteinemia. This is a distinctive entity, typically presenting with periorbital, yellowish plaques or nodules that tend to ulcerate and heal with scar formation. Lesions may also develop on the trunk or proximal limbs, especially in flexural areas (Fig. 16–2). The biopsy is characteristic (see later discussion), and the small number of patients thus far described have had a monoclonal gammopathy, many have had leukopenia, and some have had multiple myeloma or bone marrow biopsy results suggesting a lymphoproliferative disorder.

Other xanthomatous disorders may occasionally indicate an underlying plasma cell disorder. Xanthoma disseminatum is a histiocytic proliferative disorder that usually develops in patients 25 years old or younger and occurs with an increased incidence of monoclonal gammopathy or multiple myeloma (see Chapter 18 for further details) (Fig. 16–3). Generalized plane xanthomatosis has also been associated with multiple myeloma.

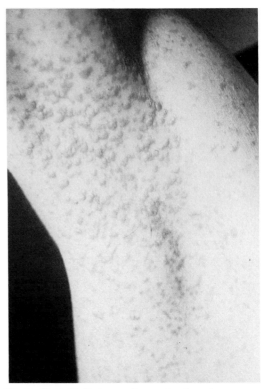

Figure 16–3. Multiple small papules in a linear array are present in this patient with papular mucinosis and paraproteinemia. (Courtesy of Dr. Joseph J. Chanda, Melbourne Beach, FL.)

Lesions in this disorder are yellow to yellow-brown, flat plaques, and when generalized, typically involve the head, eyelids, neck, and upper trunk. Very rarely, patients with multiple myeloma will have an anti-lipoprotein antibody as their monoclonal protein, and this may result in an abnormal lipid profile and occasionally in the development of xanthomas.

Benign Hypergammaglobulinemic Purpura of Waldenström. This disease is characterized by flat, petechial or small purpuric lesions on the lower extremities in association with a polyclonal hypergammaglobulinemia. New lesions may develop in cycles, and may be preceded by a burning sensation. Most patients will have a positive IgG–anti-IgG rheumatoid factor that may be difficult to detect, but that sediments in the 12–15S range on analytic ultracentrifugation. Some of these IgG rheumatoid factors have been shown to be monoclonal by specialized tests, and this may relate to the small but definitely increased incidence of multiple myeloma or other lymphoproliferative disorder that may develop in some patients after

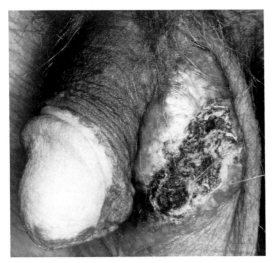

Figure 16–2. Necrobiotic xanthogranuloma is present in a patient with multiple myeloma. (Courtesy of Dr. Neil A. Fenske, Tampa, FL.)

several years of disease. Both primary and secondary forms of this disease have been described, but at least half of the patients with primary disease who were followed for 5 years developed evidence of an associated disease, occasionally malignant but usually autoimmune. Such autoimmune diseases have included keratoconjunctivitis sicca, Sjögren's syndrome, lupus erythematosus (particularly anti-Ro (SS-A) positive patients), undifferentiated connective tissue disease, or sarcoidosis.

Scleromyxedema. Scleromyxedema is a subset of lichen myxedematosus (papular mucinosis) that presents with coalescent erythematous to yellow papules and plaques, usually located on the face, that may mimic the facial features of acromegaly or generalized myxedema (Figs. 16–4 and 16–5). The patients frequently complain of an intense pruritus. These patients frequently have an associated monoclonal gammopathy and may have a very characteristic finding of a "slow gamma region" migrating protein on serum protein electrophoresis (extreme migration toward the negative elec-

trode). Evidence suggests that this unusual migration pattern is not due to a response to a common antigen, since careful studies in some patients appear to show quite different idiotype characteristics from patient to patient. Studies have shown a mucin-stimulatory effect on fibroblasts by serum from these patients, and one study has suggested but not proved that the abnormal protein is not the stimulatory factor. One report has suggested an abnormality in the F_d portion of a patient's immunoglobulin. Despite the frequent but not obligatory presence of M protein in this disease, associated lymphoproliferative malignancies have not been reported.

Other Disorders. Other cutaneous disease may have a rare but apparently real association with monoclonal protein disorders and sometimes with lymphoproliferative disease. Such diseases include scleredema adultorum, dermatomyositis, erythema elevatum diutinum, subcorneal pustular dermatosis, dermatitis herpetiformis, pyoderma gangrenosum, some forms of acquired angioedema (patients can develop a monoclonal protein with anti-C_1 esterase activity, for example), cutaneous T cell lymphoma, and Kaposi's sarcoma. Although IgG paraprotein–associated disorders are usually the most common, some of these disorders appear to have a strong IgA association, which is as yet unexplained.

Treatment

Therapy of these disorders is largely aimed at control of the underlying disease process when present. Thus, control of lymphoproliferative disease can lead to a response of the skin. In the absence of a treatable disorder, there are no specific therapies. POEMS syndrome may be treated with radiation therapy for isolated osteosclerotic lesions or with chemotherapy if systemic symptoms warrant it. Cutaneous plasmacytomas are treated with radiation and/or chemotherapy. Therapy of necrobiotic xanthogranuloma and xanthoma disseminatum is poorly effective. Therapy of hyperglobulinemic purpura in the absence of a lymphoproliferative disorder is largely symptomatic, and the therapeutic agents used to treat vasculitis should be considered (see Chapter 4). Papular mucinosis and its variants respond poorly to therapy, including

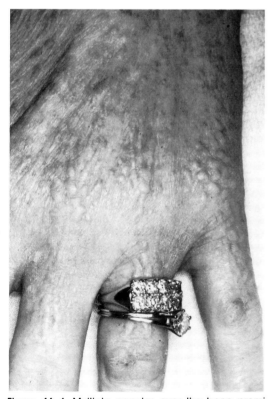

Figure 16–4. Multiple papules over the bone prominences are seen in a patient with papular mucinosis. (Courtesy of Dr. Joseph J. Chanda, Melbourne Beach, FL.)

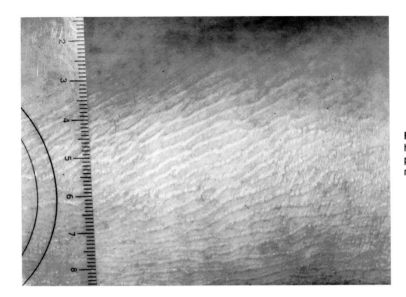

Figure 16–5. Multiple papules that have formed linear bands are present in this patient with lichen myxedematosus.

cytotoxic agents such as melphalan. It is our feeling that this "benign" process does not require aggressive therapy.

Suggested Readings

Pachman CH, Leddy JP: Cryopathic hemolytic syndromes. *In* Williams WJ, Beutler E, Erslev AJ, et al (eds): Hematology, 3rd ed. New York, McGraw-Hill Book Co., 1983, pp. 642–647.

Piette WW: Myeloma, paraproteinemias, and the skin. Med Clin North Am 70:155–176, 1986.

Watanabe S, Ohara K, Kukita A, et al: Systemic plasmacytosis: A syndrome of peculiar multiple skin eruptions, generalized lymphadenopathy, and polyclonal hypergammaglobulinemia. Arch Dermatol 122:1314–1320, 1986.

17

Amyloidosis

WARREN W. PIETTE

Amyloidosis is a general term used to describe a group of conditions characterized by the extracellular deposition of an abnormal protein that has a specific set of staining properties and a fibrillar ultrastructure. Cutaneous involvement can occur in primary systemic amyloidosis, amyloidosis associated with plasma cell dyscrasia, and localized amyloidosis. The skin is rarely involved in secondary amyloidosis.

PATHOGENESIS

The deposition of amyloid is still an incompletely understood process, but all disorders of amyloid deposition have in common the synthesis of amyloid fibrils from a precursor protein and the incorporation of a ring-shaped amyloid P component into the amyloid fibril. While most proteins in humans and other species are synthesized in an alpha helical structure, amyloid protein is among the few that are synthesized in a β-pleated structure, one extremely difficult for living systems to degrade.

With respect to the skin, there are 4 known proteins that can serve as precursors for amyloid fibrils: light chain monoclonal protein, serum protein A, pre-albumin, and keratin. The pattern of amyloid deposition directly relates to the precursor protein type. Also, the skin-relevant amyloidoses can be divided clinically into acquired systemic amyloidoses or organ-limited (skin-limited) amyloidoses.

CLINICAL FEATURES (Table 17–1)

The light chain–derived acquired systemic amyloidoses (amyloid fibril AL*) are seen in the setting of primary systemic amyloidosis or multiple myeloma. It is assumed that all AL-fibril type systemic amyloidoses are due to a monoclonal protein. In most instances, blood or urine studies for monoclonal immunoglobulin or light chain protein are positive, and even in those instances in which no monoclonal abnormality can be

---

*AL = amyloid light chain.

Table 17–1. CHARACTERISTICS OF SYSTEMIC AMYLOIDOSIS

Feature	Primary (AL)	Secondary (AA)
Age	<65	<60
Chronic inflammatory disease	Rare	Usual
Paraprotein	Almost always	Absent
Major clinical presentation	Cardiac, renal, GI	Renal
Pattern of involvement	Widespread	Widespread
Renal	Usually	Almost all
Liver	Often	Often
Spleen	Often	Often
Macroglossia	Often	Rare
Skin lesions present	Often	None
Cardiac failure	Frequent	Uncommon

detected, the problem is thought to be one of test sensitivity. A particularly amyloidogenic light chain may be so efficiently or rapidly converted to amyloid fibrils that serum or urine detection is very difficult.

The reported incidence of cutaneous lesions in AL-derived systemic amyloidosis ranges from 21 to 40%. The most common lesions include purpura, papules, plaques, and nodules, but bullous eruptions (sometimes mimicking porphyria cutanea tarda or epidermolysis bullosa acquisita), scleroderma-like skin infiltration, pigmentary changes, nail dystrophies, and alopecia have been reported. Purpura is most common (Fig. 17–1) and is usually attributed to amyloid infiltration of the dermal blood vessels and supporting tissue resulting in problems with hemostasis following mild trauma. AL amyloidosis is most prominent on the upper body. Stroking or pinching the skin usually induces purpura in lesions in these areas, and spontaneous periorbital hemorrhage is commonly seen following Valsalva-like maneuvers (coughing, vomiting) or dependency of the head. Papules and plaques are most often yellow to flesh-colored, non-pruritic, and frequently hemorrhagic. A waxy or translucent character of such papules is strongly suggestive of AL-type amyloid deposition. Papular deposition of amyloid is most common on the central face, eyelids, lips, tongue, buccal mucosa, post-auricular areas, neck, and intertriginous areas. Rarely, tissue infiltration by amyloid may present as proptosis, ophthalmoplegia, periarticular

soft tissue enlargement, or skeletal muscle pseudohypertrophy. Infiltration of lacrimal or parotid glands may cause keratoconjunctivitis sicca or may mimic Sjögren's syndrome. AL-amyloid deposition can also involve almost any internal structure, but the most characteristic associated features include peripheral neuropathy, carpal tunnel syndrome, orthostatic hypotension as a result of autonomic neuropathy, macroglossia (Fig. 17–2), congestive heart failure, and nephrotic syndrome.

Acquired systemic amyloidosis of the AA-fibril type* (secondary systemic amyloidosis) is usually seen in association with a chronic inflammatory process, such as rheumatoid arthritis, leprosy, tuberculosis, syphilis, chronic osteomyelitis, and chronic inflammatory bowel disease. It may also be associated with certain long-standing cutaneous problems such as decubitus ulcers, stasis ulcers, thermal burns, neglected basal cell carcinomas, hidradenitis suppurativa, dystrophic epidermolysis bullosa, psoriasis and psoriatic arthritis, and Reiter's syndrome. Amyloid fibrils in this setting are derived from serum protein A. This protein increases with inflammation, during pregnancy, and with advancing age. Any organ may be involved, but significant liver, spleen, and renal infiltration is most typical.

Although deposition of amyloid in the skin is common in AA amyloidosis, clinically apparent skin lesions are very rare.

---

*AA = amyloid protein.

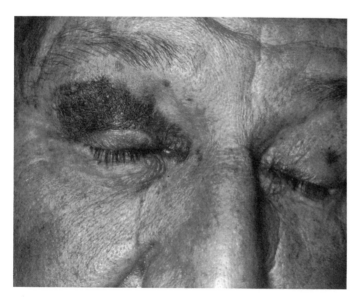

Figure 17–1. "Pinch purpura" is present in this individual with multiple myeloma. This represents amyloidosis of the skin.

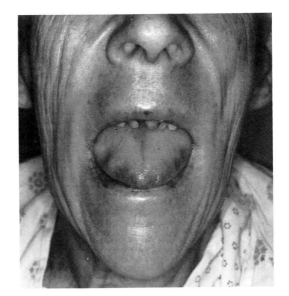

Figure 17–2. In this individual, macroglossia is present, associated with alopecia, anonychia, and pinch purpura. These findings are secondary to multiple myeloma.

Macular purpura is one of the few reported manifestations. The rarity of skin lesions in this syndrome distinguishes it from AL amyloidosis; the presence of cutaneous lesions in a patient with systemic amyloidosis strongly suggests AL rather than AA amyloidosis.

There are a number of familial syndromes that have in common the frequent deposition of amyloid in various organs. Familial Mediterranean fever, inherited in an autosomal recessive fashion, results in an AA-fibril type systemic amyloidosis apparently related to the frequent inflammatory episodes characteristic of this disease. An unknown fibril type of amyloidosis occurs in patients with the Muckle-Wells syndrome, a familial disorder characterized by repeated febrile episodes, a painful urticarial eruption, progressive deafness, and amyloid nephropathy. The remaining familial amyloidosis syndromes may differ considerably from kindred to kindred, but are usually inherited in an autosomal dominant fashion. Several types tend to share the features of peripheral polyneuropathy; autonomic nervous system dysfunction; and varying involvement of the heart, gastrointestinal tract, and eyes. Prealbumin (plasma transthyretin protein) has been shown to be the amyloid precursor protein in several of the autosomal recessive forms of familial amyloidosis. Atrophic scars, ulcerations, and/or petechiae may occur in these patients.

There are 4 types of organ-limited amyloidoses described in the skin: lichen amyloidosis, macular amyloidosis, localized amyloid deposition related to cutaneous growths, and nodular (tumefactive) cutaneous amyloidosis. Localized amyloid deposition may occur around or within a number of cutaneous growths, including actinic keratoses, basal cell carcinomas, Bowen's disease, and seborrheic keratoses; such deposition is not evident clinically. The remaining syndromes are seen uncommonly in the United States, with *lichen amyloidosis* being the most frequent. Pruritic, hyperkeratotic, flesh-colored (occasionally hyperpigmented) papules on the anterior lower extremities are the usual clinical presentation of lichen amyloidosis, though other areas may be involved. *Macular amyloidosis* is probably a variant of lichen amyloidosis, presenting as pruritic, oval, grayish brown macules on the lower extremities or back. These 3 forms of organ-limited cutaneous amyloidosis are thought to have a keratin protein as the amyloid fibril precursor, and are considered an AK-fibril type* amyloidosis. The biopsy changes in these disorders are distinctive, and they aid in distinguishing them from systemic amyloidosis.

Amyloid deposition in *nodular cutaneous amyloidosis* is thought to be derived from a light chain precursor, but this has not been proved unequivocally. This type of amyloidosis presents as nodules on the face, extremities, trunk, or genitalia. These nodules

---

*AK = amyloid keratin.

are usually flesh-colored, and frequently have overlying epidermal atrophy or features resembling anetoderma. Patients with nodular cutaneous amyloidosis require regular follow-up, since some, but not all, may develop systemic amyloidosis.

DIFFERENTIAL DIAGNOSIS

The differential diagnosis for systemic amyloidoses depends on the syndrome, but AL amyloidosis should always be considered in the differential diagnosis of cephalad-distributed waxy papules or unexplained hemorrhage induced by mild trauma. Lichen and macular amyloidosis may be confused with localized pigmentary disorders, lichen simplex chronicus, or prurigo nodularis.

HISTOPATHOLOGY

A biopsy of clinical lesions in AL-derived systemic amyloidosis should provide diagnostic evidence of amyloid deposition. Even in patients without clinical lesions, a biopsy of apparently normal skin may reveal cutaneous deposits of amyloid in up to 50% of individuals with systemic AL-type amyloidosis. Amyloid deposits are usually in the superficial dermis and in dermal vessels. Epidermal atrophy (or at least loss of rete ridges) is an associated finding. Congo red staining with green birefringence with polarized light is the most specific stain for amyloid, though other stains such as methyl violet, crystal violet, or thioflavine T may be more sensitive.

Despite the rarity of clinical lesions in AA-fibril type (secondary) systemic amyloidosis, a biopsy of apparently normal skin may yield evidence of amyloid deposition in from 7 to 40% of patients. The pattern of amyloid deposition differs from that seen with the AL type. Deposits are usually deep in the dermis and subcutaneous fat and are occasionally in a perivascular or periappendageal distribution. In the few descriptions available for plasma transthyretin (pre-albumin)–related amyloidosis, the amyloid deposition in the skin has been similar to that described for AA-fibril type amyloidosis.

Lichen amyloidosis and macular amyloidosis have a biopsy appearance unlike that of AL or AA amyloidosis. Amyloid is deposited in the papillary tips, with rete ridge elongation and sparing of dermal blood vessels, unlike that seen with the AL-type. The changes in macular amyloidosis are sometimes quite minimal. Cutaneous tumor–associated amyloidosis is sometimes quite minimal. Cutaneous tumor–associated amyloidosis is a pathologic curiosity; its recognition as an entity is important primarily to prevent its misinterpretation as evidence of a more serious amyloid disorder. The cutaneous deposits in nodular cutaneous amyloidosis may resemble both AL- and AA-fibril type disease in their distribution. Extensive dermal and subcutaneous deposits are typical, often with blood vessel wall infiltration. Also, plasma cells, giant cells, and focal calcification may be seen.

PATIENT EVALUATION

The evaluation of a patient with biopsy proven cutaneous amyloid deposition must be directed by the setting. The presence or absence of clinical lesions, the site biopsied (lesional or non-lesional skin), the presence of associated systemic findings, and the specific histologic features seen on the biopsy are all very important in determining the most appropriate evaluation for an individual patient. For example, the presence of waxy, hemorrhagic facial papules with histologic features of epidermal atrophy, significant dermal amyloid deposition, and amyloid infiltration of vessel walls is nearly diagnostic of AL-type systemic amyloidosis. In such a case, a thorough search for an associated monoclonal immunoglobulin or light chain disorder with or without multiple myeloma is mandatory. In contrast, the presence of flesh-colored, pruritic papules on the lower extremity that when biopsied show features of papillary tip amyloid deposition, sparing of vessels, and rete ridge elongation would be sufficient for the diagnosis of lichen amyloidosis and would obviate the need to search for a systemic cause.

TREATMENT

In general, treatment for AL systemic amyloidosis has been unsatisfactory, though some patients have had slowing of disease progression or even partial regression of amyloid deposition following chemotherapy for underlying myeloma or following colchicine administration. Therapy for AA systemic amyloidosis is usually directed toward the underlying disorder. Colchicine has been reported to prevent or greatly diminish AA amyloid deposition in some patients with familial Mediterranean fever, though the mechanism of action is unknown. The treatment of lichen and macular amyloidosis is often unsatisfactory. Nonetheless, attempts should be made to control the pruritus. Occasional good results have been reported with the use of topical or intralesional corticosteroid therapy, or rarely with dermabrasion.

Therapy of amyloidosis, regardless of the type, is difficult, probably owing to the insolubility of this protein.

Suggested Readings

Breathnach SM, Black MM: Systemic amyloidosis and the skin: A review with special emphasis on clinical features and therapy. Clin Exp Dermatol 4:517–536, 1979.
Kyle RA: Amyloidosis Parts 2 and 3. Intern J Dermatol 20:20–25, 75–80, 1981.
Kyle RA, Greipp PR, Garton JP, Gertz MA: Primary systemic amyloidosis. Am J Med 79:708–716, 1985.
Wright JR, Calkins E: Clinical-pathologic differentiation of common amyloid syndromes. Medicine 60:429–448, 1981.

18

The Histiocytoses

WARREN W. PIETTE

One of the most difficult and confusing endeavors in medicine is the attempt to classify disorders of the monocyte-macrophage (true histiocyte) system. This chapter is focused on providing a working classification for those histiocytic disorders that may involve the skin.

PATHOGENESIS

The pathogenesis of the histiocytic disorders is not well understood, in part because subdivisions of the monocyte-macrophage system are still rudimentary. With the possible exceptions of malignant histiocytosis (often considered a true histiocytic lymphoma), acute monocytic leukemia, and the acute disseminated type of histiocytosis X, the histiocytoses appear to be examples of unusual reactive proliferations or non-malignant neoplastic disorders of macrophage (histiocyte) cell lines. Until recently, no specific stimuli were known for any of these disorders. However, it has been found that the virus-associated hemophagocytic syndrome, which was initially believed to be a variant of malignant histiocytosis, is a reaction pattern to certain viral infections. This particular reaction pattern is more likely to occur in the setting of ongoing immunosuppressive therapy.

Because the pathogenesis of these disorders is so poorly understood, classification has depended upon clinical and pathologic features. Traditionally, these disorders have been divided into histiocytosis X (derived from the dendritic Langerhans cell) and the non-X histiocytoses.

HISTIOCYTOSIS X

Clinical Features

The syndrome of histiocytosis X has been subdivided, based on differences in clinical presentation and disease course. The most traditional division is into Letterer-Siwe disease, Hand-Schüller-Christian disease, and eosinophilic granuloma, corresponding to acute disseminated, chronic progressive, and benign localized forms of disease, respectively. Unfortunately, individual patients may have findings that do not fit neatly into a single classic type.

Letterer-Siwe disease usually begins within the first 2 years of life, often within the first 6 months. This is an acute disseminated disease, associated with fever, weight loss, and generalized lymphadenopathy. Cutaneous manifestations are common. The earliest lesions usually are reddish-brown or reddish-yellow small papules, occurring primarily on the scalp (Fig. 18–1; Plate IIIG), upper trunk, and intertriginous areas (Fig. 18–2). These lesions tend to occur in crops and may become confluent, especially on the scalp, where this condition is frequently misdiagnosed as seborrheic dermatitis. Individual lesions may develop features of scaling, crusting, pustule formation, and even hemorrhage, often in a progressive pattern. Frequently such lesions will undergo spontaneous regression, usually leaving residual scarring. Occasionally, more chronic lesions will become xanthomatous. Gingival involvement is common; mucosal ulceration or infiltration may also occur. Early in the disease course, petechial lesions may de-

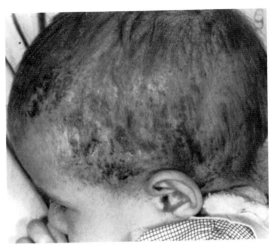

Figure 18–1. Letterer-Siwe disease. Erythematous, slightly scaly plaques are present in the scalp of this child (see also Plate IIIG).

velop because of vessel inflammation, but in advanced disease purpura and hemorrhage may result from thrombocytopenia. The disease commonly affects the lungs, liver, spleen, bone, and bone marrow. The bone lesions are osteolytic and occur primarily in the cranium, vertebrae, and the flat bones. Before methods were available to identify Langerhans cells reliably, the Letterer-Siwe syndrome probably included a number of macrophage-monocyte disorders such as acute monocytic leukemia, some lymphomas, and atypical vasculitic syndromes. Even though the outlook may be somewhat better with proper diagnosis and improved treatment, Letterer-Siwe disease is still frequently life-threatening, especially if there is splenomegaly or marrow failure (thrombocytopenia or severe anemia).

Hand-Schüller-Christian disease usually develops in children between 2 and 6 years old, and almost always presents before age 30. The triad of exophthalmos, diabetes insipidus, and bone lesions classically defines this disease subset, but few patients have all three findings. Cutaneous lesions are found in roughly one third of patients, and may resemble those seen with Letterer-Siwe disease; later in the disease course, the lesions may occur in small numbers concentrated on the lateral scalp and on the central regions of the chest and back. Mucosal involvement may be present. Unlike in Letterer-Siwe patients, hepatomegaly is rare. Pulmonary involvement and exophthalmos both occur in roughly 20% of cases. Diabetes insipidus is present in over half the patients. The most common finding is the presence of osteolytic lesions in up to 80% of patients. The lesions primarily affect the skull. The pace of Hand-Schüller-Christian disease is much slower on average than that of Letterer-Siwe disease, with about half the untreated patients dying of unrelated causes.

Eosinophilic granuloma is primarily an adult disease, typically presenting in patients between 30 and 50 years old. Men are affected more often than women. The bones and the lung are the most frequently affected sites. Lymphadenopathy is commonly present, whereas cutaneous disease is uncommon. The skull is the most common bone involved and the long bones are the least common bone location, but lesions can occur in any bone. Pulmonary nodule formation with fibrosis is the most common pulmonary complication, and is seen primarily in young white men. Cutaneous lesions are usually nodules or ulcerated nodules; similar lesions may develop on mucosal surfaces. The periorificial areas may be involved; such involvement can suggest the diagnosis, par-

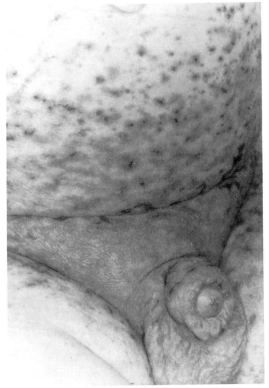

Figure 18–2. Letterer-Siwe disease. Slightly hemorrhagic erythematous papules and plaques are present in this child.

ticularly when chronic, weeping eruptions persist in and around the ear canal. Individual lesions may respond well to treatment. A chronic course with a good prognosis is typical for this disease subset.

The terms Letterer-Siwe disease, Hand-Schüller-Christian disease, and eosinophilic granuloma roughly correlate with present day concepts of acute disseminated disease, chronic progressive disease, and an often benign form of localized disease. At least two other classification systems exist for Langerhans cell disorders. One system divides these disorders into type I and type II categories, based on pathologic criteria. Type I disease is characterized by diffuse, relatively uniform infiltration of involved organs by histiocytes, and roughly corresponds with Letterer-Siwe disease. Type II disease is characterized by focal lesions in involved organs containing sheets of histiocytes in conjunction with eosinophils, giant cells, necrosis, and fibrosis. These findings are more typical of Hand-Schüller-Christian disease and eosinophilic granulomatosis. The second alternate classification system divides cases into unifocal Langerhans cell granulomatosis (seen in some forms of eosinophilic granuloma), multifocal Langerhans cell granulomatosis (seen in some forms of eosinophilic granuloma and in Hand-Schüller-Christian disease), and disseminated histiocytosis or Letterer-Siwe disease.

Differential Diagnosis

The clinical presentation of histiocytosis X can be very misleading, particularly in the older child or adult. In such patients, histiocytosis X is an uncommon disease, and even when it occurs in adults cutaneous findings are often not prominent or may mimic much more common diseases. The disseminated forms of histiocytosis X in childhood are likely to be mistaken for seborrheic dermatitis or eczema, for systemic infections (especially fungal or atypical mycobacterial), for other forms of histiocytosis, or for frank lymphoma. The classic presentation of Hand-Schüller-Christian disease is unlikely to be misdiagnosed, but xanthoma disseminatum can sometimes present in a similar fashion. The adult patient with the classic bone or pulmonary presentation of eosinophilic granuloma also presents little problem for diagnosis, but considerable confusion

may arise in those patients who have predominantly cutaneous findings, or who have ear involvement, which can easily be confused with chronic otitis media or externa.

Histopathology

Early lesions appear as localized granulomas or as areas of proliferative histiocytic response. Some but not all of the cells in the infiltrate are Langerhans cells. Lymphocytes, granulocytes, and multinucleate giant cells may be present. In older lesions, eosinophilic or granulocytic infiltration may become prominent, as may areas of necrosis. Plasma cells may also become more evident, but they are a minor component of the inflammatory response. Infiltration of the dermis adjacent to the epidermis, and often the epidermis itself, is a feature commonly seen in histiocytosis X and almost never in any of the other histiocytosis syndromes. Although some lesions may undergo xanthomatous change, most lesions will become fibrotic and eventually they will regress, leaving residual scarring.

Patient Evaluation

Evaluation of individuals with histiocytosis X must be tailored to the patient's age and to the type of presentation. In infants with acute disseminated disease, cutaneous biopsies may be sufficient to make the diagnosis if the presence of significant numbers of Langerhans cells can be confirmed. This will require a processing technique that identifies specific cell markers such as the OKT-6 monoclonal antibody stain, electron microscopy to demonstrate the presence of diagnostic Birbeck's granules, or the use of the S-100 polyclonal antibody stain. Efforts must also be directed at excluding an associated infection. For all patients, a complete history and physical examination and laboratory studies, including a complete blood count, routine serum chemistries, chest roentgenogram, and usually bone films, are required to evaluate a patient with a biopsy-confirmed diagnosis properly, even in patients with apparently localized disease. Cutaneous lesions, when present, are usually the best source of diagnostic biopsy material. Particularly in the younger patient, evaluation for subclinical diabetes insipidus may be indicated (overt diabetes insipidus in a child can be confirmed by the appropriate use of serum and urine osmolality testing).

Treatment

Therapy for histiocytosis X must be tailored to the severity of the disease and to the patient's symptoms. Patients with the Letterer-Siwe syndrome (and some patients with more extensive, symptomatic Hand-Schüller-Christian disease) usually require systemic chemotherapy, typically vinblastine or the newer, related drug VP-16, in combination with prednisone. For less acute or less extensive disease, symptomatic treatment, such as with vasopressin analogs for diabetes insipidus or local radiotherapy to selected bone lesions, is indicated. Patients with eosinophilic granuloma may respond to prednisone therapy, possibly with methotrexate or vinblastine, if systemic lesions warrant treatment. Intensive chemotherapy is most often required in the treatment of pulmonary disease. Both the risks of treatment and the high rate of eventual spontaneous remission or regression of less acute disease must be considered before therapy is begun.

NON-X HISTIOCYTOSES

Clinical Features

The clinical features of the non-X histiocytoses are summarized in Table 18–1. There is a great deal of confusion and ongoing controversy regarding the proper classification of this group of diseases. For example, cases reported of progressive nodular histiocytoma have been cited by other authors as examples of papular xanthoma. Some authors have used the term progressive nodular histiocytosis to include an entirely different clinical syndrome, which others have labeled reticulohistiocytoma multiple nodular non-X histiocytosis, or nodular cutaneous reactive histiocytosis. This same syndrome has been considered a variant of generalized eruptive histiocytoma or of multicentric reticulohistiocytosis. Therefore, any grouping of the non-X histiocytoses must be considered to be only a working classification, pending a more complete understanding of the monocyte-mac-

rophage system. A complete description of individual diseases is beyond the scope of this chapter. Only a few points regarding Table 18–1 need be added here. The issue of exactly how to separate the rare case of disseminated juvenile xanthogranuloma from slightly atypical cases of xanthoma disseminatum is an active area of discussion (Fig. 18–3; Plate III*H*). Two rare familial disorders not included in the table closely resemble multicentric reticulohistiocytosis clinically but not histologically; these are familial dermo-chondro-corneal dystrophy and familial histiocytic dermatoarthritis. Also, although listed as a variant of malignant histiocytosis in the table, cytophagic histiocytic panniculitis is considered by many investigators to be a distinct entity because of the prominent pathologic findings in the fat, and especially because atypical histiocytes have never been reported in such biopsy specimens.

Differential Diagnosis

The major area of diagnostic confusion, both clinically and histologically, for non-X histiocytoses is distinguishing them from histiocytosis X and from each other. A case in point is the entity of congenital self-healing reticulohistiocytosis, usually considered a non-X histiocytosis. It is unique among the non-X disorders in that a significant percentage of the cells in the infiltrate in such lesions are Langerhans cells. Although it may be a variant of histiocytosis X, its clinical course and pathologic features are sufficiently different to warrant its current separation.

Patient Evaluation

The proper evaluation of patients with cutaneous histiocytic disorders absolutely depends on a very careful analysis of the features of individual cutaneous lesions, paying special attention to the following: variation in lesion morphology, color, and size; cutaneous distribution of lesions; presence of ulceration or necrosis; and evidence of involution. In addition, examination of skin biopsy specimens requires special attention to the presence or absence of epidermal involvement, the exact composition of the cellular infiltrate, localization of the in-

Table 18–1. CUTANEOUS AND SYSTEMIC FINDINGS IN NON-X HISTIOCYTOSES

Disease	Age	Cutaneous Lesions	Mucous Membranes	Systemic Findings	Cutaneous Pathology	Prognosis and Treatment
Congenital self-healing reticulohistiocytosis (Hashimoto-Pritzker)	Newborn (nb)	100% skin involvement. Multiple 2 mm to 3 cm red-brown nodules, often crusted or ulcerated. Generalized distribution.	No	Usually none. May have abnormal hemograms.	Typical, large histiocytes, occasional giant cell. Lymphocytes, plasma cells common, 10–20% of cells have Langerhans cell granules. May invade epidermis.	Spontaneous regression over a 2–3 mo period.
Familial erythrophagocytic lymphohistiocytosis* (autosomal recessive)	1–6 mo (nb–3 yr)	% skin involvement unknown. Poorly described maculo-papular eruption, petechiae. Generalized distribution.	No	Anorexia, vomiting, hepatomegaly with dysfunction, splenomegaly, histiocytic meningitis, seizures, pancytopenia, immune defects, monoclonal gammopathy, hypofibrinogenemia, hyperlipidemia.	Cutaneous histology not described. Typical histiocytes with erythrophagocytosis, lymphocytes in other tissues.	Progressive course. Occasional response to variety of systemic therapies.
Virus-associated hemophagocytic syndrome (associated with CMV, EB, varicella, herpes simplex, and adenovirus)	1 yr (nb–16 yr)	20% skin involvement. Poorly described papular or maculo-papular eruption, petechiae. Generalized distribution.	No	High fever, malaise, hepatomegaly with dysfunction, splenomegaly, generalized lymphadenopathy, pulmonary infiltrates, pancytopenia, coagulation abnormalities or DIC.	Cutaneous histology not described. Elsewhere, proliferation of typical histiocytes in RE system with hemophagocytosis.	Potentially reversible, especially if associated with immunosuppressive agents that are withdrawn.
Benign cephalic histiocytosis	6–12 mo	100% skin involvement. Multiple 2–3 mm red- to yellow-brown papules, become confluent. Upper face, head, neck, shoulders.	No	None.	Slightly atypical histiocytes, rare giant cell, occasional lymphocytes or eosinophils. May infiltrate to subepidermal region.	Spontaneous regression over 2–5 yr period, often with residual pigmented, atrophic macules.

	Age	Skin involvement		Extracutaneous findings	Histology	Course
Juvenile xanthogranuloma (Fig. 18–4)	<1 yr (nb–37 yr)	100% skin involvement. Multiple 2–8 mm red-brown papules, quickly changing to yellow-brown or yellow. Scalp, face, trunk, proximal extremities. Majority have café au lait macules (or in relatives).	Rare	Extracutaneous findings rare: include neurofibromatosis, anemia, leukocytosis; lesions in bone, lung, eyes, very rarely in colon, ovaries, testes, kidney, or pericardium. Very rare cases of myelomonocytic leukemia-like disorder reported.	Early lesions: monomorphous nonfoamy histiocytes. Late lesions: foam cells, Touton and other giant cells, lymphocytes, eosinophils, and neutrophils.	Spontaneous resolution of lesions within 3–6 yrs
Generalized eruptive histiocytoma	Adult (rare, infancy to young adult)	100% skin involvement. Multiple 3–10 mm red or flesh-colored papules, develop in crops on face, trunk, proximal limbs.	Rare	General health usually normal, asymptomatic extracutaneous lesions occasionally noted.	Typical histiocytes, occasional lymphocytes, eosinophils, and neutrophils.	Spontaneous involution of individual lesions, but new lesions may arise indefinitely. Ultimately, usually subsides.
Papular xanthoma	Adult (very rare)	100% skin involvement. Multiple 2–15 mm yellow papules. No confluence, no red-brown color. Face, trunk, proximal extremities.	Yes	None	Foam cells; few typical histiocytes or giant cells.	No spontaneous involution.
Xanthoma disseminatum	Adult (Rare, child to adult)	100% skin involvement. Multiple 2–10 mm red-brown papules, evolving to yellow-brown, quickly become confluent. Trunk, face, proximal limbs, flexural and body fold areas.	Yes	Diabetes insipidus in 50%, may be transient. Upper respiratory tract infiltration can cause hoarseness or dyspnea. Eyelids, conjunctivae or cornea may be involved; growth retardation, seizures may occur.	Typical, large histiocytes, evolving into foam cells. Giant cells, lymphocytes, plasma cells, eosinophils, neutrophils often present.	Diabetes insipidus may resolve spontaneously after several years. Skin lesions may involute with scarring. General health usually good, treatment usually not effective, except for DI.

Table continued on following page

Table 18–1. CUTANEOUS AND SYSTEMIC FINDINGS IN NON-X HISTIOCYTOSES *Continued*

Disease	Age	Cutaneous Lesions	Mucous Membranes	Systemic Findings	Cutaneous Pathology	Prognosis and Treatment
Progressive nodular histiocytoma†	Child to adult (very rare)	100% skin involvement. Two types of skin lesions: multiple 2–10 mm yellow-brown papules; violaceous deep nodules with telangiectasia, occasional necrosis. Generalized distribution.	Yes	None	Typical histiocytes, foam cells, occasional giant cells. Fibrohistiocytic changes seen.	Progressive development of new lesions without involution of old.
Nodular cutaneous reactive histiocytosis (nodular non-X histiocytosis, progressive nodular histiocytosis)	Adult (very rare)	100% skin involvement. Multiple 2 mm to 3 cm red to violaceous papules, nodules, and plaques; leonine facies. Face, upper body.	No	None	Typical histiocytes massed with lymphocytes.	Electron beam therapy or chemotherapy effective if lesions require treatment.
Multicentric reticulohistiocytosis (reticulohistiocytic granuloma, diffuse cutaneous reticulohistiocytosis are skin-limited variants.)	>40 yr (rare, usually adult)	100% skin involvement. Multiple 2 mm to 2 cm translucent yellow-rose or yellow-brown papules and nodules. Mainly on fingers, hands, juxta-articular limb regions, face, occasionally trunk.	Yes	Chronic, destructive osteoarthritis, especially in hands, wrists, and knees. Fever, pleural and pulmonary lesions reported. May rarely involve eye, muscle, or cardiovascular system.	Typical, large histiocytes, with characteristic ground-glass appearance of cytoplasm; see collagenophagocytosis. Multinucleate giant cells, lymphocytes, eosinophils, neutrophils present early; later see fibrosis.	Disease often becomes inactive after several years. Treatment usually ineffective. Malignant visceral disease has been reported.

Malignant histiocytosis (histiocytic medullary reticulosis) (cytophagic histiocytic panniculitis is probable variant)	Adult (2 mo to 90 yr)	10–20% skin involvement. Few, variably sized petechiae, purpura, papules, and nodules, often with ulceration or eschar formation; eczematous lesions. Randomly distributed.	Yes	Febrile, acutely ill patients with hepatomegaly and jaundice, splenomegaly, lymphadenopathy, and pancytopenia. Some cases associated with leukemia (especially ALL), often post-chemotherapy.	Typical and atypical histiocytes with hemophagocytosis, giant cells, lymphocytes, plasma cells, neutrophils. Lymph node best tissue for diagnosis.	Fatal within months if untreated. Some patients have responded to intensive chemotherapy.
Sinus histiocytosis with massive lymphadenopathy	<20 yr (1 yr–67 yr)	10% skin involvement. Multiple <4 cm red- or yellow-brown papules or nodules; one report of massive skin infiltration. Randomly distributed.	Rare	Massive, painless cervical adenopathy; other nodes occasionally involved. Fever, leukocytosis, polyclonal hypergammaglobulinemia. 7% mortality in one large series.	Typical histiocytes, may have vesicular nuclei or foamy cytoplasm. Giant cells, lymphocytes, plasma cells, lymphophagocytosis seen. Diagnostic changes in lymph nodes.	Usually undergoes spontaneous resolution, but deaths have been reported.
Sea-blue histiocytosis	Child-young adult (rare)	<5% skin involvement. One patient had multiple, small, faintly red plaques and nodules limited to face.‡	No	Hepatosplenomegaly, thrombocytopenia common; lung, GI, nervous system lesions reported.	Typical histiocytes, sarcoid-like granulomas with giant cells, lymphocytes. Progress to fibrous stroma.	No known treatment. Apparent autosomal recessive abnormality of lipid metabolism.
Necrobiotic xanthogranuloma with paraproteinemia	Adult (40–74 yr)	100% skin involvement. <10 cm yellow or yellow-brown plaques and red nodules; overlying atrophy, telangiectasia, scarring, or ulceration. Periorbital, trunk, proximal limbs, flexures.	No	Monoclonal gammopathy, leukopenia. Some patients develop myeloma or other marrow dyscrasias.	Typical histiocytes and foam cells, organized into inflammatory granuloma with Touton's and foreign body giant cells. Necrobiosis present.	Lesions poorly responsive to most therapy. Alkylating agents useful in severe disease if WBC high enough to allow their use. Myeloma, if present, determines prognosis. (See also Chapter 16.)

Table continued on following page

Table 18–1. CUTANEOUS AND SYSTEMIC FINDINGS IN NON-X HISTIOCYTOSES *Continued*

Disease	Age	Cutaneous Lesions	Mucous Membranes	Systemic Findings	Cutaneous Pathology	Prognosis and Treatment
Erdheim-Chester disease	Adult (26–78 yr)	<10% skin involvement. Xanthelasma, proptosis, or discrete yellow-brown papules on face, lower legs. May have erythema over long bone lesions.	No	Mixed sclerotic and lytic lesions of long bones. Fever, weight loss, organ dysfunction in 30%. Extraskeletal involvement (esp. retroperitoneum, liver, lungs, heart, and kidney) in 15–25%. Two cases of diabetes insipidus.	Typical histiocytes and foam cells, often organized into inflammatory granuloma with Touton's and foreign body giant cells. No necrobiosis, lesions resolve with fibrosis.	Slowly progressive course, sometimes fatal. Poorly responsive to most therapy; some lesions may respond to radiation therapy.
Lipogranulomatosis (Farber's disease) (autosomal recessive)	Child (very rare)	100% skin involvement. Small papules to large plaques. Subcutaneous masses over wrists and ankles characteristic.	Yes	Ceramidase deficiency. Involves tendon sheaths, synovium, liver, spleen, kidney, lymph nodes, and especially CNS.	Typical histiocytes and fibroblasts in skin. Foam cells in other tissues.	Progressive course, death. No known treatment.
Gaucher's disease (autosomal recessive, 3 types, adult form has skin involvement.)	Adult (type I)	Common skin involvement. Yellow-brown, brown, or gray-brown pigmentation on face, hands, and pre-tibial area.	Yes	Glucocerebrosidase deficiency. Hepatosplenomegaly, bone lesions, pulmonary involvement in adults, with pathologic fractures due to bone lesions, and thrombocytopenic hemorrhage and neutropenic infection from hypersplenism. Yellow-brown pingueculae on bulbar conjunctivae.	Increased melanin in basal cell layer of epidermis. May see increased dermal iron on special stains.	Adult form slowly progressive. No known treatment.

Disease	Age	Skin		Features	Histology	Prognosis
Niemann-Pick disease (autosomal recessive, 4 types, infantile form has skin involvement.)	Infant	Rare skin involvement. Diffuse yellow-brown pigmentation. Xanthomas or red nodules very rarely seen in juvenile form.	No	Sphingomyelinase deficiency. Hepatosplenomegaly, rapidly progressive CNS disease in infantile form.	Increased melanin in basal cell layer of epidermis. Large vacuolated (mulberry) foam cell is characteristic, but seldom seen in skin.	Infantile form fatal by age 1–3 yr.
Tangier disease (autosomal recessive)	Child to adult	Very rare skin involvement. One patient developed truncal papules following splenectomy.	Yes	Alpha-lipoprotein deficiency. Orange-yellow striations of enlarged tonsils. Greatly decreased plasma HDL and cholesterol levels, but high tissue cholesteryl ester levels. Splenomegaly, sensory and motor neuropathies, corneal opacities.	Lipid stains of "normal" skin show lipid deposits in dermis and dermal macrophages. Tonsillar lesions have foam cells.	No evidence for predisposition to premature atherosclerotic disease.
Indeterminate cell histiocytosis (reported only recently, incidence unknown)	Adult	100% skin involvement. 5 mm to 1 cm red to brownish flesh-colored papules, plaques, or nodules on nose, ears, upper extremities, trunk, thighs.	None	1 patient developed mast cell leukemia after 6 yr.	Typical and atypical histiocytes; occasional giant cell, lymphocytes, eosinophils. Histiocytes have S-100 and OKT-6 markers but no Birbeck's (Langerhans) granules.	Both patients responded to chemotherapy. 1 patient well with >9 yr course; 1 patient well for 6 yr until leukemia developed.

*Two variants exist: a similar X-linked syndrome, and a familial histiocytosis accompanied by eosinophilia. Only the eosinophilia-related syndrome has specific cutaneous infiltration by histiocytes.
†Some authors classify these cases as papular xanthoma.
‡Facial macular hyperpigmentation of leukoderma described, but biopsies of such lesions have been non-specific.

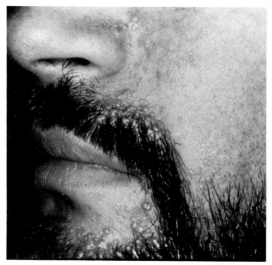

Figure 18–3. Multiple xanthogranulomas representative of non-X histiocytosis in an 18-year-old man with no evidence of internal disease (see also Plate III*H*).

filtrate to perivascular or periappendiceal locations, and special studies to evaluate the presence or absence of Langerhans cells and occasionally of specific intracellular structures such as Birbeck's granules or worm-like particles. Once proper evaluation of the cutaneous lesions has been made, a careful history and physical examination and a knowledge of the systemic findings associated with a particular syndrome can indicate the need for further diagnostic studies.

Treatment

Treatment of non-X histiocytoses is often ineffective and thus not indicated. The nat-

ural history of each syndrome, as well as available therapy, is summarized in Table 18–1. Therapeutic decisions are most critical in the setting of malignant histiocytosis and familial erythrophagocytic lymphohistiocytosis syndromes (where chemotherapy is usually indicated), in xanthoma disseminatum (where vasopressin therapy may be required), and in the virus-associated hemophagocytic syndrome (where withdrawal of any immunosuppressive therapy is usually indicated, and where specific antiviral therapy may be indicated).

Suggested Readings

Barsky BL, Lao I, Barsky S, et al: Benign cephalic histiocytosis. Arch Dermatol *120*:650–655, 1984.

Burgdorf WHC, Kusch SL, Nix TE Jr, et al: Progressive nodular histiocytoma. Arch Dermatol *117*:644–649, 1981.

Gianotti F, Caputo R: Histiocytic syndromes: A review. J Am Acad Dermatol *13*:383–404, 1985.

Gianotti F, Caputo R, Ermacora E, et al: Benign cephalic histiocytosis. Arch Dermatol *122*:1038–1043, 1986.

Groopman JE, Golde DW: The histiocytic disorders: A pathophysiologic analysis. Ann Intern Med *94*:95–107, 1981.

Magaña-García M: Pure cutaneous histiocytosis X. Int J Dermatol *25*:106–108, 1986.

Sanchez RL, Raimer SS, Peltier F, et al: Papular xanthoma; A clinical histologic, and ultrastructural study. Arch Dermatol *121*:626–631, 1985.

Taunton OD, Yeshurun D, Jarratt M: Progressive nodular histiocytoma. Arch Dermatol *114*:1505–1508, 1978.

Winkelmann RK, Hu CH, Kossard S: Response of nodular non-X histiocytosis to vinblastine. Arch Dermatol *118*:913–917, 1982.

Winkelmann RK, Kossard S, Fraga S: Eruptive histiocytoma of childhood. Arch Dermatol *116*:565–570, 1980.

19

Vascular Neoplasms

NEAL PENNEYS

There are a wide variety of tumors that are composed of vascular structures. Many of these tumors are benign, are common, and have no systemic component. For example, the capillary hemangioma (or cherry or senile angioma) occurs with aging in normal people. Certain other benign angiomatous processes, such as the port-wine stain, may occur in patients with Sturge-Weber syndrome. On occasion, large hemangiomas may be associated with hypertrophy of underlying structures or with a consumptive coagulopathy. In this chapter, however, we will focus on malignant vascular neoplasms that can present with cutaneous lesions and that include Kaposi's sarcoma, angiosarcoma, and lymphangiosarcoma of Stewart and Treves.

KAPOSI'S SARCOMA

Kaposi's sarcoma is a tumor derived from proliferating endothelial cells. Immunohistochemical evidence that has demonstrated that the atypical cells contain Factor VIII–related antigen and other antigens defined by monoclonal antibodies specific for endothelial cells supports this concept. The cause(s) of this neoplasm appear(s) to be multifactorial. Its prevalence among certain ethnic groups and its curious geographic distribution suggest genetic predisposition; however, immunosuppression and exposure to multiple infectious agents appear to also play roles in the pathogenesis of this tumor.
Clinical Features. The disease exists as two distinct forms: (1) a slowly progressive disease found in people of Mediterranean or Jewish heritage, and (2) a rapidly progressive

disease with significant mortality originally described in certain parts of central Africa but now widely found as a component of the acquired immune deficiency syndrome (AIDS). Cutaneous lesions of Kaposi's sarcoma compose a spectrum and range from macules to large tumors, and vary in hue from pink to a deep purple. Generally, skin lesions of Kaposi's sarcoma in older Mediterranean men are found initially on the soles of the feet and/or the lower legs and are deeply violaceous (Fig. 19–1). The process usually begins as a solitary lesion. As the lesions disseminate, they extend centrally toward the trunk. Intractable edema may be present as lesions extend up the legs. Skin lesions are usually asymptomatic, although a lesion will occasionally interfere with walking. Generally, progression is slow, although a rare case will have a more rapid course with dissemination. As the disease progresses, the small bowel, lungs, and other internal organs can become involved. The gastrointestinal tract is the most frequently involved site of visceral disease; however, the lesions are rarely clinically appreciated. This form of Kaposi's sarcoma, which is found primarily in older men in the United States, can be associated with other disease processes. Kaposi's sarcoma has been associated with a wide variety of lymphoreticular diseases, in particular, with lymphomas. In the slowly progressive form of Kaposi's sarcoma found primarily in older men, the course is generally of protracted extension of the neoplasm centrally toward the trunk. The majority of patients affected by Kaposi's sarcoma succumb to other disease processes and do not die as a result of the Kaposi's sarcoma.

149

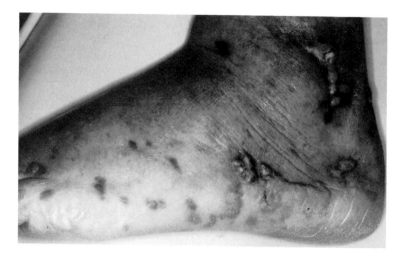

Figure 19–1. Classic Kaposi's sarcoma is present in this elderly white male. Typical nodular lesions are present on his ankle and foot.

The skin lesions of Kaposi's sarcoma associated with AIDS may be morphologically different from the form found in older individuals. These lesions may occur in any individual who is immunosuppressed. In particular, there appears to be an association with iatrogenic immunosuppression as well as with immunosuppression associated with infection by the human immunodeficiency virus (HIV, formerly known as HTLV-III). Infection with HIV appears to be acquired through sexual contact, particularly anal-receptive intercourse, and has particularly affected the gay male population. In addition, it has favored hemophiliacs, intravenous drug abusers, and Haitians.

Kaposi's sarcoma in these patients does not necessarily favor acral locations. Lesions may be solitary or widespread, macular and pink to salmon colored (Fig. 19–2). As the lesions age, the color may deepen to a brown or purple. Kaposi's sarcoma in these individuals may present with mucous membrane lesions involving oral, nasal, and conjunctival areas. Lesions may develop over short periods of time (weeks) and have unusual distributions. Generally, the skin lesions are asymptomatic. It is not unusual to detect patients who are otherwise asymptomatic who present with innocuous appearing skin lesions that upon histologic examination are identified as Kaposi's sarcoma. However, patients with AIDS and Kaposi's sarcoma may have many symptoms related to immunodeficiency, opportunistic infections, and disseminated neoplasia. There is also a well

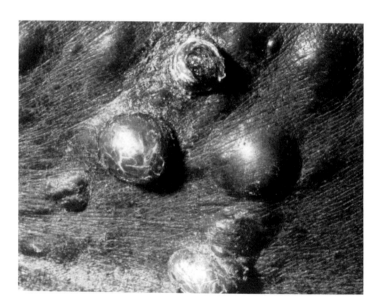

Figure 19–2. Multiple tumors are present in this Haitian male with Kaposi's sarcoma complicating acquired immune deficiency syndrome (AIDS).

known association between the development of Kaposi's sarcoma and immunosuppression after organ transplantation. Frequently, Kaposi's sarcoma will regress when immunosuppressive therapy is withdrawn in these patients.

Histopathology. Confirmation of the diagnosis in all types of Kaposi's sarcoma is made by skin biopsy, which reveals a spindle cell neoplasm containing vascular slits and extravasated erythrocytes. Cytologic atypia may not be great. In early lesions, the histologic changes may be very subtle. The nature of the infiltrating cell can be identified by appropriate immunohistochemical examination.

Patient Evaluation. When Kaposi's sarcoma presents in a gay male or in another member of a high risk group, evaluation of T cell subsets and antibody testing for exposure to HIV are indicated. Endoscopy should be performed to exclude gastrointestinal involvement. Similar studies can be performed in Kaposi's sarcoma in older individuals if appropriate symptoms such as melena indicate internal involvement. Palpable lymphadenopathy in the non-AIDS patient warrants a biopsy to rule out a coexistent lymphoma.

Treatment. Localized Kaposi's sarcoma requires no treatment. Lesions that are painful or that interfere with ambulation can be locally extirpated. Extensive Kaposi's sarcoma of an extremity can be treated with local irradiation (x-irradiation or electron beam given in low doses). Intralesional chemotherapy with vinblastine has also been useful for localized, resistant disease. Disseminated Kaposi's sarcoma may be treated with systemic chemotherapy with vinblastine, but it is often poorly responsive. Patients with iatrogenically induced Kaposi's sarcoma should have their immunosuppressive agents decreased or stopped, if possible. Kaposi's sarcoma in AIDS patients has not been responsive to therapy to date.

ANGIOSARCOMA

Angiosarcoma most frequently presents as an erythematous neoplasm of the head and neck (Fig. 19–3) with a high frequency of metastases. This tumor has a poor response to therapy.

Histopathology. Confirmation of the diag-

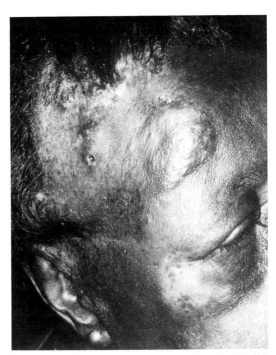

Figure 19–3. An erythematous plaque is present in this elderly black female, representative of angiosarcoma.

nosis is by skin biopsy, which reveals a malignant process composed of cells resembling atypical endothelial cells. Interlacing vascular channels may be present, a point that suggests the vascular origin of the tumor, which may otherwise be anaplastic and poorly differentiated.

Patient Evaluation. Because this tumor is aggressive and can spread to internal organs, appropriate metastatic evaluation should be performed prior to aggressive attempts to extirpate the tumor locally.

Treatment. The tumor is relatively refractory to chemotherapy and radiation therapy. Surgical extirpation is preferred if the lesion is small, but the tumor often has spread far beyond clinically recognized margins. The prognosis in these patients is guarded.

LYMPHANGIOSARCOMA OF STEWART AND TREVES

Lymphangiosarcoma of Stewart and Treves is a malignant tumor of vascular endothelium that characteristically arises in chronic lymphedema, frequently after radical mastectomy with lymph node dissection (Fig. 19–4). Although there is some contro-

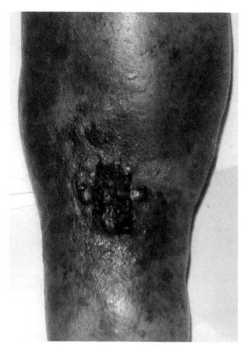

Figure 19–4. An erythematous plaque with central ulceration is present in a lymphedematous arm following breast surgery, which is representative of lymphangiosarcoma or Stewart-Treves syndrome.

versy regarding the nosology of this tumor, most experts feel that lymphatic endothelium is the site of origin.

Clinical Features. Although the lesion has been most often described in a lymphedematous limb following mastectomy, it can arise in chronic lymphedema in any location. Initially, the lesions may appear as small, translucent papules, discoloration, or discolored nodules. As the tumor enlarges, nodules can be defined more clearly. Some nodules eventually ulcerate. The tumor has a propensity to metastasize early in its course.

Histopathology. The diagnosis is confirmed by skin biopsy, which reveals a neoplasm composed of atypical endothelial cells. Interlacing vascular channels, some with the morphology of lymphatic vessels, may be present.

Patient Evaluation. Appropriate studies to exclude dissemination should precede aggressive forms of local therapy.

Treatment. Options are limited and range from amputation of the affected limb to radiotherapy and chemotherapy. The latter modalities are poorly effective.

CUTANEOUS HEMANGIOMATA AND TELANGIECTASIA

Hemangiomata are vascular malformations that may be composed of capillaries, venules, arterioles, or a mixture of vessel types. Telangiectasias are dilated and tortuous vessels. A number of internal processes and syndromes can be associated with these cutaneous vascular lesions.

A number of syndromes have angiomata or telangiectasias as a prominent component. The von Hippel–Lindau syndrome is composed of hemangioblastoma of the cerebellum, retinal angiomas, polycythemia, and occasional cutaneous vascular lesions. Klippel-Trenaunay-Weber syndrome is characterized by vascular malformation that leads to limb hypertrophy. Spinal hemangiomas may be associated with dermatomal cutaneous hemangiomas, usually unilateral and affecting the upper limb. Sturge-Weber (Dimitri's) syndrome is characterized by a unilateral vascular malformation that covers a large part of the face in the region of the ophthalmic division of the trigeminal nerve. Cerebral symptoms, including spastic hemiparesis, and a unique track-like calcification on x-ray of the skull that outlines the convolutions of the cortex are also seen. Osler-Weber-Rendu syndrome is characterized by small angiomas on the skin, mucous membranes, and the gastrointestinal and genitourinary tract. These small angiomas are of significance only in their tendency to bleed; these patients may present initially with signs and symptoms of gastrointestinal bleeding. Hemangiomata (i.e., angiokeratomas) may be markers of other syndromes, including 13, 15 trisomy, Fabry's disease, and fucosidase deficiency.

Telangiectasia is a relatively common alteration in skin and can represent a cutaneous response to a number of different stimuli. Most commonly, cutaneous telangiectasias are seen as a response to ultraviolet light exposure on sun-exposed surfaces. Certain ethnic groups are predisposed to develop these actinic changes (such as Celts). The telangiectasias associated with ataxia telangiectasia syndrome are classically on the conjunctivae, the backs of the ears, and certain flexural areas. Other features of this syndrome are cerebellar ataxia, recurrent pulmonary infections, and an increased frequency of lymphoreticular neoplasms. Telangiectasias can exist as congenital lesions with dermatomal and unilateral distributions. Mats of telangiectatic vessels can be seen on exposed surfaces in patients with chronic liver disease or with scleroderma. Lastly, telangiectasia and tortuosity of scleral vessels can be seen in chronic liver disease as well as in patients with sickle cell anemia.

Other Vascular Changes

Dilatation of superficial as well as deep vessels may be signs of underlying systemic processes. Diffuse erythema of the palms is a well known sign of chronic liver disease; however, it also occurs as a response to estrogen-containing medications, pregnancy, other chronic diseases, or subacute bacterial endocarditis, and can be familial. Dilatation of a single arteriole leads to the formation of the vascular spider, a well-recognized skin lesion that can be a marker of chronic liver disease, but may also occur as a manifestation of pregnancy or ingestion of birth control pills, and as a familial trait.

Lastly, massive dilatation of larger vessels can be the hallmark of underlying vascular obstruction such as that noted in the superior vena cava syndrome and in chronic portal hypertension.

Suggested Readings

Baes H: Angiosarcoma in a chronic lymphedematous leg. Dermatologica 134:331–336, 1967.

Cox FH, Helwig EB: Kaposi's sarcoma. Cancer 12:289–298, 1959.

Friedman-Kien AE, Laubenstein LJ, Rubenstein P, et al: Disseminated Kaposi's sarcoma in homosexual men. Ann Intern Med 96:693–700, 1982.

Harwood AR, Asorba D, Fofstader SL, et al: Kaposi's sarcoma in recipients of renal transplant. Am J Med 67:759–765, 1979.

Laskas JJ Jr, Shelley WB, Wood MG: Lymphangiosarcoma arising in congenital lymphedema. Arch Dermatol 111:86–89, 1975.

Maddox JC, Evans HL: Angiosarcoma of skin and soft tissue. Cancer 48:1907–1921, 1981.

Reed WB, Kamath HM, Weiss L: Kaposi's sarcoma, with emphasis on the internal manifestations. Arch Dermatol 110:115–118, 1974.

Stewart FW, Treves N: Lymphangiosarcoma in postmastectomy lymphedema. Cancer 1:64–68, 1948.

Wilson Jones E: Malignant angioendothelioma of the skin. Br J Dermatol 76:21–23, 1964.

Wilson Jones E: Malignant vascular tumors. Clin Exp Dermatol 1:287–312, 1976.

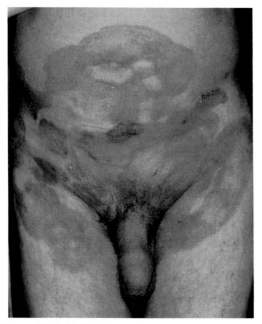

Figure 20–3. Multiple irregular erythematous plaques are present in a man with mycosis fungoides (see also Plate IVA).

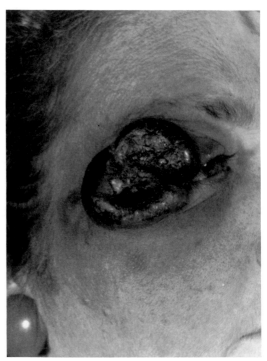

Figure 20–5. A large tumorous lesion has developed in this patient with mycosis fungoides.

tumors may develop within these plaques (Fig. 20–4), and such lesions may ultimately become eroded or even deeply ulcerated (Fig. 20–5). It may be difficult to determine whether a lesion is best described as an indurated plaque or as an early nodule, and for this reason the Mycosis Fungoides Co-operative Group has adopted the minimum standard of 3 cutaneous tumors (nodules) for assignment of a patient to a tumor category. The infiltrative plaques or nodules may

result in a leonine facies (Fig. 20–6), as is sometimes seen in leprosy or chronic lymphocytic leukemia. Patients with mycosis fungoides may present with tumor stage lesions without antecedent macules or plaques; this presentation has been called tumeur (tumor) d'emblee (Fig. 20–7).

Patients with mycosis fungoides may develop a generalized erythroderma, but erythroderma owing to cutaneous T cell lymphoma usually occurs *de novo* in the setting of Sézary's syndrome. This syndrome, characterized by erythroderma, leukocytosis with circulating Sézary's cells (lymphocytes with hyperconvoluted or cerebriform nuclei), adenopathy, and hepatosplenomegaly, is usually considered a leukemic variant of mycosis fungoides. Severe pruritus is common in patients with Sézary's syndrome and can be severe enough to provoke suicide.

Lesions in mycosis fungoides patients typically evolve from a variety of non-specific, pre-diagnostic lesions to biopsy-confirmed macular and papular stages. Some patients may ultimately develop cutaneous nodules or erythroderma.

Another disease usually classified as a variant of mycosis fungoides is *pagetoid*

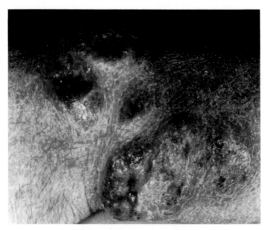

Figure 20–4. Multiple nodular lesions have developed in this patient with mycosis fungoides.

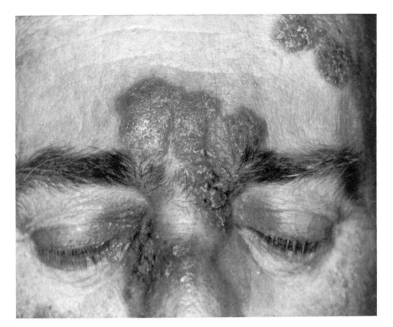

Figure 20–6. Early onset of leonine facies in this individual with mycosis fungoides.

reticulosis. Clinically, this typically presents as a scaling, erythematous, slowly changing polycyclic plaque (Fig. 20–8). The term pagetoid reticulosis refers to the characteristic pagetoid infiltration of epidermis by large, atypical cells not usually seen in mycosis fungoides. A solitary lesion on a distal extremity is typical of the localized form (*Woringer-Kolopp disease*). At least some patients with such a lesion do develop clear-cut evidence of cutaneous T cell lymphoma elsewhere, though there is some debate concerning the inevitability of this transition. A more generalized type of pagetoid reticulosis, characterized by multiple lesions with similar clinical and histologic findings, has been termed the Ketron-Goodman type. It is generally accepted as an unusual variant of cutaneous T cell lymphoma.

The syndrome of *alopecia mucinosa,* characterized clinically by flesh-colored to erythematous follicular papules or boggy, indurated plaques and histologically by

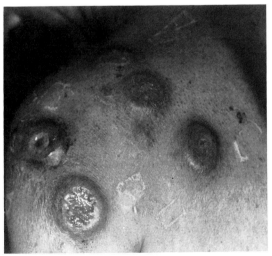

Figure 20–7. Rapid onset of multiple tumors in a patient with mycosis fungoides represents the tumeur d'emblee.

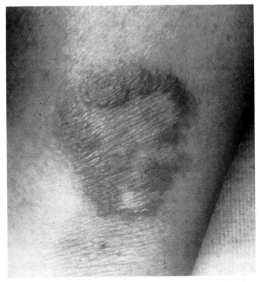

Figure 20–8. Localized intraepidermal mycosis fungoides, also known as Woringer-Kolopp disease.

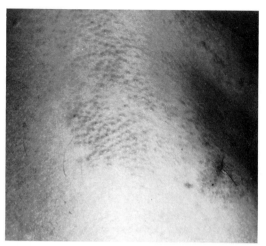

Figure 20–9. Papular lesions of alopecia mucinosa existed in this patient with mycosis fungoides. This is the same patient as pictured in Figure 20–6.

follicular mucinosis, can be seen as an isolated finding or in conjunction with other diseases, including mycosis fungoides (Fig. 20–9). If a patient has alopecia mucinosa in association with mycosis fungoides, a biopsy of the lesion will usually show not only the changes of follicular mucinosis but also those of mycosis fungoides. Without histopathologic changes at least suggestive of mycosis fungoides in a biopsy of a patient with alopecia mucinosa, prolonged follow-up for the development of mycosis fungoides is probably not needed.

Mycosis fungoides is usually a slowly progressive disease; many patients eventually die of causes unrelated to their T cell lymphoma. Enlargement of the peripheral lymph nodes is usually the first site of clinically evident extracutaneous disease, and symptomatic visceral involvement is a late manifestation, if it develops at all. Of patients dying because of their disease, roughly half do so because of septicemia or serious infection, with the skin being the site of initial infection. Disseminated disease resulting in inanition or serious organ dysfunction accounts for most of the remaining deaths that are due to cutaneous T cell lymphoma.

Clinical staging systems for mycosis fungoides are useful in estimating prognosis and in planning therapy, but the number of different staging systems used previously makes comparisons of different study results difficult. A revised staging system adopted by the Mycosis Fungoides Cooperative Group is outlined in Table 20–1, along with survival figures for a study by that group involving 340 patients classified by that staging system. The type and extent of skin disease and the number of sites of palpable lymphadenopathy are the most important variables in this and in most other staging systems designed to assess prognosis of cutaneous T cell lymphoma.

The presence of early cutaneous involvement by a leukemia or lymphoma is strongly suggestive of a T cell origin for that neoplasm. Although T cell neoplasms probably account for approximately 20% of all leukemias and lymphomas, they may account for 50% or more of all such tumors presenting in the skin. Many of these T cell tumors are not mycosis fungoides or Sézary's syndrome, and are usually easily distinguished

Table 20–1. CLINICAL STAGING SYSTEM FOR MYCOSIS FUNGOIDES
(MYCOSIS FUNGOIDES COOPERATIVE GROUP)*

Clinical Stage	Clinically Enlarged Skin Category	Nodal Sites†	Approximate 5-yr Survival (%)
1	T_0 No clinically or histopathologically suspicious skin lesions	0–1	80
	T_1 Papules, plaques, or eczematous patches (<10% body surface)		
2	T_0–T_1	2–8	60
	T_2 Same as T_1, but >10% body surface	0–1	
3	T_2	2–8	50
	T_3 At least 3 tumors with or without other cutaneous changes	0–8	
4	T_4 Erythroderma (Sézary's syndrome) with or without other skin changes	0–8	40

*Analysis of 340 patients; only 10 patients were T_0 category. (Adapted from Lamberg, SI, et al: Ann Intern Med *100*:187, 1984.)

†Nodal sites included left and right cervical, left and right axillary, left and right groin, epitrochlear, and submandibular.

from them by their clinical and histopathologic pattern in the skin. Included among such neoplasms are T cell chronic lymphocytic leukemia, peripheral T cell lymphomas, adult T cell leukemia-lymphoma of Japan, T cell lymphoblastic lymphoma, adult T cell lymphoblastic lymphoma, multilobated cutaneous T cell lymphoma, and a variety of "histiocytic" or large cell lymphomas of T cell origin. It is also important to point out that there is accumulating evidence that at least some conditions diagnosed as angioimmunoblastic lymphadenopathy are actually angiocentric T cell lymphomas, and the possibility exists that angioimmunoblastic lymphadenopathy is actually a polyclonal B cell reaction to a monoclonal T cell disorder and may progress to an overt malignancy in some patients (see also Chapter 15).

In general, the more closely the malignant T cell phenotype resembles that of mycosis fungoides, and the more indolent the disease, the more closely the clinical and histologic picture will resemble that of mycosis fungoides. Much more has been learned about T cell disorders as a result of the improved capability to distinguish T cells from B cells, and also since the discovery of the HTLV-I retrovirus responsible for the adult T cell leukemia-lymphoma endemic in Japan and in scattered areas worldwide. The HTLV-I retrovirus is also responsible for some sporadic cases of peripheral T cell lymphomas and T cell leukemias.

Some cases of adult T cell leukemia-lymphoma of Japan bear a close resemblance to mycosis fungoides and Sézary's syndrome, because of a high incidence of clinical skin involvement with epidermotropism and the presence of Pautrier-like abscesses on histologic examination. Many reports of cutaneous involvement in chronic T cell lymphocytic leukemia are, in retrospect, probably descriptions of this HTLV-I–associated syndrome. Despite the resemblance of this syndrome to classic cutaneous T cell lymphoma, a more aggressive course; prominent, early bone marrow, spleen, and other organ involvement; differences in histologic appearance; and the presence of HTLV-I antibodies make this a distinctive entity.

Chronic lymphocytic leukemia of T cell origin is an uncommon leukemia, accounting for only 2% of chronic lymphocytic leukemias in one survey series. Early cutaneous infiltration manifesting as papules, plaques, or erythroderma is common in this disorder, though early reports tended to overestimate the frequency of cutaneous involvement because of inclusion of the Japanese T cell leukemias. The histologic picture is usually that of a subepidermal, band-like lymphocytic infiltrate, but unlike mycosis fungoides there is usually sparing of the uppermost dermis and no epidermotropism. The clinical picture is atypical for cutaneous T cell lymphoma because of the presence of splenomegaly and of early prominent bone marrow involvement.

Peripheral T cell lymphomas represent a broad spectrum of clinical and histologic findings, but in general they are characterized by generalized lymphadenopathy, hepatic and splenic enlargement, an increased frequency of hypercalcemia and lytic bone lesions, frequent autoimmune cytopenias, an aggressive course, and often by polymorphous cellular infiltrate. Some patients with angioimmunoblastic lymphadenopathy or lymphomatoid granulomatosis have been reclassified as having peripheral T cell lymphomas, and some patients with HTLV-I–associated lymphoma fit this syndrome. When cutaneous involvement does occur, it may be due to non-specific infiltration, a monomorphous infiltration of abnormal cells, or a polymorphous infiltration with some features of Hodgkin's disease or angioimmunoblastic lymphadenopathy. Except for some HTLV-I–associated lymphomas, epidermotropism is not seen.

Other non-epidermotropic T cell tumors include T cell lymphoblastic lymphoma, acute T cell lymphoblastic leukemia, and usually "histiocytic" or large cell tumors whose T cell origin may be unsuspected prior to cell marker studies. Because of this, cell marker studies should be performed in any patient with leukemia or lymphoma with early cutaneous findings.

Multilobated cutaneous T cell lymphoma is a type of lymphoma with prominent extranodal distribution, particularly in the skin and subcutaneous tissues. On histologic examination, there is epidermal and superficial dermal sparing and a deeper dermal and subcutaneous lymphocytic infiltrate with scattered, large cells with characteristic multilobated nuclei. The clinical findings and disease course closely resemble those of Crosti's reticulosis, an entity reported primarily in the European literature. These two diseases may be identical, but the cell origin of Crosti's reticulosis remains controversial.

DIFFERENTIAL DIAGNOSIS

An often confusing variety of conditions are mentioned in the context of diseases that may have a risk of progression to mycosis fungoides. Usually included in this category are acute and chronic pityriasis lichenoides, large plaque parapsoriasis, poikiloderma vasculare atrophicans, retiform parapsoriasis, and actinic reticuloid.

Both acute and chronic forms of pityriasis lichenoides exist and are very rarely associated with the development of a lymphoma. Acute pityriasis lichenoides is a condition that may itself be chronic, but in which lesions undergo a typical acute evolution from papules to hemorrhagic or superficially necrotic papules and then heal with variable degrees of scarring. Chronic pityriasis lichenoides is characterized by erythematous, often hyperpigmented papules or plaques that tend to be asymptomatic but recalcitrant to treatment. The skin lesions of lymphomatoid papulosis may resemble those of either acute or chronic pityriasis lichenoides clinically. However, histologically they have one of two types of atypical cells accounting for at least 10% of the dermal infiltrate. One type of atypical cell is a large cell with a hyperchromatic cerebriform nucleus and sparse cytoplasm; it is a helper T cell. The other type of atypical cell is even larger, with a polymorphous nucleus and abundant cytoplasm; it is thought to be similar to cells of the dendritic macrophage series (e.g., interdigitating reticulum cell). This "histiocyte" may be multinucleated or closely resemble a Reed-Sternberg cell. Lymphomatoid papulosis may actually represent a syndrome in which some patients have a monoclonal T cell proliferation that rarely develops into a T cell lymphoma, and others have an apparently reactive macrophage proliferation that may develop an associated lymphoma (especially Hodgkin's) but that typically has a benign, resolving course. Regressing atypical histiocytosis probably represents a variant of the histiocytic subset of lymphomatoid papulosis.

The term parapsoriasis includes a group of disorders that have no relationship to psoriasis. Small plaque parapsoriasis is im-portant because it may be confused with acute or chronic pityriasis lichenoides or with large plaque parapsoriasis, but it has no known malignant potential. Small plaque parapsoriasis is characterized by erythematous yellow or brown, slightly scaly plaques developing primarily on the trunk and proximal extremities. The plaques are usually small, almost always less than 5 cm in diameter. Digitate dermatosis is a variant in which elongated plaques develop, often in a palisading formation on the trunk. When such plaques are sufficiently yellow, the term xanthoerythroderma perstans has been used.

Large plaque parapsoriasis is characterized by poorly defined erythematous macules or plaques, usually greater than 10 cm in diameter. Typical features include hypo- and hyperpigmentation, telangiectasia, fine scaling, and areas of epidermal atrophy. Lesions occur most frequently on flexural surfaces, the breasts, buttocks, and thighs. The term poikiloderma vasculare atrophicans has been used to describe this constellation of findings, but the term poikiloderma was first coined to describe the areas of atrophy, pigmentary change, and telangiectasia seen in some patients with dermatomyositis. The size and distribution of the lesions and the clinical setting are therefore important in making the diagnosis of large plaque parapsoriasis. Such distinctions are important because large plaque parapsoriasis progresses to mycosis fungoides in up to 20% of cases. Retiform parapsoriasis is a variant of large plaque psoriasis that is distinguished by a net-like coalescence of small, scaly papules in areas of severe epidermal atrophy, pigmentary changes, and telangiectasia. This variant is much more strongly associated with progression to mycosis fungoides than simple large plaque parapsoriasis alone.

Actinic reticuloid is a severe, persistent photodermatitis of older men associated with intractable pruritus. Erythematous, flat-topped papules or plaques that appear primarily on the exposed skin may mimic mycosis fungoides; occasional episodes of erythroderma may occur, further confusing the diagnosis. A dense polymorphous infiltrate containing atypical lymphocytes is found on biopsy examination; this infiltrate may extend deeply around the adnexal structures. The epidermal infiltration by lymphocytes may resemble Pautrier's microabscesses. Finally, Hodgkin's disease and large cell lymphoma have been very rarely reported as associated neoplasms.

HISTOPATHOLOGY

Histologic findings suggestive of mycosis fungoides or Sézary's syndrome must always be interpreted in conjunction with the clinical findings to prevent misdiagnosis. However, in very early mycosis fungoides it can be most difficult both clinically and histologically to find unequivocal evidence for the diagnosis of cutaneous T cell lymphoma. This accounts for the often very long prediagnostic phase of this disease. To maximize the chance for proper diagnosis, multiple cutaneous biopsies should be taken in any patient suspected of having mycosis fungoides or Sézary's syndrome, since very similar appearing clinical lesions may have very different histologic pictures. Features suggestive of cutaneous T cell lymphoma include a polymorphous, band-like upper dermal infiltrate consisting mainly of lymphocytes and histiocytes, epidermotropism (lymphocyte infiltration of the epidermis) in the absence of spongiosis (epidermal edema), and especially epidermal collections of hyperchromatic mononuclear cells. As clinical lesions evolve from macular to papular or plaque stage lesions, such findings become more common, so that a definite histologic diagnosis can usually be made from plaque stage lesions. If a patient progresses to the tumor stage, however, the histologic picture may change to that of a monomorphous, large cell lymphocytic infiltrate without evidence of epidermotropism or Pautrier's abscesses. Interestingly, a response to therapy may be followed by the return of the histologic picture of epidermotropism. The histologic picture of Sézary's syndrome is identical to that of mycosis fungoides in the plaque stage; multiple biopsies may be required here, also, to obtain a diagnostic histopathologic finding. In addition, an elevated number of circulating atypical lymphocytes with characteristic hyperconvoluted or cerebriform nuclei is required for the diagnosis of Sézary's syndrome.

PATIENT EVALUATION

Unlike most leukemias and lymphomas, classic cutaneous T cell lymphoma is usually clinically limited to the skin for a long time, and seldom shows significant marrow infiltration by leukemic cells until quite late in the course, even in the setting of Sézary's syndrome. Because of this, the clinical staging of such patients differs from that for other leukemias and lymphomas. At a minimum, a complete history and physical examination, a skin biopsy or biopsies, a chest radiograph, a blood count with differential, and a biopsy of palpable lymph nodes when such are present are required for staging.

Extracutaneous involvement is unusual in early stages of mycosis fungoides, and when extracutaneous involvement develops, the peripheral lymph nodes are usually involved first, followed by the liver and lung involvement. Bone marrow involvement is uncommon, even in Sézary's syndrome; therefore, the finding of significant bone marrow infiltration by lymphoma should indicate the need to consider alternative diagnoses.

TREATMENT

In order to achieve a cure in patients with either mycosis fungoides or Sézary's syndrome, one of two conditions must be met: (1) either the disease must be localized to the skin and local therapy must be effective in eradicating the localized disease, or (2) systemic therapy must be available that is curative for the disseminated disease. The research on cell trafficking in cutaneous T cell lymphoma indicates that from very early in the disease, the lymphoma cells freely travel from the skin to lymph nodes or through the blood stream and then return to the skin as a preferential homing site. This means that local therapy, no matter how effective, is unlikely to be curative. Despite occasional reports of cure of mycosis fungoides in early stages by electron beam therapy, it is precisely in the earliest stages that an unquestioned diagnosis of malignancy is most difficult to make. Based on the knowledge gained from clinical trials in other lymphomas such as Hodgkin's disease, the best chance for cure rests with the earliest administration possible of effective therapy. However, despite a number of aggressive single and multiple agent chemotherapy trials and the development of more specific anti–T cell chemotherapeutic agents, no good evidence for cure of the systemic disease exists. The appropriate choice of therapy for an individual patient must balance these considerations against the usually slow and often unpredictable disease course.

Topical chemotherapy has been a common and usually effective local therapy for palliation of macular and plaque type mycosis fungoides. Topical nitrogen mustard (mechlorethamine) is the most commonly used drug. It is relatively safe, and can be used at home by the patient. The major side-effect is the development of contact dermatitis, which can be either a primary irritant reaction or a true allergic eczematous dermatitis. Dry skin (depending on the vehicle used for administration) may also develop, and perhaps there is a long-term slight risk of developing a skin cancer of epidermal cell origin. When topical nitrogen mustard is ineffective or not well tolerated, topical carmustine (bischloroethylnitrosourea [BCNU]) may be used; unlike topical nitrogen mustard, its systemic absorption through the skin can be sufficient to result in delayed bone marrow suppression. The total daily dose applied to the skin must therefore be carefully monitored.

The use of ultraviolet B phototherapy has been occasionally useful for treatment of cutaneous T cell lymphoma, but PUVA (psoralen–ultraviolet A) therapy is now used much more frequently. This therapy requires the administration of methoxsalen as a systemic photosensitizer followed by the administration of ultraviolet A light approximately 2 hours later. The patient must be protected from environmental sources of ultraviolet A for 24–48 hours following methoxsalen administration. This therapy is often quite effective for thin, superficial lesions of cutaneous T cell lymphoma, but requires treatments 3 or 4 times weekly. Side-effects include the risk of a severe sunburn-like reaction if the patient is improperly protected from ultraviolet A radiation, a slightly increased risk of developing superficial epidermal skin cancers, and the possible risk of cataracts if the lens and cornea are improperly protected during and after therapy.

Radiation therapy is very effective in inducing regression of cutaneous lymphoma lesions; it is especially useful for nodular lesions that often do not respond to phototherapy or topical chemotherapy. Electron beam therapy is particularly useful for treatment of cutaneous T cell lymphoma, because treatment can be limited to the upper dermis and epidermis, reducing the deeper injury that occurs with conventional radiotherapy. Electron beam therapy can also be given as a single total body administration of 3000 rads in 200 rad daily fractions. It should be remembered that the conventional cutaneous side-effects of radiation therapy can follow electron beam therapy in spite of the small depth dose. Therefore, unless reproducible, convincing evidence can be obtained for the claimed curative effect of electron beam therapy, it probably should be reserved for patients in whom topical chemotherapy or phototherapy has been unsuccessful.

A variety of agents such as bacille Calmette-Guérin (BCG) ointment, dinitrochlorobenzene (DNCB), and purified protein derivative (PPD) have been used to induce a cutaneous inflammatory reaction. The result of these treatments is unpredictable, and they may cause more cutaneous symptoms than the underlying disease; therefore, the use of such regimens is limited.

As mentioned previously, a variety of single agent and multiple agent chemotherapy protocols have been ineffective in inducing complete, permanent remissions of mycosis fungoides or in Sézary's syndrome, although the short-term response is often dramatic, even in advanced disease. Newer agents with more selective anti–T cell effects have given disappointing results. For example, tilorone is ineffective in cutaneous T cell lymphoma. Although the adenosine deaminase inhibitor 2′-deoxycoformycin can induce temporary remissions, its use is often associated with severe central nervous system and renal toxicity and the risks of long-term immunosuppression. Cyclosporin A has also had limited success in T cell lymphomas, but its use is associated with a number of side-effects, including a generalized capillary leak phenomenon, renal injury or failure, and immunosuppression. Some reports have also suggested the possibility of inducing a more aggressive course of disease with this agent. The retinoid group of drugs (etretinate, 13-cis-retinoic acid) has been reported to have some effect on cutaneous T cell lymphomas, and the ongoing research to provide newer types of retinoid-related drugs may provide hope for even more effective compounds. Anecdotal reports also exist for an effect of the antiviral compound acyclovir on cutaneous T cell lymphomas, but there is as yet no rationale for its use in this disease.

Despite its apparent similarity to mycosis fungoides, Sézary's syndrome is notorious for its relative lack of response to many of these previous therapies. Leukapheresis has been effective in relieving pruritus and reducing scaling and erythema refractory to other therapy; it usually must be continued indefinitely and is an expensive, time consuming procedure. Another promising therapy directed at circulating cells is extracorporeal photopheresis, in which oral psoralen is administered to a patient to induce systemic ultraviolet A photosensitivity, and then the blood is exposed to ultraviolet A during extracorporeal circulation. This allows a much higher dose of ultraviolet A to be used than could be administered in standard PUVA therapy. This procedure is still experimental, but early results are promising.

The use of biologic response modifiers and antilymphocyte sera is another area of promising research. Thus far, the most promising agent for disseminated disease is high dose recombinant leukocyte A interferon. This therapy is currently very expensive and is complicated by its considerable toxicity.

The choice of therapy for a patient with mycosis fungoides or Sézary's syndrome must be tailored to the individual patient, and will have to be adjusted as new advances in therapy are designed. In most instances, the aim of therapy must be palliation, and the use of aggressive systemic therapy should probably be confined to patients with advanced disease or in controlled trials.

Suggested Readings

Abel EA: Clinical features of cutaneous T-cell lymphoma. Dermatol Clin 3:647–664, 1985.

Edelson RL: Cutaneous T-cell lymphoma: Mycosis fungoides, Sézary syndrome, and other variants. J Am Acad Dermatol 2:89–106, 1980.

Lamberg SI, Green SB, Byar DP, Block JB, et al: Clinical staging for cutaneous T-cell lymphoma. Ann Intern Med 100:187–192, 1984.

Tigelaar RE: Lymphocyte traffic and the skin. Dermatol Clin 3:569–585, 1985.

Toback AC, Edelson RL: Pathogenesis of cutaneous T-cell lymphoma. Dermatol Clin 3:605–614, 1985.

Vonderheid EC, Micaily B: Treatment of cutaneous T-cell lymphomas. Dermatol Clin 3:673–687, 1985.

21

Cutaneous Melanoma and Pigmented Lesions

JOSEPH L. JORIZZO

There has been a steady increase in the incidence of melanoma throughout the world over the past half century. Data from the National Cancer Institute suggest that an 80% increase in the incidence of melanoma occurred in the United States between 1973 and 1980. An increase in understanding of the biology of melanoma has changed the emphasis and approach to the topic of melanoma from late-stage, dismal-prognosis, and palliation to early detection and good hope for cure. Therefore, it is imperative that the primary care physician increase his or her skill in the recognition and clinicopathologic understanding of early melanoma and the precursor lesions dysplastic and congenital nevi.

MELANOMA

Epidemiology

The published facts are striking: At the current rate of increase of incidence of melanoma, 1 in 185 Americans will develop melanoma during their lifetime and 1 in 400 Americans will die of the disease. In 1980, there were 13,600 new cases of melanoma and melanoma accounted for 1% of all cancer deaths. The dramatic increase in the incidence of melanoma in the United States and worldwide appears confined to whites, especially those whose ancestry is Northern European. Hispanics, blacks, and Asian Americans have a much lower incidence of melanoma than do individuals of Northern European ancestry. There is a strong correlation between a history of easy sun burning and/or difficulty in suntanning and melanoma. However, the office worker with intermittent sun exposure may be more at risk than the outdoor worker with regular sun exposure. Genetic factors other than skin type (i.e., propensity to tan versus burn after ultraviolet light exposure) may also be involved but are poorly identified at present.

Hormonal factors have been implicated in melanoma because of the rarity of melanoma before puberty and because of less well accepted reports of increased incidence of melanoma in women who use oral contraceptives and reports of exacerbation or onset of melanoma with pregnancy. The role of hormonal factors is poorly understood. Although various dietary factors have been implicated, there is currently no definite association between diet and melanoma.

Clinical Aspects

A tremendous advance since the late 1960s has been the suggestion by Clark and colleagues and modification by Breslow and coworkers that cutaneous melanomas be divided into 4 distinct clinicopathologic types (fourth type added more recently) and histologically measured by depth of invasion and thickness to obtain proper prognostic information. The existence of 4 distinct types of melanoma has been challenged, but is accepted by the majority of experts as at least representing points on a spectrum of cutaneous melanoma. The 4 types of cutaneous melanoma are lentigo maligna, superficial spreading, nodular, and the more recently described acrolentiginous melanoma.

The most common sites of melanoma on the skin in whites are the back, anterior torso, upper extremities, and head and neck in males. In females, the back, lower legs, upper extremities, and head and neck are the most common sites.

The National Cancer Institute (Office of Cancer Communication, National Cancer Institute, Bethesda, MD 20892) publishes a list of melanoma warning signs, of which all primary care physicians should be aware. The signs include large size (greater than 5 mm), multiple colors (brown, white, pink, but especially black), irregular border (notched or angular), abnormal surface (scale, ooze, bleeding), unusual sensation (pruritus or pain), and abnormal surrounding skin (spread of pigment to adjacent skin or loss of pigment or presence of inflammation). A complete cutaneous examination is an important part of any physical examination. Owing to the large clinical error in diagnosis of the earliest lesions of melanoma, suspicious lesions must be excised for histologic examination.

Clinical differences exist among the 4 types of cutaneous melanoma. Superficial spreading melanoma is the most common type. These lesions may occur on any part of the body. Variation in color is a hallmark. White areas often correspond histologically with areas of tumor regression, red areas with inflammation, and blue-black areas with deeper tumor penetration (Fig. 21–1; Plate IVB). The border is usually irregular, corresponding to horizontal growth. These lesions may grow in a horizontal growth phase for 5–10 years before becoming vertically invasive. Thus early, thin superficial spreading melanomas are often curable with complete surgical excision.

Lentigo maligna melanoma occurs in the large, light brown patches on sun-exposed skin (usually face of elderly individuals) (Fig. 21–2; Plate IVC) that were previously called Hutchinson's freckles (Fig. 21–3). This lesion can persist in a horizontal

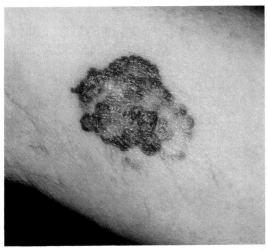

Figure 21–1. An irregular margin with multiple colors of black, blue, slight red, and white are seen in this superficial spreading melanoma (see also Plate IVB).

growth phase for even 30 years. Lesions may be many centimeters in diameter before a vertical growth phase supervenes.

Nodular melanoma may also occur anywhere on the skin surface. These lesions begin directly in a vertical growth phase. The color is relatively uniform and dark. They appear as nodules that may be sharply delineated (Fig. 21–4). Amelanotic nodular melanomas may present as flesh-colored nodules.

Acrolentiginous melanomas arise on the palms, on the soles, and on subungual skin and mucous membranes. These lesions also

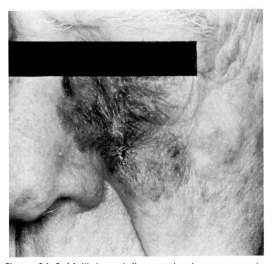

Figure 21–2. Multiple variations and colors are seen in this elderly man with lentigo maligna melanoma (see also Plate IVC).

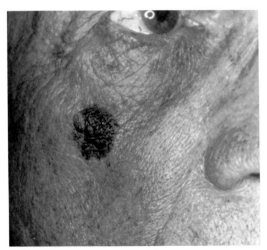

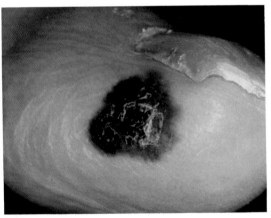

Figure 21–5. Acrolentiginous melanoma (see also Plate IVD). (Courtesy of Dr. Neil A. Fenske, Tampa, FL.)

Figure 21–3. A earlier lesion represents lentigo maligna; if left alone, progression to lentigo maligna melanoma would occur.

have a horizontal growth phase. This is the predominant form of melanoma in blacks and occurs in all ethnic groups (Fig. 21–5; Plate IVD).

Late stage melanoma frequently metastasizes to the skin. These lesions are often pigmented and present as multiple cutaneous nodules.

Pathology

Superficial spreading melanoma is characterized by atypical melanocytes that in-

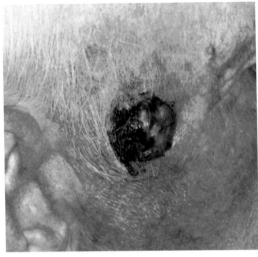

Figure 21–4. Nodular lesion of melanoma.

vade up into the epidermis from the basal cell layer. Lateral spread of the lesion is usually limited to 3 rete ridges on either side of the invasive component. Areas of dermal invasions are usually surrounded by a mononuclear cell infiltrate.

Lentigo maligna melanoma is characterized by extensive lateral spread of melanocytic atypia along the basal cell layer. There is usually evidence of solar degeneration in the upper dermis.

Nodular melanoma is dominated histologically by invasive vertical growth of atypical melanocytes. Adjacent epidermis is remarkably normal in appearance.

Acrolentiginous melanomas show features of both superficial spreading and lentigo maligna melanoma histologically. Lymphocytic infiltration may be striking.

Once the diagnosis of melanoma has been determined, Clark's level and Breslow's thickness must be ascertained, as these have major prognostic significance. Clark's levels are as follows: Level 1—tumor cells in the epidermis only; Level 2—tumor cells in the papillary dermis; Level 3—tumor cells filling and expanding the papillary dermis and at the interface of the papillary and reticular dermis; Level 4—tumor cells invading the reticular dermis; Level 5—tumor cells in subcutaneous fat. Breslow's thickness is the most accurate guide to prognosis, particularly owing to a large variation in prognosis within Clark's Level 3 (i.e., thick versus thin Level 3). Breslow's thickness is measured with the ocular micrometer on a microscope in millimeters from the granular layer in the epidermis to the deepest invasive part of the tumor. There is a direct inverse correlation between 5-year survival and tumor thickness.

Prognosis and Prevention

A 1985 estimate predicted that 18,000 Americans would develop melanoma in 1985 and that 6000 of those individuals would die from their disease. Current understanding regarding prognostic factors in melanoma was advanced by computer analysis of data from 1130 consecutive patients with melanoma from the New York University Melanoma Cooperative Group.

Lesion thickness, as discussed previously in relation to Clark's levels and Breslow's thickness, is the best correlate of 5-year survival in melanoma. Five-year survival in the aforementioned study was as follows: lesion less than 0.85 mm thick, 99%; 0.86–1.69 mm, 94%; 1.70–3.59 mm, 81%; and >3.60 mm, 49%. It is important to realize that 5-year survival is not the same as cure in melanoma.

Stage I disease (localized to skin only) has a prognosis related to lesion thickness. Patients with stage II disease (regional lymph nodes) and stage III disease (disseminated) have a poor prognosis.

Anatomic site and patient age are also prognostic variables. Melanomas in the head and neck, trunk, hands, and feet have the worst prognosis. Patients over age 50 have a worse prognosis than those under age 50. Other factors, such as ulceration, regression, and histologic presence of microscopic satellites, are less clearly associated with prognosis.

To reduce the incidence and increase the cure rate of melanoma, a concerted effort must be made to educate the public to reduce exposure to ultraviolet light and to teach health care providers and the public to identify thin, potentially curable, melanomas. The public and health care providers must also both be educated in the detection of precursors to melanoma (i.e., dysplastic nevi and congenital nevi). Catchy slogans such as "Slip, Slap, Slop" (slip on clothing, slap on a hat, slop on sunscreen) have been used to promote public awareness of the need for sun protection in melanoma prevention programs.

Treatment

Surgical excision is the critical form of therapy for primary melanoma. The classic 5-cm margin of excision was arbitrary and has been challenged. Lesions less than 1 mm thick are currently treated by local excision, and thicker lesions are excised with a 3-cm margin and grafting at many centers. Because the type of therapy is so dependent on accurate histologic assessment, complete local surgical excision is recommended for diagnosis.

The issue of prophylactic lymph node dissection is also a source of controversy. The proponents of this approach argue that 5–50% of patients who have a prophylactic lymph node dissection have nodal involvement. Opponents point to the morbidity of the procedure and to the role that normal nodes may have in immune surveillance. There is a tendency in the United States to perform lymph node dissection in lesions of intermediate (0.76–3.99 mm) thickness, with the argument that thinner lesions probably have not affected the nodes and thicker ones may have spread beyond the nodes. Clinically enlarged lymph nodes are usually excised. A surgical approach to therapy is often beneficial even in advanced disease. Many examples of prolonged survival after surgical removal of isolated metatases have been reported.

In general, response rates of patients with advanced melanoma to single agent or combination chemotherapy is poor. DTIC (dacarbazine) and vindesine (a semisynthetic vinca alkaloid) have both been reported to give up to 25% response rates as single agents. These responses are, in general, short lived. Isolation perfusion, in which the artery supplying a limb affected by melanoma is perfused with a chemotherapeutic agent, is an adjuvant to surgery. Antiestrogen therapy has been used as a form of palliative hormonal therapy.

Melanoma is, in general, a radioresistant tumor. Lentigo maligna melanoma may be more sensitive, but in general radiation therapy is used to palliate painful bone metastases and can be used in conjunction with high dose corticosteroid therapy to treat cerebral metastases.

Melanoma is a tumor that can recur after a disease free interval of many years. Also, there have been many instances of dramatic spontaneous regressions. These factors and others have made melanoma a popular field for the use of immunotherapy. Bacille Cal-mette-Guérin (BCG) vaccine, transfer factor, interferon, and the recent use in animals of melanoma-associated materials have not been accompanied by impressive success heretofore in the treatment of melanoma.

CONGENITAL NEVI

A congenital nevus is a melanocytic ham-artoma that is present at birth. Many patients are confused and believe that most of their many acquired nevi are congenital. How-ever, most of those acquired nevi appeared between the ages of 2 and 30. Small congen-ital nevi (less than 1.5 cm) may be confused clinically with acquired nevi. Medium (1.5–20.0 cm) and large congenital nevi are larger and usually more hairy than acquired nevi. Histologically, congenital nevi are deeper and more infiltrative than acquired nevi.

Large congenital nevi (greater than 20 cm) may be associated with a 5–20% risk of melanoma over a patient's lifetime. Al-though there is controversy about the risk of melanoma in congenital nevi, most derma-tologists and pediatricians recommend the prophylactic excision of these lesions.

DYSPLASTIC NEVUS SYNDROME

Patients with multiple large nevi and mel-anomas and with strong family histories of melanoma have been reported since the early 1800s. The term familial dysplastic nevus syndrome has recently been applied

to these families. The frequency is not yet known, although estimates predict that more than 30,000 Americans have the syndrome. The syndrome may be inherited as an auto-somal dominant trait with reduced pene-trance.

Clinically, there are several features that distinguish dysplastic nevi (Fig. 21–6; Plate IVE) (Table 21–1). Unlike normal acquired nevi, several of these lesions may develop into melanomas in a single patient.

The histopathologic features of dysplastic nevi have been summarized as follows: nu-clear atypia (dysplasia) of melanocytes, der-mal lymphocytic host response, and lamellar fibroplasia. These histopathologic features are now being identified in individuals with clinically dysplastic nevi who do not come from families with a history of melanoma and do not have melanomas themselves. The true implications of nevi with these histo-pathologic features are not yet fully appre-ciated. In families with at least 2 blood relatives with melanoma, an individual with dysplastic nevi may have a 300-fold in-creased risk of developing melanoma. Pa-tients with dysplastic nevi must be followed by complete cutaneous examinations aided by serial photography. Lesions even mildly suspicious for melanoma must be excised. These patients should also have monthly self-examination, reduced sun exposure, twice yearly examination by a dermatologist, and examination of first degree relatives. Dysplastic nevi that occur sporadically have a lower risk for developing into melanoma than those that occur in individuals with at least 2 blood relatives with cutaneous mel-anoma.

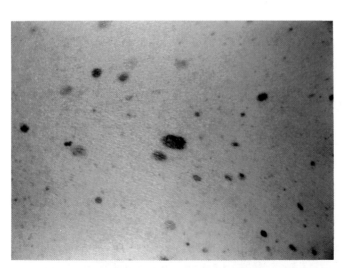

Figure 21–6. Multiple irregular pigmented lesions are seen in a patient with a familial dysplastic nevus syndrome (see also Plate IVE).

Table 21–1. CLINICAL FEATURES OF ACQUIRED NEVI AND DYSPLASTIC NEVI

	Usual Acquired Nevi	Dysplastic Nevi
Color	Uniformly tan or brown. Moles look alike.	Mixture of pink, tan, brown, and black. Variability of color from lesion to lesion.
Shape	Round with defined border.	Irregular.
Surface	Smooth. Flat to raised.	Smooth, scaly, rough, or pebbly.
Size	Usually about 5 mm or less.	>5 mm or even >10 mm.
Number	10–40 scattered over body.	Normal number to >100.
Location	Usually above waist and not on scalp, breasts, or buttocks.	Generalized, including scalp, breasts, and buttocks.

Modified from *About Dysplastic Nevi*, a publication from the National Cancer Institute, Bethesda, MD 20892.

SOME OTHER PIGMENTED LESIONS

To be more confident in evaluating pigmented lesions to diagnose melanoma, the non-dermatologist must become familiar with a host of other pigmented lesions. Some of these lesions are briefly mentioned.

Acquired Nevi. These lesions represent small hamartomas of rounded melanocytes called nevus cells. They develop during childhood and young adulthood. In general, these lesions are associated with a low risk for melanoma.

Mongolian Spot. These are the rounded blue-black macular lesions often seen at birth in black or Asian, and less commonly white, infants. The vast majority regress spontaneously. These benign lesions are probably related to a delay of migration of melanocytes into the epidermis.

Blue Nevi. These often solitary, blue lesions have a very low malignant potential. They are hamartomas of melanocytes in the dermis.

Nevi of Ota and Ito. These lesions resemble blue nevi histologically. The former lesion (Ota) occurs in the distribution of the trigeminal nerve. These are benign dermal melanocytoses.

Lentigo Simplex. These hyperpigmented macular lesions may occasionally resemble junctional nevi. They are benign. Histologically, there is an increase in basal melanocytes.

Lentigo Senilis (Solar Lentigo). These "liver spots" are larger than lentigo simplex lesions and occur in a photodistribution. Histologically, they are similar to lentigo simplex but show more elongation of the epidermal rete ridges.

Ephelides (Freckles). These small, tan macules occur on sun-exposed skin. They fade during the winter months and are benign.

Becker's Nevus. Adolescent males may experience the onset of a tan, hypertrichotic macular hamartoma on the shoulder. Histologically, the rete ridges are elongated and there are increased melanocytes in the basal layer. There is no malignant potential.

Café-au-lait Spots. These "coffee with cream" colored macules are benign. They may be a marker for neurofibromatosis.

Dermatofibroma. These dermal nodules are benign fibroblast tumors. There is often associated epidermal hyperpigmentation.

Other Lesions. Other lesions that must be considered in the differential diagnosis of melanoma are halo nevi, Spitz's nevi (once called benign juvenile melanoma), pigmented actinic keratoses, pigmented basal cell carcinomas, pigmented squamous cell carcinomas, seborrheic keratoses, pyogenic granulomas, angiokeratomas, venous lakes, and tinea nigra palmaris.

Suggested Readings

Breslow A: Thickness, cross-sectional areas and depth of invasion in the prognosis of cutaneous melanoma. Ann Surg *172*:902–908, 1970.

Clark WH Jr, From L, Bernardino EA, Mihm MC: The histogenesis and biologic behavior of primary human malignant melanomas of the skin. Cancer Res *29*:705–726, 1969.

Greene MH, Clark WH Jr, Tucker MA, et al: Acquired precursors of cutaneous malignant melanoma: The familial dysplastic nevus syndrome. N Engl J Med *312*:91–97, 1985.

Mackie RM, Young D: Human malignant melanoma. Int J Dermatol *23*:433–443, 1984.

Mihm MC, Clark WH Jr, From L: The clinical diagnosis, classification and histogenic concepts of the early stages of cutaneous malignant melanoma. N Engl J Med *284*:1078–1082, 1971.

Rigel DS, Friedman RJ (eds): Symposium on melanoma and pigmented lesions. Dermatol Clin *3*:(2):1–365, 1985.

IV

CUTANEOUS ENDOCRINOLOGY AND METABOLIC DISEASE

22

Diabetes Mellitus

JOSEPH L. JORIZZO

Diabetes mellitus is a common medical disease with sequelae that affect almost every organ system. The skin is no exception, with up to one third of patients with diabetes mellitus estimated to have various cutaneous associations. Although some cutaneous conditions seen in patients with diabetes are idiopathic, a number of associations are directly attributable to various aspects of the diabetes. Some examples are as follows: conditions related to microangiopathy (e.g., necrobiosis lipoidica diabeticorum, diabetic dermopathy), related to tendency toward infections (e.g., furunculosis, extensive dermatophytosis, and refractory candidiasis), related to vascular insufficiency (e.g., peripheral gangrene), related to neuropathy (e.g., neurotropic ulcers), related to altered metabolism (e.g., eruptive xanthomas), and related to complications of treatment (e.g., insulin lipoatrophy).

GENERAL DISEASE ASSOCIATIONS

Rubeosis

A characteristic chronic flushed appearance to the face and neck, and even of the extremities, in patients with diabetes mellitus has been termed rubeosis. There may be reduced vasoconstrictor tone in affected vessels, which allows for pooling of blood in the dermal venous plexus. Histopathologic assessment reveals no abnormality. Dramatic facial redness has been shown to occur in up to two thirds of hospitalized patients with diabetes mellitus. The condition is improved by better diabetic control and may be worsened by vasodilators, including alcohol and caffeine.

Diabetic Dermopathy

The presence of atrophic hyperpigmented patches, primarily on the lower legs, in patients with diabetes mellitus has been well appreciated since the mid-1960s. Although the condition occurs in a majority of elderly patients with diabetes mellitus, it is not specific for diabetes. Diabetic dermopathy may be due to diabetic microangiopathy, and it appears to correlate with the presence of retinopathy, neuropathy, and nephropathy, although all studies have not confirmed this correlation. The lesions are distinct from those of necrobiosis lipoidica diabeticorum in that they lack the distinctive collagen changes seen in the latter condition. Diabetic dermopathy appears to be an inflammatory condition that begins as a cluster of erythematous papules that coalesce. Histopathologic examination of the early lesions shows thickening of blood vessels with a perivascular lymphocytic infiltrate. Lesions may be induced by trauma. No treatment is required.

Diabetic Bullae

The association of tense bullae, primarily on the lower extremities, and diabetes mellitus has long been appreciated. The histopathology and pathogenesis of these bullae have been debated. Earlier studies suggested an intraepidermal location, whereas subsequent electron microscopic studies more strongly support a dermal-epidermal junction blister (i.e., lamina lucida) with the basal lamina on the floor of the blister. The blisters are non-scarring clinically. Reports of a reduced threshold for suction blister formation in insulin dependent diabetics support a theory of a primary weakness in dermal-epidermal adhesion. The description of a thickened, reduplicated basement membrane zone also supports this concept. Immunopathologic studies to rule out autoimmune bullous dermatoses are required and are negative in patients with diabetic bullae.

Necrobiosis Lipoidica Diabeticorum

Necrobiosis lipoidica diabeticorum is clinically characterized by well-circumscribed, yellow-brown patches with pronounced epidermal atrophy (Fig. 22–1; Plate IVF). The active border is raised and erythematous. Lesions may occur anywhere, but favor the legs. Ulceration is common (Fig. 22–2). Histopathologically, lesions progress from an early neutrophilic vascular reaction with progressive degeneration of collagen to a palisading granuloma with marked dermal sclerosis and destruction of adnexal structures.

Whereas about one third of patients with necrobiosis lipoidica diabeticorum have frank clinical diabetes mellitus, about one third have only glucose intolerance and one

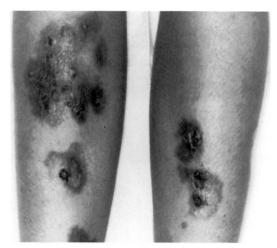

Figure 22–2. Ulcerating necrobiosis lipoidica diabeticorum.

third have totally normal glucose tolerance tests. Patients with necrobiosis lipoidica diabeticorum should be evaluated and followed for the development of diabetes mellitus.

Excellent control of the diabetes is unfortunately not associated with improvement in the necrobiosis lipoidica diabeticorum. Although the etiology of this cutaneous disorder remains unknown, debate has centered on an immune complex–mediated vasculitis with secondary collagen degeneration versus a cell-mediated immune reaction.

Intralesional corticosteroid therapy may be effective in preventing expansion of lesions. Aspirin and dipyridamole may be effective; however, they have not been convincingly demonstrated to be so in a double blind study. Maintenance therapy with pentoxifylline (Trental), a vasodilator, has also been anecdotally praised as a therapy for this condition. Semipermeable membrane dressings (e.g., OpSite, Vigilon, Duoderm) are helpful in treating painful ulcerating necrobiosis lipoidica diabeticorum. Surgical excision of lesions may be associated with their recurrence.

Disseminated Granuloma Annulare

Granuloma annulare is a condition that is clinically characterized by rings of dermal papules that have histologic similarities to the palisading granulomas of necrobiosis lipoidica diabeticorum. Although simple localized granuloma annulare is not associated with diabetes mellitus, there has been con-

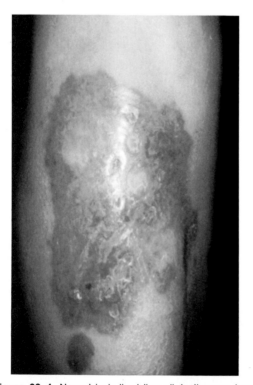

Figure 22–1. Necrobiosis lipoidica diabeticorum (see also Plate IVF).

troversy in several published series about the association of disseminated (generalized) granuloma annulare with diabetes mellitus. If provocative testing is used, many, or even most, patients with generalized granuloma annulare will be shown to have at least glucose intolerance.

Cutaneous Perforating Diseases

Kyrle's disease and perforating folliculitis are conditions characterized by hyperkeratotic papules and nodules in which histopathologic assessment confirms basophilic debris in the dermis with evidence of transepidermal elimination. Although these conditions are usually quite rare, their incidence in diabetic patients undergoing renal dialysis may approach 5–10%. Although the mechanism of this eruption in these patients is unknown, trauma to the dermis by scratching may be a large contributing factor. Treatment is primarily for the pruritus. Ultraviolet B light therapy (as described in Chapter 10, Generalized Pruritus) has been used. Topical tretinoin (Retin-A) has been used to treat the perforating lesions with some success.

Vitiligo

Vitiligo is an autoimmune disease characterized by macular patches of total depigmentation. Melanocytes are absent from affected patches. Vitiligo occurs with greater frequency than expected in maturity onset diabetics. In insulin dependent diabetics, the vitiligo may be associated with anti-insulin and other autoendocrine antibodies.

Scleredema and Sclerotic Skin Changes

Scleredema (formerly called scleredema adultorum of Buschke) is a distinctive clinical entity characterized by dramatic induration of the skin of the neck and upper back. Histologically, the induration can be shown to be caused by dermal deposition of glycosaminoglycans (e.g., hyaluronic acid). Although a reversible form of the disorder is associated with antecedent streptococcal infection, the diabetic type of scleredema is usually chronic. This phenomenon may be similar to the more prevalent waxy induration of the skin of the extremities seen in insulin dependent diabetics. These patients have limited joint mobility. The mechanism of glycosaminoglycan accumulation is unknown. The process does correlate with the duration of diabetes mellitus and with the presence of microvascular disease. There is no specific therapy.

Acanthosis Nigricans and Lipodystrophy

Acanthosis nigricans is characterized by a typical velvety epidermal thickening with hyperpigmentation primarily in the axillary, inguinal, and neck folds. Although severe acanthosis nigricans can be associated with advanced malignant tumors such as adenocarcinomas, it has been well associated with insulin resistance and diabetes mellitus. It has been postulated that many obese patients with what was previously labeled "pseudoacanthosis nigricans" may actually have insulin resistance. Insulin-like growth factors have been postulated to account for the epidermal proliferation. Insulin resistance can occur in a number of clinical settings. The type A abnormality occurs in women with acanthosis nigricans and insulin resistance that is due to insulin receptor abnormalities. These young, tall, hirsute women usually have polycystic ovaries. Type B subjects have acanthosis nigricans and insulin resistance owing to antibodies to insulin receptors. These patients are usually older women with arthralgias, alopecia areata, proteinuria, and antinuclear and anti-DNA antibodies.

A host of generalized and partial lipodystrophies are associated with insulin resistance and with acanthosis nigricans (Fig. 22–3). These syndromes may be congenital or acquired, familial or sporadic, generalized or complete. One form of acquired partial lipodystrophy is not associated with acanthosis nigricans. Women with this form have low serum C3 levels. A C3 nephritic factor is present in serum and produces nephrotic syndrome.

VASCULAR CHANGES

Diabetes mellitus is a disease with profound effects on both large and small blood

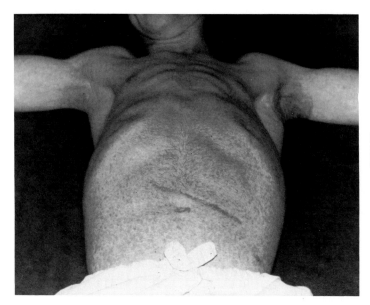

Figure 22–3. Acanthosis nigricans and lipodystrophy in this patient with diabetes.

vessels. Diabetic microangiopathy is characterized histologically by endothelial cell proliferation and basement membrane thickening affecting arterioles, venules, and capillaries. This small vessel vasculopathy may account for the acral erysipelas-like erythema described in elderly diabetics. This non-inflammatory, well-marginated erythema may evolve into superficial gangrene.

Dry gangrene in diabetics, especially of the feet, may be due to larger vessel obstruction. However, small vessel involvement usually plays an important adjunctive role. The diabetic patient with gangrene of a foot that has strong peripheral pulses is an all too familiar consequence of small vessel involvement in diabetes.

Large vessel atherosclerosis of leg vessels is greatly increased in incidence in the diabetic patient population.

With the large and small vessel peripheral vascular disease and the frequency of peripheral gangrene and leg ulcers, patients with diabetes mellitus require meticulous foot care. Tinea pedis must be aggressively treated. The diabetic patient may develop macerated toe webs as a result of secondary bacterial infection of tinea pedis. A soft tissue abscess followed by osteomyelitis followed by need for amputation may be the sequelae. The slightest cutaneous injury, especially when located acrally, must also be treated aggressively to prevent serious infection. Toenails must be trimmed straight across to prevent the development of in-

grown toenails, which can become infected. Intermittent claudication and particularly foot pain at rest should be evaluated in conjunction with a vascular surgeon. Treatment of vascular ulcers is with aggressive use of topical and at times systemic antibiotics. The semipermeable membrane dressings are also helpful in treating these ulcers. Unfortunately, amputation of an extremity may be required when vascular flow is inadequate and cannot be surgically restored or when osteomyelitis and other infection cannot be controlled.

INFECTIONS

There is some current debate as to whether well-controlled patients with diabetes mellitus have an increased risk of infections in general. Many investigators, however, do believe that cutaneous infections are more prevalent and more difficult to eradicate in the diabetic host. It is unclear whether diabetic patients may be more susceptible to infections or less well able to eradicate established infections. Local and serum hyperglycemia may have direct promoting effects and may modulate the inflammatory response of the host.

The poorly controlled diabetic patient is particularly at risk for developing severe acute mucocutaneous candidal infections. Oral thrush and angular cheilitis and candidal vaginitis and balanitis can become plaguing, recurrent problems. These mucosal infections often respond to topical therapy with nystatin or the imidazoles and to better diabetic control. Refractory disease may necessitate therapy with oral ketoconazole. Candidal paronychia is characterized by chronic nail matrix dystrophy (as manifested by horizontal ridging of the entire nail plate) and loss of the cuticle. Secondary acute staphylococcal paronychia may occur as a complication. Anticandidal topical therapy and attention to keeping the local area dry must be continued for several months for a normal nail plate to grow.

There is controversy as to whether patients with diabetes mellitus have an increased incidence of dermatophytosis. Dermatophytosis, especially of the feet, can have devastating consequences in the diabetic patient, as discussed previously, and should be treated aggressively with topical imidazoles whenever scaling of the toe webs recurs after an initially documented tinea pedis infection.

Erythrasma is an infection with *Corynebacterium minutissimum*, which is especially prevalent in intertriginous areas of obese diabetic patients. Wood's light examination confirms the diagnosis if a coral fluorescence (owing to a porphyrin produced by the organism) is seen. Topical therapy with erythromycin or clindamycin, as formulated to treat acne, is often adequate to eradicate the infection. Compresses, drying powders, and meticulous local hygiene as well as improved diabetic control reduce the risk of recurrence.

Impaired neutrophil function in poorly controlled diabetics may account for the increased difficulty in eradicating infections with *Staphylococcus aureus* and with beta-hemolytic streptococci. Impetigo, cellulitis, ecthyma and folliculitis, furuncles, and carbuncles may occur. The diagnosis in each instance is confirmed by clinical evaluation and by Gram's stain and culture of the organism. In addition to local compresses, systemic antibiotic therapy to cover both organisms is usually indicated. Erythromycin or, for more aggressive infections, a penicillinase resistant penicillin is often appropriate. Newer substitutes are available. Surgical incision and drainage are often required to treat furuncles and carbuncles.

Diabetes with ketosis that is debilitating puts the patient at risk for life-threatening mucormycosis (Fig. 22–4). Various fungi of

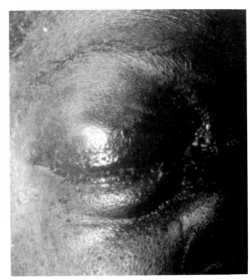

Figure 22–4. Swelling of the upper eyelid is present in this patient with mucormycosis.

the *Phycomycetes* group produce necrotizing infection, especially in the nasopharyngeal area, that may lead to cerebral involvement and death. Prompt intensive supportive care and intravenous therapy with amphotericin B are required.

NEUROCUTANEOUS COMPLICATIONS

Motor neuropathy in diabetic patients may predispose such individuals to ulceration, especially of a toe affected by various secondary deformities (Fig. 22–5). Autonomic neuropathy may be associated with localized anhidrosis. Peripheral sensory neuropathy may predispose a patient to the development of a neurotrophic ulcer. These ulcers are often particularly deep and refractory to therapy. Special custom-made footwear is an important part of preventive and ongoing management. Débridement of these ulcers by a surgeon is often required.

ASSOCIATIONS RELATED TO ALTERED METABOLISM

Eruptive Xanthomas

Patients with diabetes mellitus may occasionally develop a sudden eruption of yellow-red papules (Fig. 22–6; Plate IVG). These lesions histologically show infiltra-

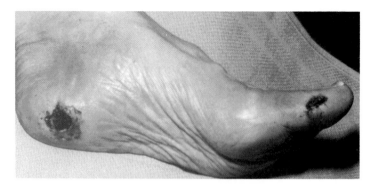

Figure 22–5. Diabetic neuropathy with neurotrophic ulcers.

tion of the dermis with macrophages filled with lipid, called foam cells. Eruptive xanthomas occur in the setting of grossly uncontrolled diabetes in a patient who has become extremely hypertriglyceridemic. The lesions resolve with reduction of the triglyceride levels through diabetic control.

Yellow Skin

Many patients with diabetes mellitus have elevated serum carotene levels, and up to 10% of diabetics have secondary yellowish discoloration of skin. The elevation of carotene may relate to its impaired hepatic con-

version. Treatment of this cosmetic problem involves reduction of dietary intake of foods high in carotene, such as oranges, yellow fruits and vegetables, egg yolks, and butter.

CUTANEOUS COMPLICATIONS OF ANTIDIABETIC THERAPY

Insulin allergy is more commonly seen with beef insulin than with pork insulin. There are documented examples of insulin allergy by the following mechanisms: immediate hypersensitivity reactions that cutaneously manifest as urticaria; serum sickness–like reactions, often characterized by

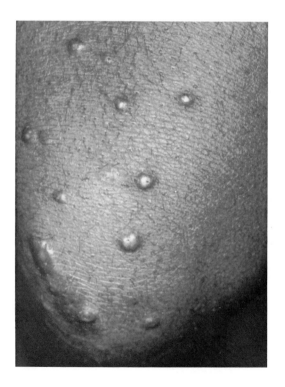

Figure 22–6. Multiple eruptive xanthomas in poorly controlled diabetic (see also Plate IV *G*).

vasculitic or by purpuric urticarial lesions; and delayed hypersensitivity reactions, which may present as localized nodules.

Insulin lipodystrophy is less common than insulin allergy. Atrophic patches develop at sites of injection, usually 1–2 years after starting insulin therapy. This reaction is not believed to be immunologically mediated, although the exact mechanism is unknown.

Oral Hypoglycemics

Cutaneous reactions that can occur with other drugs, such as macular erythemas, urticaria, and erythema multiforme, also occur with the oral hypoglycemic medications. In addition, the following drugs can produce special reactions: tolbutamide (photosensitivity), and chlorpropamide (disulfiram-alcohol–like reactions and photosensitivity).

Suggested Readings

Huntley AC: The cutaneous manifestation of diabetes mellitus. J Am Acad Dermatol 7:427–455, 1982.

Ober KP: Acanthosis nigricans and insulin resistance associated with hypothyroidism. Arch Dermatol 121:229–231, 1985.

Rosenbloom AL, Silverstein JH, Lezotte DC, et al: Limited joint mobility in childhood diabetes mellitus indicates increased risk for microvascular disease. N Engl J Med 305:191–194, 1981.

Sibbald RG, Schachter RK: The skin and diabetes mellitus. Int J Dermatol 23:567–584, 1984.

Stawiski MA, Voorhees JJ: Cutaneous signs of diabetes mellitus. Cutis 18:415–421, 1976.

Toonstra J: Bullosis diabeticorum: Report of a case with a review of the literature. J Am Acad Dermatol 13:799–805, 1985.

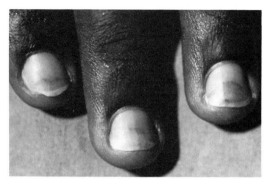

Figure 23–2. Onycholysis associated with thyrotoxicosis.

changes disappear after effective treatment of the disease. Alopecia areata, like vitiligo, occurs in an increased incidence in patients with hyperthyroidism, especially Graves' disease. Onycholysis and koilonychia (Plummer's nails) are the most common nail changes associated with hyperthyroidism (Fig. 23–2). The nails have also been described as being soft and friable. Nail changes occur in only 5% of patients with hyperthyroidism. There may be swelling of the neck as a result of gland enlargement, and the skin may be warmer in this area (Fig. 23–3). Gynecomastia may be seen in approximately 5% of males with hyperthyroidism.

Two additional but often very obvious clinical manifestations of hyperthyroidism owing to Graves' disease are ophthalmopathy and pre-tibial myxedema, including thy-roid acropachy. The ophthalmopathy varies from mild (exophthalmos) to severe (proptosis) and may include edema and vascular congestion of the sclerae (chemosis), as well as impairment of extraocular muscle function. Exophthalmos occurs in the majority of patients with Graves' disease, expecially in those with associated pre-tibial myxedema (Fig. 23–4). It may be the first sign of the hyperthyroid state and it may begin unilaterally, although it is usually bilateral. Common complaints of patients with exophthalmos are protruding eyes, easy tearing, photophobia, and the sensation of grit in the eyes. When severe, the exophthalmos can lead to the development of corneal ulcerations, diplopia, and panophthalmitis with loss of visual acuity. Infiltration of the retro-orbital tissues and extraocular muscles by plasma cells, lymphocytes, and mucopolysaccharide appears to produce the exophthalmos, but the precise cause is unknown. It is generally felt that the process is autoimmune and due to an exophthalmos-producing factor.

Pre-tibial myxedema is an uncommon manifestation of Graves' disease, occurring in 1–3% of cases. Pre-tibial myxedema was originally believed to be caused by LATS. The actual mechanism is not completely understood, but it appears that fibroblasts from the shins, the usual location for the disease, are specifically stimulated by some yet to be defined pre-tibial myxedema factor. It frequently begins weeks to years after

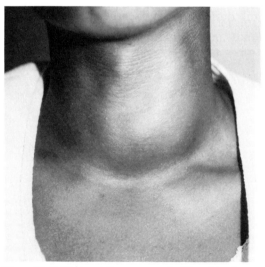

Figure 23–3. Neck swelling as a result of thyroid enlargement in a patient with thyrotoxicosis.

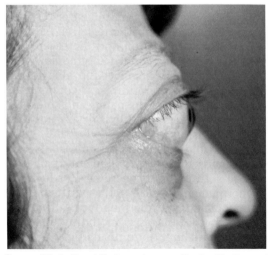

Figure 23–4. Exophthalmos in a patient with Graves' disease.

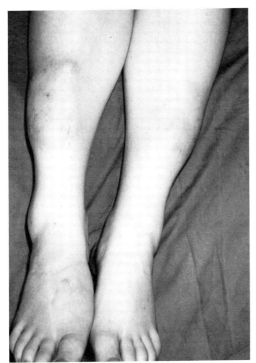

Figure 23–5. Early pretibial myxedema manifested as infiltrative plaques in a woman 7 years after thyroid-ectomy for Graves' disease.

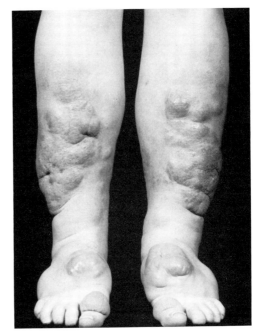

Figure 23–6. Same patient as in Figure 23–5, four years later, with extensive pretibial myxedema.

surgical or radioactive iodine therapy for thyrotoxicosis, and thus it often occurs in the absence of chemical hyperthyroidism. The disease begins with the gradual development of bilateral, asymmetric, raised firm plaques or nodules on the shins (Fig. 23–5). The plaques may be pink, violaceous, or flesh-colored and may have a waxy or translucent quality. Large, grotesque, and cumbersome lesions may develop in extreme cases, and the lesions may coalesce, progressing to a picture resembling elephantiasis verrucosa nostras (Fig. 23–6). The hands may be involved (Fig. 23–7) and, very rarely, there may be associated clubbing of the digits and diaphyseal proliferation of the periosteum in acral and distal long bones, a condition known as thyroid acropachy. The clinical course of pre-tibial myxedema is variable, but spontaneous remissions do occur. The disease persists for years in the majority of patients.

HYPOTHYROIDISM

Hypothyroidism (myxedema) results from a deficiency of thyroid hormone and, like

hyperthyroidism, is most common in females, especially those between the ages of 40 and 60. Over 95% of cases are classified as primary or idiopathic (usually acquired but, occasionally, congenital), and 5% are

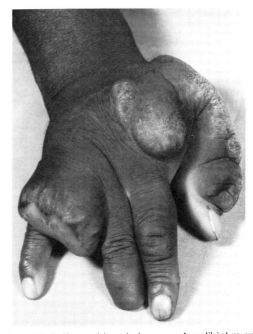

Figure 23–7. Unusual hand changes of pretibial myxedema in a male with severe exophthalmos associated with Graves' disease.

due to pituitary or hypothalamic dysfunction. The majority of cases of primary acquired hypothyroidism are due to Hashimoto's thyroiditis or idiopathic myxedema (believed to be an end-stage of Hashimoto's thyroiditis), and to thyroid destruction following ^{131}I therapy or subtotal thyroidectomy for hyperthyroidism. Only rarely does myxedema result from iodine deficiency (endemic goiter) or drugs (such as lithium carbonate, thiourea drugs, sulfonamides, etc.). The term thyroiditis includes such rare disorders as acute suppurative thyroiditis (usually as a result of bacteria or fungi), subacute granulomatous or lymphocytic thyroiditis, and chronic sclerosing thyroiditis of Riedel, but the large majority of cases are known as Hashimoto's, or chronic lymphocytic, thyroiditis. This latter disease is a leading cause of hypothyroidism, occurring in approximately 2% of affected women, although not all patients with Hashimoto's thyroiditis are symptomatic or require treatment. The disease is believed to be autoimmune, as many of the patients have serum autoantibodies that react with thyroglobulin or thyroid microsomes. Patients also show evidence of cell-mediated immunity directed against the thyroid. There also appears to be a strong genetic predisposition for Hashimoto's thyroiditis for individuals with the HLA-B8 and DR3 haplotype.

The clinical manifestations of hypothyroidism can be attributed to a deceleration of cellular metabolic processes and to myxedema, the accumulation of acid mucopolysaccharide in various organs, especially the skin, vocal cords, and oropharynx. When the deficiency occurs in infancy, as seen with thyroid dysgenesis, cretinism results. This disease, which is relatively uncommon except in goitrous regions of the world, usually becomes evident clinically by 6 weeks of age. Early symptoms of cretinism are often non-specific and include lethargy, feeding difficulty, constipation, persistent neonatal jaundice, and, in one third of patients, respiratory distress as a result of myxedema of the oropharynx and larynx. The classic manifestations of enlarged tongue, abdominal distention, umbilical hernia, puffy facies, dry hair and skin, and hypotonia are usually not evident before 3–4 months of life. Growth and mental retardation, the two most significant points for consideration in early diagnosis and therapy, develop even later. The cretinoid facies may suggest the diag-

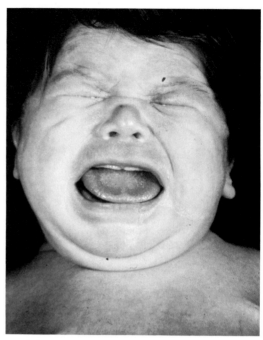

Figure 23–8. Typical facial features of cretinism.

nosis and include sparse hair, narrow forehead, puffy eyes and cheeks, depressed nasal bridge, pug nose, thick neck, and protruding tongue (Fig. 23–8).

Hypothyroidism in the older child and adult is characterized clinically by weakness and fatigue; constipation; modest weight gain with anorexia; cold intolerance with decreased sweating; a husky voice; muscle cramps; swelling of the hands, face, and extremities; and changes in the skin, hair, and nails (Table 23–2). This condition is

Table 23–2. DERMATOLOGICAL MANIFESTATIONS OF HYPOTHYROIDISM

Skin	Dry, rough or coarse; cold and pale; puffy, boggy, or edematous (myxedema)
	Yellow discoloration as a result of carotenemia
	Ichthyosis and palmoplantar hyperkeratosis
	Easy bruising (capillary fragility)
	Eruptive and tuberous xanthomas (rare)
Hair	Dull, coarse, and brittle
	Slow growth (increase in telogen, or resting, hairs)
	Alopecia (lateral third of eyebrows, rarely diffuse)
Nails	Thin, brittle, striated
	Slow growth
	Onycholysis (rare)

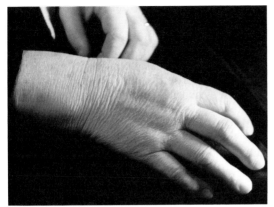

Figure 23–9. Puffy and pale hand in a woman with primary hypothyroidism.

also known as myxedema, owing to the increase of dermal acid mucopolysaccharides, primarily hyaluronic acid, which have a high affinity for water. The accumulation of mucin and water leads to edema or puffiness that is most obvious in the skin but that also occurs in internal organs. The tongue is often enlarged, and the voice is usually hoarse from edema of the oropharynx. The speech is often slowed in conjunction with slowing of body motion or activity in general. The skin is boggy but non-pitting, especially around the eyes, lips, and over acral parts (Figs. 23–9 and 23–10). In addition to being

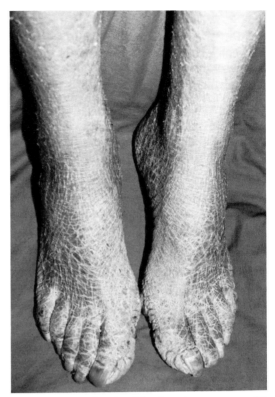

Figure 23–11. Ichthyosis of the legs in a woman with severe hypothyroidism.

puffy, the skin is often cold, pale, rough, and dry. There may be a yellowish discoloration owing to carotenemia, which results from decreased conversion of carotene to vitamin A in the liver. Ichthyosis and hyperkeratosis, especially of the soles, may be remarkable in severe cases (Fig. 23–11). Bruising, owing to increased capillary fragility, occurs in some patients, and tuberous and eruptive xanthomas may be seen rarely as a result of an abnormality in lipid metabolism.

The hair is dull, coarse, and brittle in hypothyroidism, and the growth rate is slowed with an increase in telogen, or resting, hairs. Alopecia may be diffuse, but, classically, there is a loss of the lateral third of the eyebrows. The nails grow slowly and may be thin, brittle, and striated. Onycholysis, which occurs more frequently with hyperthyroidism, has been reported in a few patients with myxedema.

Extracutaneous features of hypothyroidism are numerous and include pleural and pericardial effusion, a decrease in heart rate and cardiac output, a narrow pulse pressure,

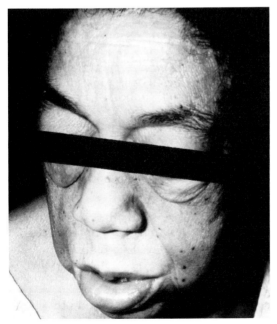

Figure 23–10. Edematous or puffy eyelids, swollen lower lip, and droopy facial appearance in a woman with myxedema.

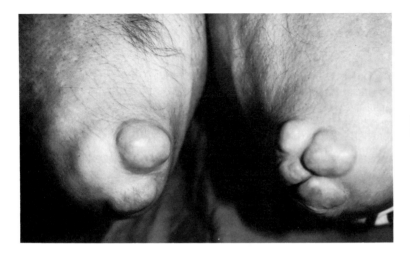

Figure 24–2. Tuberous xanthomas of the elbows.

knees, and buttocks. They are painless, and they frequently coalesce to form large, globular masses (Figs. 24–2 and 24–3). Their presence usually suggests an elevation of serum cholesterol, but they may also be seen with triglyceride elevation. Patients with tuberous and tendinous xanthomas have an extremely high incidence of atherosclerotic vascular disease.

Planar Xanthomas. Planar xanthomas are, by far, the most commonly encountered xanthomas. These yellow, soft, macular to barely palpable lesions occur in 3 forms: xanthelasmas, xanthoma striatum palmare, and diffuse plane xanthoma. Xanthelasmas occur around the eyelids, especially on the medial canthal skin (Fig. 24–4; Plate V*A*). At least 50% of patients with xanthelasmas

will have normal plasma lipid levels. When the lipids are abnormal, the cholesterol level is usually elevated. This is especially true of younger patients. An associated finding in many of these patients is corneal arcus (Fig. 24–5), which, in the older population, may occur in the setting of normal lipids as well. The flat, yellow to orange lesions in the palmar creases occur only in patients with abnormal serum lipids, including elevation of cholesterol and triglyceride. Patients with diffuse plane xanthomas, especially noted on the neck, face, upper trunk and arms, may or may not have normal lipid levels, but they frequently have been found to have paraproteinemia, including multiple myeloma.

Eruptive Xanthomas. Eruptive xanthomas

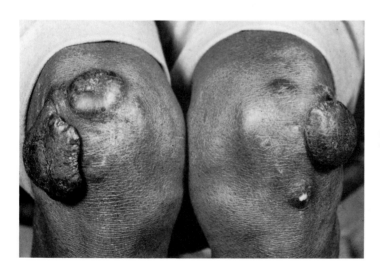

Figure 24–3. Tuberous xanthomas over the knees.

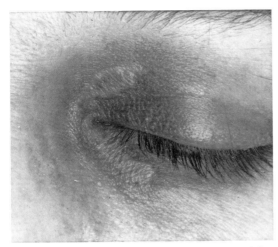

Figure 24–4. Planar xanthomas (xanthelasmas of the eyelids) (see also Plate VA).

appear suddenly, usually in crops, and, unlike the other forms of xanthomas, they may be pruritic. Eruptive xanthomas are characterized by their yellow color, small size (1–4 mm in diameter), palpability, and the erythematous halo around their base. They occur most commonly over pressure points and extensor surfaces of the arms, legs, and buttocks (Figs. 24–6 and 24–7). Rarely, they may be diffusely scattered over the trunk or on the mucous membranes. They occur exclusively in association with elevated triglycerides. A frequent circumstance is their occurrence with hypertriglyceridemia secondary to uncontrolled diabetes mellitus.

Therapy of the diabetes mellitus can lead to resolution of the xanthomas.

DISORDERS OF LIPID METABOLISM

The disorders of lipid metabolism with cutaneous manifestations are primarily the hyperlipoproteinemias (hyperlipidemias), and they have been defined as primary (genetic) or secondary to other diseases (Tables 24–1 and 24–2). At times, it is very difficult to differentiate primary from secondary hyperlipoproteinemias because of similar clinical and laboratory findings. Distinguishing between these 2 categories is important for therapeutic reasons. Xanthomas represent the major cutaneous change of lipid disease and are especially important because their recognition can lead to the investigation, diagnosis, and treatment of the various hyperlipidemias. This is significant because abnormalities of plasma lipoproteins can result in the predisposition to premature coronary artery disease, pancreatitis, and neurologic disease. Various classification schemas have been proposed, based primarily on the genetics of the syndromes and the lipoprotein patterns (Table 24–1). However, numerous synonyms have been used to describe the different disorders, making precise classification difficult. The diagnosis is based on the history (including the family history); presence, type, and distribution of xanthomas; fasting levels of serum triglyc-

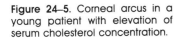

Figure 24–5. Corneal arcus in a young patient with elevation of serum cholesterol concentration.

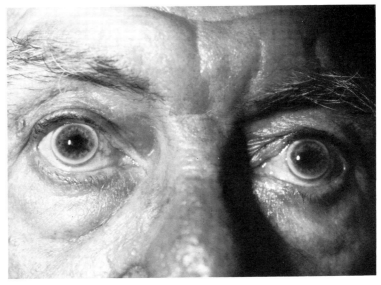

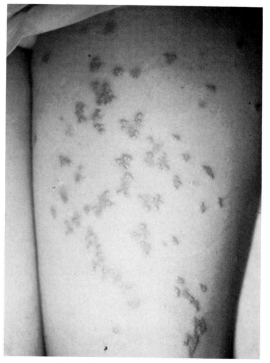

Figure 24-6. Eruptive xanthomas.

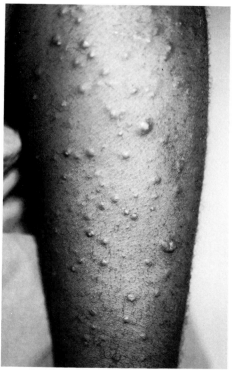

Figure 24-7. A cluster of eruptive xanthomas on the anterior thigh.

eride and cholesterol; and the "refrigerator test." In this test, plasma or whole blood is stored in the refrigerator overnight. If a creamy layer forms over clear plasma beneath, chylomicrons are present (Fig. 24–8). The entire plasma is turbid when there is a high concentration of VLDL or IDL* (Fig. 24–9). Clear plasma rules out disorders of chylomicrons, VLDLs, and IDLs. Pathophys-

*Abbreviations: VLDL = very-low-density lipoprotein; LDL = low-density lipoprotein; IDL = intermediate-density or remnant lipoprotein.

iologically, the disorders are due to increased production or deficient removal of the various lipoproteins (chylomicrons, VLDL, LDL, and IDL). The estimated frequency of occurrence of the primary hyperlipidemias ranges from relatively common (1:100 for type III familial dysbetalipoproteinemia) to extremely rare (1:1,000,000 for the autosomal recessive apoprotein CII deficiency).

Hyperchylomicronemia. Two genetically determined defects of triglyceride removal lead to hypertriglyceridemia and hyperchy-

Table 24–1. PRIMARY HYPERLIPOPROTEINEMIAS

Elevated Lipoprotein Class	Synonyms and Primary Disorders
Chylomicrons	Type I, familial lipoprotein lipase deficiency, familial apoprotein C-II deficiency
Chylomicrons and VLDLs*	Type V, familial combined hyperlipidemia
VLDLs	Type IV, endogenous familial hypertriglyceridemia
LDLs†	Type II-a, familial hypercholesterolemia, familial combined hyperlipidemia
LDLs and VLDLs	Type II-b, familial multiple lipoprotein–type hyperlipidemia, combined hyperlipidemia
IDLs‡	Type III, remnant hyperlipidemia, familial dysbetalipoproteinemia

*VLDL = very-low-density lipoprotein
†LDL = low-density lipoprotein
‡IDL = intermediate-density or remnant lipoprotein

Table 24–2. SECONDARY HYPERLIPOPROTEINEMIAS

Cholestatic liver disease
Diabetes mellitus
Drugs: estrogens, isotretinoin, corticosteroids
Hypothyroidism
Pancreatitis
Paraproteinemia: multiple myeloma, Waldenström's
   macroglobulinemia, cryoglobulinemia, lymphoma
Renal disease: nephrotic syndrome and uremia

lomicronemia, and they are the autosomal recessive lipoprotein lipase deficiency (also known as type I or Bürger-Grütz disease) and familial apoprotein CII deficiency. However, the vast majority of patients with high levels of chylomicrons and triglycerides have acquired or secondary forms of hyperlipidemia. Pancreatitis and bouts of abdominal pain are common in severe type I disease, often beginning in early childhood. In addition, the children develop hepatosplenomegaly, eruptive xanthomas, and lipemia retinalis, especially when the triglyceride levels exceed 4000 mg per dl. Premature

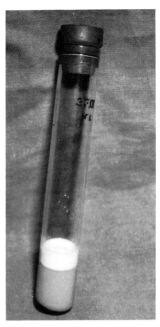

Figure 24–9. "Refrigerator test" on whole blood revealing that the entire plasma is turbid, indicating an elevation of VLDL or IDL.

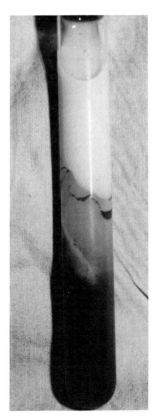

Figure 24–8. "Refrigerator test" on whole blood revealing a creamy layer over clear plasma, indicating the presence of chylomicrons.

atherosclerotic vascular disease does not occur in type I disease. Patients with absence of lipoprotein lipase activator (apoprotein CII) first develop symptoms after adolescence. Patients with type V disease have elevation of both chylomicrons and VLDLs, so-called familial combined hyperlipidemia. Symptoms usually begin in adult life, and, as is true for many patients with primary hyperlipidemia, secondary factors, such as alcohol intake, obesity, associated renal disease, or diabetes mellitus, are frequently involved in the exacerbation of the disease.

Increased VLDLs. Endogenous familial hypertriglyceridemia (type IV disease) results primarily from accelerated production of VLDL in the liver. This autosomal dominant disorder is common. Symptoms first appear in adulthood, frequently being precipitated by the ingestion of large amounts of carbohydrate or alcohol. Not uncommonly, patients with this disorder are obese, diabetic, and hyperuricemic. In addition, these patients appear to have an increased risk of coronary heart disease. Eruptive xanthomas are common, and xanthoma striatum palmares can be seen as well. As mentioned previously, VLDLs may be elevated along with chylomicrons in type V disease. Patients with elevation of both VLDL and LDL have type II-b disease. In type II-b disease, some patients have elevated triglyceride in addition to higher cholesterol levels, but the VLDL level is insufficient to produce milky or turbid plasma as determined by the "refrigerator test."

Increased LDLs. LDLs (beta-lipoproteins) alone are elevated in the plasma in type II-a disease (familial hypercholesterolemia) and are elevated with VLDLs in type II-b disease. There are several different phenotypic genetic conditions of familial hypercholesterolemia, and the severity of the clinical manifestations varies considerably. Xanthomas, especially the tendinous and tuberous types, are very prominent, and there is a significant increase in the incidence of coronary heart disease, often beginning in early adulthood.

Elevated IDLs. Patients with high levels of cholesterol and triglyceride, carried in remnant lipoproteins (IDLs), have type III or broad-beta disease (familial dysbetalipoproteinemia). Type III hyperlipoproteinemia is inherited as an autosomal dominant disease, although similar remnant lipoprotein accumulation in the plasma has been seen as a secondary phenomenon in hypothyroidism. The disorder appears to be related to a defect in the removal of these remnants from the circulation. Clinically, patients with broad-beta disease are usually obese, glucose intolerant, and have xanthomas (tuberous in 80%, xanthoma striatum palmare in 64%, and tendinous in 25%), as well as peripheral and coronary vascular disease.

Secondary Hyperlipoproteinemias. The diagnosis of a specific type of hyperlipoproteinemia cannot be made on the basis of the clinical type of xanthoma found in a patient because these same xanthomas occur in various lipid disorders, primary or secondary. Secondary or acquired hyperlipidemias result from disease in various organs (liver, kidney, thyroid, pancreas, etc.) and are due to a disturbance in the metabolism of triglycerides and cholesterol. In fact, the majority of cases of xanthomatosis are secondary rather than the primary familial disorders listed in Table 24–1. Eruptive xanthomas may appear when hypertriglyceridemia develops in patients with diabetes mellitus that is uncontrolled, as well as in patients with the nephrotic syndrome. Tuberous and eruptive xanthomas can be seen in patients with hypothyroidism, but only rarely. Infants with biliary atresia and adults with biliary cirrhosis may develop any of

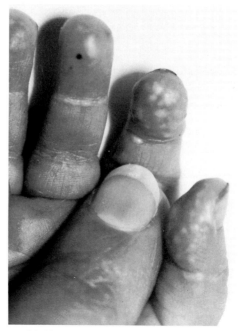

Figure 24–10. Xanthomas on the fingers of an infant with biliary atresia.

the 4 types of xanthomas (Fig. 24–10). Diffuse plane xanthomas are associated primarily with malignancies of the reticuloendothelial system, including multiple myeloma and lymphoma, as well as with various other paraproteinemias.

Normolipemic Xanthomatosis (see also Chapter 18). Xanthomas may occur in disorders with histiocytic proliferation and secondary uptake of fat rather than with an error of lipid metabolism. Blood lipid levels are normal in these disorders, which include nevoxanthoendothelioma, xanthoma

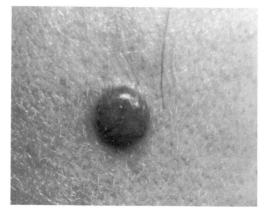

Figure 24–11. Nevoxanthoendothelioma (juvenile xanthogranuloma) on the face of a young woman.

disseminatum, and cerebrotendinous xanthomatosis, among others. This group of diseases is collectively known as the normolipemic xanthomatoses. Nevoxanthoendothelioma, also known as juvenile xanthogranuloma, is a benign proliferation of lipid laden histiocytes occurring primarily in infancy and usually characterized by one or a few nodules that are yellow-brown in color and that vary in size from a few millimeters up to several centimeters in diameter (Fig. 24–11). They are especially common on the scalp, face, or extensor extremities, and, although they usually disappear spontaneously in several months, they may persist for many years. Involvement of visceral organs is rare, but the lesions may occur in the iris and ciliary body of the eye, as well as in the lung, liver, heart, and oropharynx. Xanthoma disseminatum is a very rare and unusual disease characterized by xanthomatous nodules in the axillae, the antecubital and popliteal fossae, and the intertriginous areas, as well as in the oropharynx and the upper respiratory tract. The disorder is benign, self-limited, and has a good prognosis. Approximately twenty cases of familial cerebrotendinous xanthomatosis have been described. Deposition of cholestanol and cholesterol in all tissues of the body begins in childhood. Xanthomas in the Achilles tendon are characteristic, but the major damage results from sterol deposition in the brain and lungs.

Hypolipoproteinemias. Abnormally low levels of cholesterol and triglyceride may be observed in patients with malabsorption, parenchymal liver disease, or cachexia, but primary or familial cases of hypolipoproteinemia are extremely rare and include such diseases as Tangier disease (alpha-lipoprotein deficiency), hypo- or abetalipoproteinemia, and lecithin-cholesterol acyltransferase deficiency. Cutaneous lesions are not specific in these disorders, but patients with Tangier disease have very characteristic yellow-orange tonsils.

THERAPY

The therapy of disorders of lipid metabolism depends on the underlying lipoprotein abnormality and is directed toward returning the lipids to normal levels. There is no effective therapy for the normo- or hypolipemic conditions, and dietary manipulation and drugs are the mainstays of therapy for primary hyperlipidemias. An attempt should be made to find some underlying secondary disease causing the hyperlipidemia. Therapy can be very effective in clearing the xanthomas, but the goal is to attempt to reverse or slow the associated atherosclerotic process, the most serious complication of lipid disorders. Full discussion of therapy is beyond the scope of this chapter.

Suggested Readings

Frederickson DS, Lees RS: A system for phenotyping hyperlipoproteinemia. Circulation 31:321–327, 1965.

Havel RJ: Approach to the patient with hyperlipidemia. Med Clin North Am 66:319–333, 1982.

Kottke BA, Zinsmeister AR, Holmes DR Jr, et al: Apolipoproteins and coronary artery disease. Mayo Clinic Proc 61:313–320, 1986.

Love JR, Dubin HV: Xanthomas and lipoproteins. Cutis 21:801–805, 1978.

Parker F: Xanthomas and hyperlipidemias. J Am Acad Dermatol 13:1–30, 1985.

Schafer EJ, Levy RI: Pathogenesis and management of lipoprotein disorders. New Engl J Med 312:1301–1310, 1985.

25

Androgen-Related Disorders

JOSEPH L. JORIZZO

A consideration of the dermatological signs of internal diseases that includes a discussion of endocrinology must include the role of androgens in hirsutism, acne, and androgenic alopecia. Although these conditions most frequently occur as cutaneous diseases in isolation, they can be a feature of androgen excess. A complete review of diseases producing androgen excess is more appropriate to an endocrinology textbook. Conditions that must be considered in the female patient with androgen excess include polycystic ovary, ovarian hyperthecosis, ovarian androgen producing tumor and other ovarian syndromes, virilizing adrenal hyperplasia, Cushing's syndrome, adrenal androgen producing tumor, and hyperprolactinemia.

HIRSUTISM

A practical clinical definition of hirsutism is an excess of terminal hair in a pattern not normal in the female. This may be a significant psychosocial problem to the patient, owing to the cosmetic implications of hirsutism. The physical finding of hirsutism can be a sign of underlying systemic disease that should often warrant a complete history, physical examination, and appropriate laboratory evaluation by the patient's physician.

Increased terminal hair usually develops at the following sites in a female with hirsutism: upper lip, cheeks, chin, back, thighs, arms, central chest, and suprapubic area. It should be emphasized that normal women have hair over most of their bodies and that between one quarter and one third of normal young women may have some facial, chest, or suprapubic hair.

Before puberty, most of the body is covered with the fine vellus hair ("peach fuzz"). Terminal hairs are the coarse, longer, pigmented hair such as those that occur on the scalp and eyebrows. Sex hormone–responsive hair follicles account for the androgen-promoted conversion of vellus hair into terminal hair at certain sites.

Additional important definitions when hirsutism is reviewed are hypertrichosis and virilism. Hypertrichosis refers to an increase in hair growth on all body areas, not just in androgen dependent areas. Virilism is the full syndrome of masculinization, which includes hirsutism but which also includes deepening voice, increase in muscle mass, breast involution, acne, androgenic alopecia, and enlargement of the clitoris.

Pathogenesis

Although hirsutism may be due to normal variation or to familial tendency, the development of more sensitive assay techniques has revealed abnormalities of androgen metabolism in these patients. In women, the ovary and adrenal glands are the sources of androgen. As in men, peripheral conversion of androgens to more active forms occurs. Adrenal androgens include androstenedione, testosterone, dehydroepiandrosterone

(DHEA), and DHEA sulfate. Androstenedione and the more potent androgen testosterone are produced by the ovary. Androstenedione is converted peripherally to testosterone. Dihydrotestosterone, a reduction product of testosterone that is produced from peripheral conversion, is the androgen that principally affects the pilosebaceous unit. Another androgen produced peripherally is androstanediol. Sex hormone–binding globulin (SHBG) is increased by estrogens, and its level in serum is inversely related to testosterone's metabolic clearance rate. Free (unbound ≈1% total) testosterone levels are the best correlates of androgen excess. Androgen synthesis in both ovaries and adrenals is stimulated by luteinizing hormone (LH) and adrenocorticotropic hormone (ACTH). There is little negative feedback from androgens to these pituitary hormones.

Hirsute women often have an elevated production rate of testosterone and an increased metabolic clearance rate of testosterone with decreased SHBG. Virtually all hirsute women therefore have elevated free testosterone levels, but less than half have elevated total testosterone levels. Whether the source of increased testosterone is ovarian or adrenal is the cause of much debate. End organ effects such as the sensitivity of individual hair follicles to androgens are very important in the development of hirsutism. Racial and genetic factors probably have their influence at this level. Androgen dependent follicles have higher levels of 5-alpha-reductase, the enzyme that converts testosterone to dihydroxytestosterone. Levels of DHEA or DHEA sulfate and androstenedione levels may be elevated in adrenal masculinizing diseases. Ovarian disease is characterized by elevated free testosterone levels (total testosterone may be normal) and by elevated androstenedione levels.

Patient Evaluation

The evaluation of the patient with hirsutism is summarized in Table 25–1. The physician must exclude a neoplastic cause of hirsutism as a main goal of evaluation of the hirsute patient. A history of gradual onset and the absence of masculinization are findings against a neoplastic origin for hirsutism. Women with hirsutism who do not have

Table 25–1. SCREENING OF THE PATIENT WITH HIRSUTISM

A. History and physical examination
   If there is a clinical impression of acromegaly, Cushing's syndrome, or major menstrual disturbance, the patient should be referred to an endocrinologist or a gynecologic endocrinologist.
B. Laboratory screening for malignancy
   1. Plasma testosterone
      If >2.0 mg/ml, refer patient for further evaluation with suppressive tests and imaging procedures to exclude tumor (usually gonadal).
   2. Dehydroepiandrosterone sulfate
      If >9000 mg/ml, refer patient as for elevated plasma testosterone (tumor in this instance, however, is usually adrenal).

regular menstrual periods should be referred to a gynecologic endocrinologist for evaluation. Careful assessment for signs of Cushing's syndrome is important. The patient's medications should be checked for drugs associated with hirsutism (e.g., phenytoin, diazoxide, minoxidil, progestins, corticosteroids, and danazol).

Laboratory evaluation should include a check of plasma free testosterone and DHEA levels. If these are significantly elevated (testosterone greater than 2.0 mg/ml, DHEA sulfate greater than 9,000 mg/ml), a tumor is likely. Further endocrinologic evaluation of patients with these high levels is mandatory. Other laboratory assessment is guided by the history and physical examination. Only when screening history and physical examination are negative for masculinization, Cushing's syndrome, and acromegaly and when screening laboratory evaluation does not suggest a tumor can a diagnosis of nonendocrine hirsutism be considered.

Treatment

The importance of cosmetic therapy should not be minimized in the treatment of hirsutism. Options include shaving (which does not make hair more coarse or faster growing), plucking or waxing (these methods are effective temporarily, but are painful), bleaching, depilatory creams (which may cause irritation), and electrolysis (which is expensive and may produce mild scarring).

In theory, one could use low doses of systemic corticosteroids to produce feedback suppression of adrenal androgen and systemic oral contraceptive therapy to suppress ovarian androgens. In most cases, one therapy or the other is sufficient. A low progestin oral contraceptive can be prescribed with appropriate follow-up, or low dose dexamethasone can be prescribed. Serum free testosterone levels can be monitored during therapy, which should be for at least 1 year.

Peripheral androgen blockers round out the therapeutic options. Cyproterone acetate has been used in Europe as an antiandrogen that blocks both androgen synthesis and peripheral androgen receptors. It is used in association with oral contraceptives in female patients. Spironolactone and cimetidine have been used in the United States for this purpose. Spironolactone is an antagonist of peripheral androgen receptors. The patient must be treated for at least 6 months to determine if therapy is effective. Good double-blind studies are not yet available using these treatments.

ACNE VULGARIS

Although acne is essentially a normal variant rather than a disease during the adolescent period, it can cause significant cosmetic and psychosocial morbidity. Acne, like hirsutism, can be a feature of virilization.

Pathogenesis

The most important factor in the pathogenesis of acne is sebum production. The sebaceous glands are stimulated by androgens from the testes in males and from the adrenal glands and ovaries in females. Differential peripheral conversion of testosterone to dihydrotestosterone at the sebaceous gland level explains why glands in the "sebaceous areas" (e.g., face, upper back, chest, etc.) enlarge dramatically at puberty, whereas those in other areas (e.g., the dorsum of the hand) do not. Endocrine factors reviewed for hirsutism are relevant for women with acne.

Other factors in the pathogenesis of acne include obstruction of the pilosebaceous ducts and colonization of the follicular ducts with *Propionibacterium acnes*. In areas with large sebaceous glands, great quantities of sebum are obstructed in their outflow from the sebaceous duct. Local bacteria make sebum more irritating, they are directly chemotactic, and they activate complement via the alternative pathway. This combination of events is postulated to produce both the noninflammatory, obstructive (i.e., comedonal) lesions of acne and the inflammatory papules, pustules, and cysts.

Clinical Aspects and Patient Evaluation

The clinical lesions of acne consist of noninflammatory lesions, called comedones, and of the following inflammatory lesions: papules, pustules, and cysts. These lesions are located primarily on the face, chest, and back.

Acne can be a feature of the same types of endocrine disorders discussed with hirsutism (Fig. 25–1). Unless other features of adrenal, ovarian, or other endocrine dysfunction are present, the mere presence of acne lesions alone should not prompt an endocrinologic evaluation.

There is great debate about the androgen status of clinically normal women with acne. Some investigators have clearly shown no elevation of plasma free testosterone levels or of DHEA sulfate concentrations in women with acne. Other investigators suggest that this may not be true. Studies suggest an increase in plasma 3-alpha-androstanediol glucuronide concentrations in women with acne compared with age-matched controls.

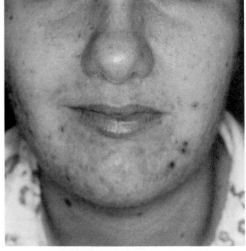

Figure 25–1. Polycystic ovarian disease is present in this individual with acne and slight amount of hirsutism. (Courtesy of Dr. Joseph Chanda, Melbourne, FL.)

Therapy

Traditional therapies for acne include topical tretinoin for comedonal lesions; and topical and systemic antibiotics, topical benzoyl peroxide, and oral isotretinoin for inflammatory lesions. Investigators who believe that increased androgens at a serum or target level relate to the pathogenesis of acne advocate suppressive therapy, such as with low dose oral dexamethasone. Suppressive therapy with corticosteroids is not a common practice among dermatologists.

ANDROGENIC ALOPECIA

Both men and women may experience the not uncommon, non-scarring, patterned form of alopecia known as androgenic alopecia (or male-pattern baldness). In this condition, terminal hair follicles are converted into vellus-like follicles ("peach fuzz"). The process occurs gradually over a number of years, with affected follicles on the fronto-temporal and vertex areas producing progressively finer, shorter hair.

Adequate androgen levels and a genetic predisposition are required for the process of androgenic alopecia to occur. Eunuchs and males castrated before puberty do not develop baldness even if there exists a strong genetic predisposition. The exact mechanism of the alopecia is unknown. It appears that end organ androgen responsiveness is very important, because hair transplanted from unaffected sites to affected sites does not convert to vellus hair.

The diagnosis is based on clinical features supported by a family history and on the exclusion of other forms of alopecia by careful scalp examination. An evaluation for endocrinologic abnormalities is not indicated unless there are signs of significant acne, hirsutism, and virilization in a female patient or other signs of endocrine disease in a male.

There is no current effective therapy for androgenic alopecia. Topical agents such as the antihypertensive agent minoxidil have caused much excitement, but do not appear to offer a miracle cure for this problem. Wigs, creative hairstyling, and hair transplantation are useful cosmetic solutions for selected patients.

Suggested Readings

Braithwaite SS, Jabamoni R: Hirsutism. Arch Dermatol 119:279–284, 1983.

Cunliffe WJ: Acne vulgaris: Pathogenesis and treatment. Br Med J 1:1394–1396, 1980.

DeVillez RL: Topical minoxidil therapy in hereditary androgenic alopecia. Arch Dermatol 121:197–202, 1985.

Kligman AM: An overview of acne. J Invest Dermatol 62:268–287, 1974.

Kvedar JC, Gibson M, Krusinski PA: Hirsutism: Evaluation and treatment. J Am Acad Dermatol 12:215–225, 1985.

Rittmaster RS, Loriaux DL: Hirsutism. Ann Intern Med 106:95–107, 1987.

26

Adrenal Disease and Other Endocrine Disorders

KENNETH E. GREER

ADRENAL DISEASES WITH CUTANEOUS MANIFESTATIONS

The adrenal glands are composed of two types of tissues, an outer, fatty layer (adrenal cortex) and an inner medulla (adrenal medulla). Hormones secreted from the cortex (steroids) are essential for life and provide resistance to various stresses and maintain the activity of a number of enzyme systems. They can be divided into 3 principal groups: glucocorticoids, mineralocorticoids, and sex steroids. The major disorders of the adrenal cortex arise from deficiency or excess of the various hormones. Cutaneous changes are most obvious in Cushing's syndrome, a disorder that is due to chronic excess of glucocorticoids; in various virilizing disorders, owing to excess adrenal androgen; and in Addison's disease, which results from a deficiency of all 3 classes of steroid hormones. The hormones from the medulla are the catecholamines, especially norepinephrine and epinephrine, the latter constituting 75% of the total. These hormones, along with dopamine, are vital for the function of the sympathetic nervous system. The major disease of the adrenal medulla with skin manifestations is pheochromocytoma.

Cushing's Syndrome

In 1932, Harvey Cushing described the disorder of glucocorticoid excess based on 12 patients with pituitary tumors. Today the most common cause of the disorder (also known as hypercortisolism) is iatrogenic Cushing's disease as a result of the widespread systemic use of glucocorticoids, such as prednisone and dexamethasone. Endogenous glucocorticoid excess can result from a pituitary or extrapituitary tumor secreting excess adrenocorticotropic hormone (ACTH) or from adrenal tumors, which may be benign or malignant. Over two thirds of all cases of endogenous hypercortisolism are due to an adenoma or microadenoma of chromophobe or basophile cells of the pituitary gland, and only 15–20% are from adrenal tumors. The adrenal tumors may be bilateral, although 90% are unilateral. The majority are malignant and are very difficult to treat. Finally, more than 25 different types of extrapituitary tumors causing ectopic Cushing's syndrome have been described, but small cell carcinoma of the lung is by far the most common.

The 3 most common clinical features of Cushing's syndrome are obesity, hypertension, and a plethoric, or red, face. The habitus is very characteristic and is largely due to the fact that there is redistribution of fat, so that the cheeks are full and round (moon facies), the abdomen is protuberant, and the limbs are often spindly; also, there are prominent fat deposits over the upper back (buffalo hump) and supraclavicular areas (Figs. 26–1 to 26–3). Hypertension results from cortisol excess, increasing the sensitivity of

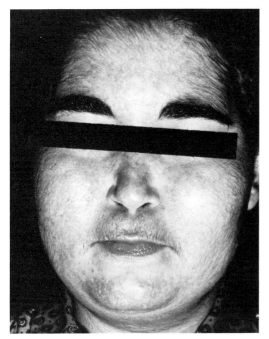

Figure 26–1. Round facies, telangiectasias, and hirsutism in a woman with Cushing's disease.

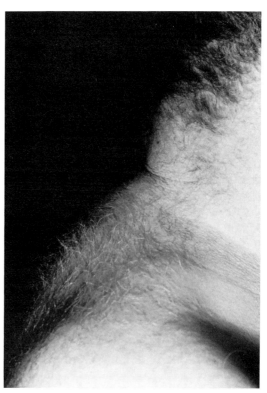

Figure 26–3. "Buffalo hump" and hypertrichosis in a male with Cushing's syndrome.

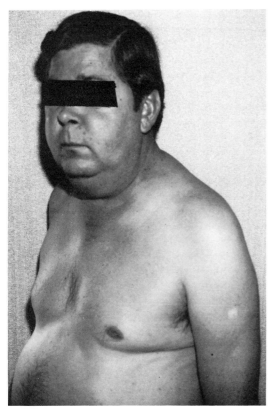

Figure 26–2. Central obesity of Cushing's syndrome.

the arterial system to neural and humoral pressor stimuli. Some patients have erythrocytosis, which, along with the hypertension and prominent telangiectasias, produce the facial plethora. Over 90% of patients with Cushing's syndrome will have impaired carbohydrate tolerance, but only 20% have overt diabetes mellitus. Two thirds of patients complain of muscle weakness, and the majority of women will have oligomenorrhea. The disease occurs more commonly in women, especially in the third and fourth decades. Easy bruising, backache, increased bone fragility as a result of osteoporosis, hirsutism and/or virilism, and mental disorders are quite common also. Hypokalemia, hypercalcemia, and renal stones are seen occasionally.

The outward appearance and cutaneous manifestations of fully developed Cushing's syndrome are characteristic and are strongly suggestive of the diagnosis (Table 26–1). In addition to the fatty changes and facial plethora, hypertrichosis may be very prominent, especially in females. There is often an obvious increase in lanugo hair on the face and upper extremities, but, occasionally, coarse and pigmented hair is present

Table 26–1. CUTANEOUS MANIFESTATIONS OF CUSHING'S SYNDROME

Typical habitus with fat redistribution
Facial plethora
Broad, purple striae and easy bruising
Thin, fragile, and shiny skin
Hirsutism
Steroid acne
Addisonian type hyperpigmentation
Tinea versicolor or tinea corporis

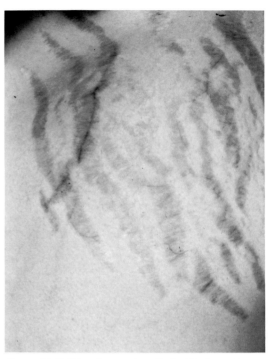

Figure 26–5. Striae in a male with Cushing's syndrome.

(Fig. 26–1). The accentuation of the hair as well as the occasional exacerbation of acne occurs largely as a result of an associated excess of androgens. However, steroid acne, characterized by widespread perifollicular papules and pustules without comedones and cysts, appears to be due to excess glucocorticoids (Fig. 26–4). An acneiform eruption is especially common in exogenous or iatrogenic Cushing's syndrome. Striae result from a fragmentation of elastic fibers and from thinning of the collagen in the dermis. They are most noticeable over the abdomen, under the arms, and on the hips (Fig. 26–5). The striae are often broad and purple and are identical to the striae that can be produced by the use of potent topical corticosteroids under occlusion material for several weeks. The skin is often shiny, atrophic, and fragile and is easily denuded. Minor trauma readily produces ecchymoses, and wound healing after surgery or trauma is slowed. Approximately 6% of patients with Cushing's syndrome have addisonian-like hyperpigmentation, presumably related to increased levels of ACTH. The pigmentation is especially likely to occur in patients with ectopic ACTH secreting tumors. Infections with *Pityrosporon orbiculare* (tinea versicolor) (Fig. 26–6) or *Trichophyton rubrum* (tinea pedis, corporis, or cruris and onychomycosis) are not uncommon, and these superficial fungal diseases may be more widespread in patients with Cushing's syndrome.

The diagnosis of Cushing's syndrome and the differential diagnosis of the various forms of the disease can be straightforward in some instances, but often they are very confusing. Detailed flow sheets or algorithms have been developed to assist the clinician in this effort, but they are beyond the scope of this chapter. The evaluation usually involves both laboratory and radiographic studies. Treatment may be difficult and largely depends on the specific form of Cush-

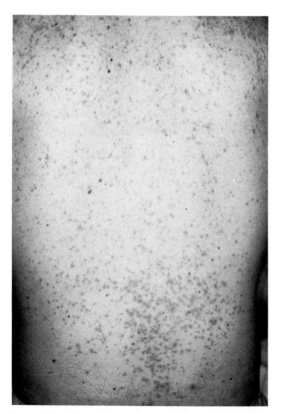

Figure 26–4. Steroid acne in an adolescent male with iatrogenic Cushing's syndrome.

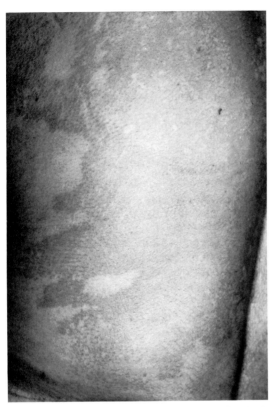

Figure 26–6. Widespread tinea versicolor in Cushing's syndrome.

ing's disease. The goal is to reduce the hormone levels to normal and to eradicate any associated tumors. Cushing's disease, which is usually due to a tumor of the pituitary, is most frequently treated by surgery or irradiation of the pituitary gland. The cure rate is between 70 and 90%. Surgery is the treatment of choice for patients with adrenal tumors producing Cushing's syndrome, but cure is not often possible. There are medications that may help suppress adrenal steroid production or reduce tumor size that may be used adjunctively with surgery. The response in patients with ectopic ACTH secreting tumors depends largely on the type of tumor and whether or not it has spread or involves vital organs by the time the diagnosis is established. If the tumor can be eradicated, the prognosis is usually quite good.

Addison's Disease (Adrenal Insufficiency)

Addison's disease is a rare disorder resulting from deficient production of adren-ocortical hormones. Frequently, it is due to idiopathic atrophy of the adrenal cortex. The mechanism for this form of adrenal insufficiency is believed to be autoimmune. Other causes of Addison's disease include various granulomatous diseases and infections (including tuberculosis or histoplasmosis); infiltrative diseases (such as amyloidosis or metastatic carcinoma); and adrenal destruction from surgical or medical adrenalectomy, hemorrhage, and infarction. These conditions causing "primary" adrenal failure far outnumber "secondary" causes, which are due to ACTH deficiency and occur with diseases of the pituitary and hypothalamus, as well as after the long-term systemic administration of daily corticosteroids. The distinction between primary and secondary adrenal failure is more important than simply as a determinant of the cause, as primary adrenal failure, or Addison's disease, is commonly associated with deficiency of other adrenal steroids, especially aldosterone. One important diagnostic point, however, is that ACTH levels are usually markedly elevated in primary adrenal failure and low or undetectable in secondary disease.

The clinical features of Addison's disease include weakness and weight loss, seen in virtually 100% of patients, as well as hypotension, gastrointestinal symptoms, and hyperpigmentation. The onset of various symptoms is related to the cause, as infarction or hemorrhage produces sudden, unexpected hypotension, whereas the clinical manifestations develop insidiously in chronic idiopathic adrenal failure. Insufficient levels of cortisol result in anorexia, weakness, hyponatremia, and a decreased ability to withstand stress. Inadequate aldosterone concentration results in urinary loss of sodium with subsequent loss of extracellular fluid. This leads to weight loss, a fall in blood pressure, decreased renal blood flow and azotemia, generalized weakness, and postural hypotension. The most prominent cutaneous sign of Addison's disease is hyperpigmentation, which is due to melanocyte stimulation by high levels of ACTH. Hyperpigmentation is absent in secondary adrenal failure. The skin darkening is generalized, although it is accentuated in sun-exposed areas. It is frequently prominent in scars, in the creases of the palms, and on the lips and oral mucosa (Figs. 26–7 and 26–8). Nevi and freckles become more intensely pigmented, and linear pigment lines may appear on the finger-

porphyrin in red blood cells, plasma, and/or stools. Collection of material for analysis must be performed in a light-free area to avoid inactivation of protoporphyrin as a result of exposure to ultraviolet light from the environment.

Therapy. Avoidance of sunlight and the use of opaque sunscreens and protective clothing are helpful in these patients. The disease is due to exposure to rays in the ultraviolet A and visible light range, and most sunscreens are poorly effective in this particular range. Interestingly, as patients age, symptoms seem to abate.

Another therapeutic maneuver that has been of some benefit is the use of oral beta-carotene. Beta-carotene is a carotinoid pigment that is present in most green plants. Beta-carotene (Solatene) is given orally in a dosage of 60–180 mg per day, based upon the age and weight of the patient. The onset of action of beta-carotene is slow. Often several months pass before patients notice a decrease in their symptomatology.

PORPHYRIA CUTANEA TARDA

Porphyria cutanea tarda (PCT) was first described in the 1930s by Waldenström and is by far the most common disorder of porphyrin metabolism. The disease is a photocutaneous syndrome that may be classified as an hepatic porphyria because the overproduction of porphyrins occurs in the liver. The primary defect in PCT is a decreased activity of the enzyme uroporphyrinogen decarboxylase (URO-D). This defect allows for the accumulation of precursors, in particular, uroporphyrin, and occasionally coproporphyrin.

Pathogenesis. In the normal circumstance regarding heme synthesis, URO-D affects the sequential decarboxylation of uroporphyrinogen to coproporphyrin. Decreased URO-D activity in the liver seems to be the fundamental biochemical abnormality in all patients with PCT. In some families inheritance of this defect is by an autosomal dominant mode, and children thus may present with cutaneous disease. Apparently, homozygous inheritance of the genetic defect results in a profound diminution of URO-D activity and eventuates in the recently described entity hepatoerythropoietic porphyria. However, there are multiple pa-

tients who do not have a family history of PCT, and are classified as having sporadic PCT. This group includes patients exposed to halogenated hydrocarbons, to environmental toxins, to alcohol, to iron overload, and to estrogen-related compounds.

In PCT, porphyrin excretion is chiefly uroporphyrin with some slight increase in coproporphyrin. Porphobilinogen is not elevated in the urine and thus is not of diagnostic value in these patients. Ionic iron has been shown to inhibit the enzyme uroporphyrinogen III cosynthetase. This enzyme is responsible for the conversion of uroporphyrinogen I to uroporphyrinogen III. This may help explain why removal of iron or why excess iron is involved in improvement or worsening, respectively, of PCT in the affected patient.

Porphyrins that accumulate absorb light in an energy band known as Soret's band, which ranges from 400 to 410 mm. This band is near the junction of long-wave ultraviolet A light and visible light. The absorption of this light allows the porphyrin molecule to become excited. In the presence of oxygen, this excited molecule degrades and releases energy that involves hydrogen peroxide and lipid peroxides. These peroxides can lead to cellular degeneration. Inflammation is believed to be mediated through the complement pathway. Although the photosensitivity is better understood, an explanation on a biochemical basis for hypertrichosis, skin fragility, and eventual sclerodermoid changes is not available.

Clinical Manifestations. The cutaneous manifestations of PCT allow most dermatologists to diagnose this disease without a great deal of difficulty. The skin disease is manifested by fragility of the skin, formation of vesicles and often bullae, hypertrichosis, hyperpigmentation, eventual sclerodermoid changes, scarring in a photodistribution, and the formation of small cystic lesions known as milia.

The skin lesions occur in light-exposed sites, which in women include the lower legs and feet. Often patients do not recognize that their disease is induced by sunlight; rather, they believe that trauma is the initiating factor in the formation of their blisters. The vesicles and bullae form in a subepidermal region; however, they are still fragile (Fig. 27–3). Eventually, scarring and formation of milia will occur in the photodistri-

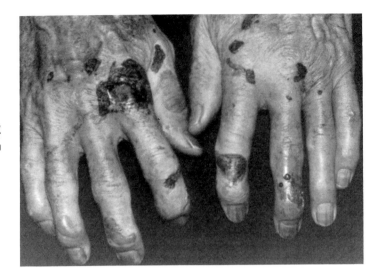

Figure 27-3. Multiple erosions, scarring, milium, and several blisters are present in this patient with porphyria cutanea tarda.

buted blister sites (Fig. 27–4). In addition, facial hypertrichosis is a striking sign of PCT (Fig. 27–5), and, at times, it can be the presenting complaint. Hypertrichosis may occur with other abnormalities, particularly those related to abnormal androgen production. Hyperpigmentation is also present in PCT, often on exposed surfaces only, in contradistinction to the hyperpigmentation that may be seen with hemochromatosis or Addison's disease, which occurs in a generalized fashion.

Various hepatic abnormalities have been described in patients with PCT. Some authorities believe PCT to be one of the less common skin markers of internal neoplasms; in particular, hepatic tumors, both benign, malignant, and metastatic, have been described in association with PCT. Hepatic disease is common in patients with PCT. There is a strong association with chronic alcohol ingestion and, thus, with alcohol-induced hepatitis or cirrhosis. It has been estimated that as many as two thirds of patients with PCT may eventually develop cirrhosis confirmed by liver biopsy.

In addition to hepatic abnormalities, patients with PCT (as well as some of the other porphyrias) more frequently manifest various types of lupus erythematosus. Patients with discoid lupus erythematosus, subacute cutaneous lupus erythematosus, and sys-

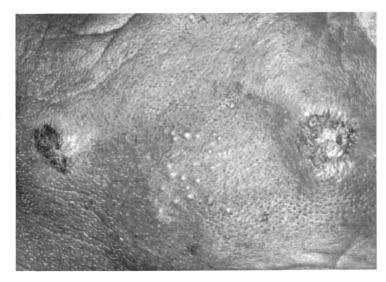

Figure 27-4. Small milial cysts as well as erosive lesions on the face of this patient with porphyria cutanea tarda. (Courtesy of Dr. Neil A. Fenske, Tampa, FL.)

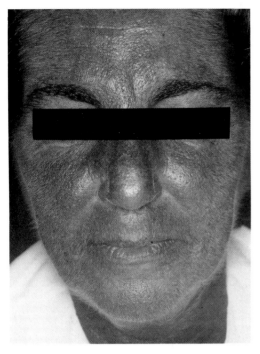

Figure 27–5. Superficial hypertrichosis in porphyria cutanea tarda. Also, note hyperpigmentation.

temic lupus erythematosus have been described who also have PCT. Often the association is only recognized after therapy with an antimalarial agent for the lupus erythematosus precipitates the porphyria.

Etiologic Associations. PCT occurs in both inherited and acquired forms. Exposure to a number of environmental factors has been known to trigger the onset of disease in many patients. In particular, alcohol ingestion, estrogen therapies, iron therapy, and ingestion of aromatic hydrocarbons have been linked to the development of PCT. On rare occasions, PCT has been linked to granulomatous hepatitis, hepatic sarcoidosis, hepatitis B infection, and various hepatic tumors.

Evaluation. Patients suspected of having PCT should be carefully examined, and quantitative tests for urinary porphyrins should be ordered. These tests are also useful in following the patient's course. In addition, tests of liver function and potentially a liver biopsy should be considered. Certain patients may manifest overt diabetes mellitus; thus, a fasting blood glucose determination is indicated. As previously mentioned, several patients with various lupus erythematosus subsets and PCT have been described; thus, antinuclear antibody and related testing should be considered.

Differential Diagnosis. The list of differential diagnoses of PCT is not vast. The vesicular component with scarring, milia formation, and hyperpigmentation may occur in hereditary coproporphyria, in variegate porphyria, in hepatoerythropoietic porphyria, in patients with chronic renal failure who are on hemodialysis, in epidermolysis bullosa acquisita, or in bullous amyloidosis. Lastly, there are a group of patients who have a condition known as pseudoporphyria, which may be induced by various drugs, including nalidixic acid, tetracycline, furosemide, or naproxen. Appropriate testing of urinary, fecal, and plasma porphyrin levels can separate these subgroups. Sclerodermoid changes may occur in PCT, and these conditions must be differentiated from systemic sclerosis, vinyl chloride ingestion, eosinophilic fasciitis, and conditions that produce sclerodermatous skin changes.

Treatment. The treatment of PCT involves the removal of any known factor that may trigger the disease. In particular, all alcohol ingestion should be stopped, and the taking of estrogen compounds and any iron therapy should be discontinued.

Phlebotomy is the first line of therapy and appears to be widely used as well as safe in controlling the disease process. Phlebotomy can be performed on an outpatient basis, removing 1 unit of blood weekly or biweekly until either the urinary porphyrin content returns to normal or the hemoglobin decreases below 10 gm per dl. Clinical improvement usually begins within 2–4 months after phlebotomy is begun. Phlebotomy is effective not only for the vesicular component of PCT, but also may eventually result in slow improvement in hypertrichosis as well as in hyperpigmentation. Sclerodermoid changes do not seem to be improved by phlebotomy. An alternative to phlebotomy therapy is the use of low dose oral antimalarials, either chloroquine phosphate or hydroxychloroquine sulfate. These agents must be given in very low doses, begun initially with careful monitoring to avoid acute toxicity from rapid discharge of porphyrins from the liver. In addition, patients with PCT who have renal failure have benefited from plasmapheresis.

Suggested Readings

Bickers DR: Porphyria. Basic science aspects. Derm Clin 4:277–290, 1986.

Grossman ME, Poh-Fitzpatrick MB: Porphyria cutanea tardia: Diagnosis, management, and differentiation from other hepatic porphyrias. Derm Clin 4:297–309, 1986.

Harber LC, Bickers DR: Photosensitivity Diseases: Principles of Diagnosis and Treatment. Philadelphia, WB Saunders Co., 1981.

Poh-Fitzpatrick MB: The erythropoietic porphyrias. Derm Clin 4:291–296, 1986.

V

CUTANEOUS GASTROENTEROLOGY

28

Cutaneous Diseases Associated with Gastrointestinal Abnormalities

JOHN J. ZONE

There are a number of situations in which diseases of the gastrointestinal tract are associated with cutaneous diseases. This discussion includes cutaneous associations of the following disorders: gastrointestinal hemorrhage, polyposis, malabsorption, and inflammatory bowel disease.

GASTROINTESTINAL HEMORRHAGE

Extensive gastrointestinal hemorrhage may occasionally be related to systemic disorders that are easily recognized by their cutaneous findings. Pseudoxanthoma elasticum and Rendu-Osler-Weber syndrome will be discussed.

Pseudoxanthoma Elasticum

Pseudoxanthoma elasticum is a genetic disorder characterized by progressive calcification of elastic fibers in the skin, retina, and blood vessel walls. Clinical findings usually begin in the second decade. Affected skin reveals progressive yellowish coalescent papules on the neck, axilla, and groin, which may give a peau d'orange appearance and eventually cause the skin to appear loose and wrinkled (Fig. 28–1; Plate VB).

The earliest eye changes are angioid streaks that present as linear and branching networks of grayish discoloration around the optic disc. They are larger in caliber than blood vessels and represent a rupture in the elastic lamina of Bruch's membrane of the retina. Both scarring and hemorrhage lead to a loss of visual acuity. Fragmentation of the elastic media of mid-sized blood vessels may produce bleeding or occlusion of blood vessels, such as those of the gastrointestinal tract, coronary artery system, and extremities. Gastrointestinal hemorrhage is the most common hemorrhage observed, and it may be fatal. Pregnancy may accentuate degenerative disruption of elastic tissue and may particularly predispose the patient to upper gastrointestinal bleeding.

Pathogenesis

Pseudoxanthoma elasticum is a genetic disorder in which there is both recessive and dominant inheritance. Distinct clinical patterns were noted in various kindreds described by Pope in 1974. This implies that several different genes and metabolic products might be responsible for a final common clinical syndrome involving the calcification of the elastic fibers and resultant tissue damage and destruction.

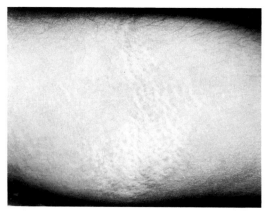

Figure 28–1. Pseudoxanthoma elasticum (see also Plate V*B*).

The earliest detectable change on electron microscopy is calcification of normal appearing elastic fibers. There is then calcification of elastic fibers in the lower dermis and subsequent calcification and destruction of all dermal elastic fibers with the resultant laxity and yellowish discoloration of the skin. Submucosal vessels of the gastrointestinal tract develop fragmentation of the elastic media with subsequent rupture of vessels. Gastrointestinal bleeding may occur in areas affected by other diseases such as peptic ulcer disease, but it may also occur spontaneously in normal mucosa. Reports suggest an increased risk of gastrointestinal hemorrhage during pregnancy. This is thought to be due to an increased progression of vascular degeneration during pregnancy, but the mechanism for this is unknown. Peripheral arteries in the extremities may become so calcified that there is an actual reduction of pulses.

Classification

Pseudoxanthoma elasticum occurs in about 1 in 160,000 births. Pope has classified pseudoxanthoma elasticum on the basis of the segregation patterns derived from pedigree studies of British patients. He divided the pedigrees into autosomal dominant or autosomal recessive by standard criteria. He then arbitrarily divided both dominant and recessive on the basis of clinical characteristics. The following classification system is now used: dominant 1 (on the basis of 12 cases), dominant 2 (52 cases), recessive 1 (54 cases), and recessive 2 (3 cases). An adaptation of his clinical summary is presented in Table 28–1. Recessive 2 is the most distinctive form. There is complete cutaneous infiltration, lemon yellow elastic degeneration of the skin, and absence of systemic disease. Recessive 1 represents all recessive cases without these unique clinical findings and occupies an intermediate position clinically between the 2 dominant groups. It resembles the dominant 1 group

Table 28–1. PERCENTAGE OF PATIENTS WITH SPECIFIC CLINICAL CHARACTERISTICS OF PSEUDOXANTHOMA ELASTICUM

Characteristics	Dominant 1	Dominant 2	Recessive 1	Recessive 2
Peau d'orange and flexural rash	100	24	77	—
Macular rash	—	70	13.9	—
General increase of extensibility	8	66	3.9	—
General cutaneous pseudoxanthoma elasticum	—	—	—	100
Angina	56	—	—	100
Claudication	56	—	—	—
Hypertension	75	7.8	19.7	—
Hematemesis	8	3.8	15.8	—
Ophthalmic abnormalities				
Severe choroiditis	75	7.8	35	—
Angioid streaks	34	47	47	—
Washed-out pattern	—	12	1.9	—
Peau d'orange	—	8	—	—
Prominent choroidal vessels	—	18	—	—
Myopia	24	48	5.8	—
High, arched palate	—	54	11.9	—
Blue sclerae	8	41	9.8	—
Loose jointedness	—	35	5.8	—

Adapted from Pope FM: Two types of autosomal recessive pseudoxanthoma elasticum. Arch Dermatol *110:*209, 1974.

described in the following discussion, although vascular and retinal degeneration are much milder than in the dominant groups. Hematemesis is common, especially among affected females. Pope divided the 2 dominant groups based on 2 families he had studied and on the basis of published cases. Dominant 1 group showed flexurally distributed peau d'orange pseudoxanthomatous rash, severe vascular complications (such as angina, coronary artery disease, and claudication), and a severe, degenerative retinopathy with early blindness. The dominant 2 group was much less severely affected. They had an atypical canary yellow macular rash, or sometimes no rash at all. There were minimal vascular complications and very mild retinal changes. Chorioretinitis was rare in this group, but peau d'orange skin patterns and prominent choroidal vessels were common. Increased cutaneous extensibility; blue sclerae; a high, arched palate; and myopia were also seen.

Patient Evaluation

The diagnosis of pseudoxanthoma elasticum is most likely to be suggested by eye findings in the second decade of life, by premature vascular disease, or by a positive family history. The earliest ophthalmologic findings are usually angioid streaks. Scarring and hemorrhage may lead to a loss of visual acuity, which is a common presenting symptom. If pseudoxanthoma elasticum is suspected, detailed examination by an ophthalmologist is essential. Because eye changes are seen early in life, funduscopic examination is also required to screen relatives of known patients.

Skin biopsy is essential in suspected cases or in potentially involved family members. Faint basophilic staining of elastic fibers may be observed in specimens stained with routine hematoxylin and eosin stains. Involved skin shows characteristic black staining of clumped elastic fibers with orcein or Verhoeff's stain. Staining for calcium frequently shows significant elastic tissue calcification. Although such findings are classically present in involved skin, clinically normal appearing skin of the axilla may show similar findings. Such a biopsy may confirm a diagnosis of pseudoxanthoma elasticum in patients with angioid streaks and minimal cutaneous findings.

Patients with pseudoxanthoma elasticum need to be evaluated closely for evidence of vascular complications. Clinical evidence of melena should be pursued immediately with endoscopy and barium contrast studies because of the potentially catastrophic nature of gastrointestinal bleeding. Symptoms of angina are common, and the potential for myocardial infarction requires close follow-up of the patient. Claudication is a common symptom of arterial insufficiency. Radiographs of the extremities will reveal characteristic calcification. In summary, close attention needs to be paid to the vascular complications of this disease, as they are potentially fatal.

Differential Diagnosis

The characteristic yellowish papules of pseudoxanthoma elasticum may be confused with solar elastosis. The neck is a common site for both problems, but pseudoxanthoma elasticum also occurs in the axilla, groin, and popliteal and antecubital fossae. Solar elastosis produces abnormal elastic tissue that is histologically detected as dense masses in the upper dermis that do not take up stains for calcium. Pseudoxanthoma elasticum shows irregular clumps of elastic tissue in the mid- to lower dermis. Eruptive xanthomas may also present as yellowish papules, but they usually affect the buttocks and thighs. Xanthelasma characteristically involves the eyelids. Histologically, xanthomas demonstrate foam cells filled with lipid droplets that stain positively for fat.

Angioid streaks are valuable markers for the diagnosis of pseudoxanthoma elasticum, but are not pathognomonic findings. Similar findings are seen in Paget's disease of the bone and in sickle cell disease. The former condition shows characteristic roentgenographic abnormalities with increased bone formation, bowing of the tibia and femur, enlargement of the skull, and elevation of serum alkaline phosphatase. Patients with sickle cell disease show anemia and characteristic abnormalities of the peripheral blood smear. Other abnormalities that have been reported to be associated with angioid streaks include Ehlers-Danlos syndrome, hyperphosphatasemia, and trauma. These are much less frequent associations, however, and may even be attributed to chance. No fundamental pathogenetic relationship among the disorders causing angioid streaks has been established.

langiectasia, but occurs in an autosomal dominant inheritance pattern.

Sunlight and ionizing radiation produce localized linear telangiectasias in exposed areas. Traumatic lesions are usually linear or occasionally spider-like and localized. Rosaceal telangiectasias are linear, are limited to the face and nose, and spare mucous membranes. Cherry angiomata usually occur on the chest, are more papular, and are rare on the lips and mucous membranes. Nevoid telangiectatic syndromes are characterized by segmented involvement of body areas with reticular vascular proliferation. Chronic liver disease is characterized by spider angiomata with a characteristic central arteriole and branching. Ataxia telangiectasia patients have facial telangiectasia in combination with progressive cerebellar ataxia and recurrent respiratory symptoms in early childhood.

Angiokeratomas may be associated with a variety of clinical syndromes, and are usually keratotic papules that blanch poorly on diascopy. Idiopathic solitary lesions occur on the penis and scrotum. Angiokeratomas associated with Fabry's disease are usually truncal and not mucosal.

Patient Evaluation

If the characteristic telangiectasias are present on the skin or mucous membranes, detailed family history and history of bleeding episodes are essential. Examination of asymptomatic family members may be helpful. Clinical telangiectasias may be minimal, especially in children and adolescents; therefore, close physical examination is essential. Recurrent epistaxis at a young age may precede obvious telangiectasias by many years, and this makes family history especially important.

The source of melena should be aggressively sought. Recurrent epistaxis may be responsible. Hematemesis or nasogastric intubation positive for blood should prompt endoscopy. Signs of hematochezia justify colonoscopy. Selective angiography may be of help if brisk bleeding is present. Evaluation of the fate of infused labeled red blood cells may be a valuable test. Demonstration of the lesions of HHT at surgery without prior localization is difficult, even during episodes of massive bleeding. Barium contrast studies of the bowel are of no help.

All affected patients should be screened for pulmonary arteriovenous fistulae by chest x-ray. Arterial oxygen desaturation is frequent if significant shunting has occurred. Evidence of vascular malformations of the central nervous system should be pursued vigorously if focal symptoms are present.

Treatment

Epistaxis can usually be controlled with nasal packing or with electrocautery. Systemic estrogen therapy has been said to produce squamous metaplasia of mucosal surfaces, thereby making lesions more resistant to trauma. The placement of a skin graft intranasally to protect fragile telangiectatic vessels from local trauma has been helpful. Prophylactic lubrication of the nasal mucosa may also help.

Gastrointestinal bleeding responds to electrocautery or to laser via endoscopy if the site of bleeding can be identified. If these treatments are unsuccessful, surgical intervention is necessary.

Significant arteriovenous fistulae in any location are usually well controlled by resection. Recent work with silicone and latex balloon embolization may significantly decrease the morbidity in pulmonary arteriovenous malformations.

POLYPOSIS

Gastrointestinal polyps may be adenomatous in origin, in which case they have proven malignant potential. In contrast, hamartomatous polyps represent malformation of the connective tissue of the intestinal mucosa and have little pre-malignant potential. One to several adenomatous polyps occur in 10% of adults. The term "polyposis" refers to multiple polyps (greater than 100), and the condition carries a proportionately greater risk of adenocarcinoma. Familial polyposis coli is characterized by autosomal dominant inheritance of colorectal polyposis alone. Gardner's syndrome is characterized by an autosomal dominant inheritance of colorectal polyposis with the additional findings of multiple epidermoid cysts (Fig. 28–3), subcutaneous fibromas, desmoid tumors, and osteomas.

Pathogenesis

Kindred studies of Gardner's syndrome show an autosomal dominant inheritance with a penetrance of essentially 100% when

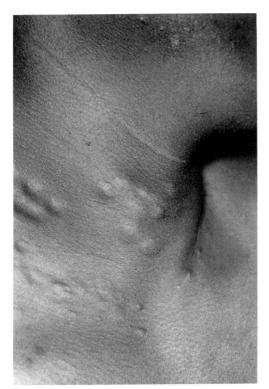

Figure 28–3. Gardner's syndrome. Multiple epidermal cysts are present in this patient with adenomatous colonic polyps.

kindreds are closely examined. However, there may be considerable variation in expressivity of the gene. The sexes are affected equally, and the chromosomes are structurally normal. The gene frequency at birth has been calculated to be 1 in 14,000. It seems likely either that the mutant gene is producing growth stimulating molecules affecting multiple tissues or that the gene somehow causes cells of various body areas to respond vigorously to normal growth stimuli.

Controversy exists as to the genetic relationship between familial polyposis coli and Gardner's syndrome. Some investigators have suggested that the two are one disease with variable phenotypic expression. However, close phenotypic evaluation of the kindreds suggests that they are genetically distinct entities. Whether gene interaction is involved has also been questioned. The final answer will not be available until the gene is identified.

Classification

Familial polyposis coli was originally separated from Gardner's syndrome solely on the basis of the cutaneous findings in Gardner's syndrome. Adenomatous polyps from both sources seem to be histologically, pathologically, and developmentally similar. There is great variation in the age of onset and in the number and location of polyps in both disorders. It may be impossible to diagnose intestinal polyposis before the age of 16, but the extracolonic manifestations of Gardner's syndrome can be recognized in infancy or early childhood. The original Gardner's syndrome description included osteomas, epidermal inclusion (epidermoid) cysts, and subcutaneous fibromas in combination with intestinal polyposis. Osteomas, particularly of the facial bones and jaw, may be palpable or seen in adults, but young children may have many small 3–5 mm cysts on the chest, back, and upper arms. Subcutaneous encapsulated fibromas range in size and occur on the scalp, shoulders, arms, and back.

Since the original description, desmoid tumors and dental abnormalities have been added to Gardner's syndrome. Desmoid tumors represent benign, diffuse proliferation of soft fibrous tissue. They are abdominal wall tumors that may grow to several centimeters in size. They frequently occur at sites of trauma or surgery, but may arise *de novo*. Mesenteric fibrosis occurs in a similar fashion. The dental abnormalities include odontomas as well as unerupted and supernumerary teeth. A variety of other benign cutaneous tumors have been associated with Gardner's syndrome, but not with high enough frequency to contribute to the diagnosis.

Differential Diagnosis

Differentiation between Gardner's syndrome and sporadic epidermoid cysts and fibromas is primarily based on the large numbers of lesions and on a positive family history in Gardner's syndrome patients. The presence of desmoid tumors should prompt consideration of the diagnosis.

Several other skin conditions are associated with polyps. Hamartomatous polyps are malformations of the intestinal mucosa that have undergone excessive growth. They may be isolated or multiple and are not premalignant. Peutz-Jeghers syndrome consists of hamartomatous gastrointestinal polyps and spotty melanin pigmentation on the lips, buccal mucosa, palms, and soles. These hamartomatous polyps may occur in any part of the gastrointestinal tract but are particularly common in the small intestine. Obstruction and intussusception may occur. Multiple hamartoma syndrome (Cowden's disease) is characterized by warty papules and nodules on the mucosal and cutaneous surfaces of the mouth, forearms, and face. Hamartomatous gastrointestinal polyps may also occur. The Cronkhite-Canada syndrome consists of polyposis of the stomach, small intestine, and colon. The "polyps" represent thickened areas of mucosa. Nail atrophy, alopecia, and skin pigmentation also occur.

Patient Evaluation

Patients with cutaneous findings suggestive of Gardner's syndrome should have a detailed family history taken in hope of confirming the diagnosis. Facial bone roentgenograms may demonstrate osteomas. Colonoscopy and biopsy can then confirm the diagnosis. Examination of the colon in high risk individuals should be routine during childhood.

Treatment

Untreated patients with Gardner's syndrome have nearly a 100% chance of eventually developing colon cancer. Malignant changes have been reported as early as age 9, and the incidence of carcinoma in preadolescent polyposis patients is about 5%. Consequently, colectomy is recommended at the earliest possible age. Close surveillance by a gastroenterologist is essential.

Desmoid tumors are considered benign, but their infiltration into surrounding muscle and fascia may be problematic and may require excision, which is technically difficult because of poorly defined margins. Epidermal cysts and fibromas can be removed surgically if desired. There appears to be no increased risk of malignant degeneration in such lesions.

ASSOCIATION BETWEEN ACROCHORDONS AND COLONIC POLYPS

Acrochordons, or simple skin tags, occur as multiple, fleshy papules or filiform growths, especially on the neck, axilla, and groin. They are traditionally considered to be of little clinical significance. Studies by Leavitt and colleagues, Chobanian and coworkers, and Beitler and colleagues have demonstrated a significant incidence of adenomatous colonic polyps among those patients who also had skin tags. However, these studies evaluated only subjects with suspected colonic disease who were selected for colonoscopy. Conclusions on the association between colonic polyps and skin tags in the general population are therefore invalid.

The frequency of skin tags is age-dependent, and age-matched controls are essential for conclusions on the use of this sign in the general population. Prospective study of a large unselected population will be necessary to evaluate the clinical usefulness of this association. No information on the potential predictive value of number and location of skin tags is currently available. The huge number of patients with skin tags makes it impossible to recommend exploratory colonoscopy on the basis of cutaneous skin tags of any type in the absence of colonic symptoms and signs. Clinical recommendations will have to await the eventual unfolding of this interesting clinical story.

MALABSORPTION

Malabsorption may be associated with characteristic cutaneous findings, as in the case in dermatitis herpetiformis and zinc deficiency. In such cases, the pathognomonic cutaneous findings usually allow for diagnosis of the bowel abnormality. These two disorders will be discussed in detail. Less specific cutaneous signs of malabsorption are frequently present independent of the cause of the malabsorption. These include stomatitis and glossitis, which are believed to be related to vitamin B deficiencies; angular cheilitis; purpura as a result of vitamin C and vitamin K deficiencies; asteatotic, eczema-like eruptions of uncertain cause; patchy hyperpigmentation; and slowed nail and hair growth as well as alopecia probably secondary to protein malnutrition (see Chapter 31).

Acrodermatitis Enteropathica

Acrodermatitis enteropathica is characterized by the selective deficiency of zinc. Clas-

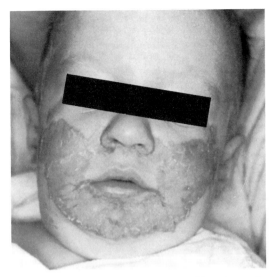

Figure 28–4. Acrodermatitis enteropathica (see also Plate VD).

sic cases are genetic in origin, but an acquired form may develop in patients who are treated with total parenteral nutrition deficient in zinc or may occur in association with gastrointestinal malabsorption syndromes. Clinical findings usually begin after infants are weaned. They consist of acral, perioral, and perirectal vesiculobullous, pustular, and eczematous skin lesions (Figs. 28–4 and 28–5; Plate VD). Alopecia, diarrhea, growth retardation, neuropsychiatric disorders, and recurrent infections develop subsequently if the disorder goes unrecognized. Zinc supplementation is curative.

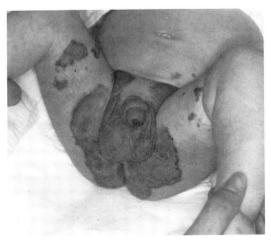

Figure 28–5. Acrodermatitis enteropathica.

Pathogenesis

Acrodermatitis enteropathica is a genetic disorder transmitted as an autosomal recessive trait. Absorption of dietary zinc is limited to 2–3% of intake, although the exact mechanism of malabsorption of zinc in these patients is unknown. Serum zinc levels are persistently low. Administration of large amounts of oral zinc will reverse the clinical findings. Zinc metalloenzymes are also low. The onset of symptoms usually occurs within the first few months of life and is frequently associated with the change from breast feeding to cow's milk. It is believed that low molecular weight zinc binding ligands are responsible for the superior absorption of zinc from human milk. Zinc deficiency in infants has also been reported in which there apparently was defective mammary gland zinc secretion.

The exact metabolic pathogenesis of individual cutaneous and systemic lesions is poorly understood. Zinc is needed in various metalloenzymes for protein and DNA synthesis and for cell division. The biologic effects of zinc are so protean that it is unlikely that a single biochemical pathogenesis will be identified for acrodermatitis enteropathica.

Zinc deficiency has profound effects on the immune system, including effects on T cell helper function, T cell suppressor function, and natural killer cell activity. Zinc also affects neutrophil chemotaxis. These abnormalities may be responsible for significant problems with intercurrent infection.

Classification

In addition to the inherited form of zinc deficiency, there are a variety of other causes. These are listed in Table 28–3. Dietary zinc deficiency is prevalent in underdeveloped countries and may be present to moderate degrees in the United States, es-

Table 28–3. CAUSES OF ZINC DEFICIENCY

Genetic acrodermatitis enteropathica
Dietary
Following excessive alcohol ingestion
Malabsorption
Following intestinal surgery
Total parenteral nutrition
Following penicillamine therapy
Chronic renal disease

pecially in infants. Consumption of unrefined cereals containing high levels of phytate renders zinc unavailable for absorption. Alcohol intake induces hyperzincuria by poorly understood mechanisms.

Zinc deficiency occurs in patients with steatorrhea from any cause. Fat malabsorption produces an alkaline environment in the bowel, and zinc forms insoluble complexes with fat and phosphates resulting in an increased loss of zinc in the stool. Exudation of large amounts of zinc protein complexes into the intestinal lumen may also contribute to the decrease in plasma zinc concentration that occurs in patients with inflammatory bowel disease. Zinc deficiency has also been reported following intestinal bypass surgery, presumably by similar mechanisms.

Failure to include zinc in fluids for total parenteral nutrition may cause severe zinc deficiency with clinical features that resemble these seen with the congenital types of acrodermatitis enteropathica. Severe zinc deficiency has also been reported following therapy with penicillamine or other chelating agents.

Differential Diagnosis

Classic acrodermatitis enteropathica is clinically characteristic when the perioral, perirectal, and digital areas are all involved. Incomplete expression may produce confusion with perioral dermatitis, hand dermatitis, candidiasis, and pustular psoriasis. The additional findings of alopecia and diarrhea in zinc deficiency minimize the clinical confusion. The histologic appearance of acrodermatitis enteropathica is non-specific. The vesicle is intraepidermal in location, and neutrophils may infiltrate the epidermis with extensive crusting.

Patient Evaluation

Measurement of zinc levels in plasma is diagnostic, provided the sample is not hemolyzed or contaminated. Particular care needs to be taken to ensure that test tubes and other measurement equipment are free of zinc. Zinc levels in red blood cells and hair may also be assessed to determine body zinc status, but these are generally less reliable tests. Urinary excretion of zinc is usually decreased as a result of zinc deficiency

from malabsorption. Determination of 24-hour urinary zinc may be of help in diagnosing hyperzincuria and plasma zinc deficiency caused by excessive alcohol intake and chronic renal disease.

Alkaline phosphatase is a zinc dependent enzyme and is frequently depressed in the serum of zinc deficient subjects. Carboxypeptidase and thymidine kinase may have similar depressions, but are less easily measured.

Treatment

Deficiency of zinc can be corrected easily by oral supplementation. If the intake of animal protein is adequate, 15–30 mg daily of zinc sulfate may be adequate. If dietary protein intake is predominantly in the form of cereals, 50–200 mg daily may be needed.

Response to therapy is dramatic. Skin lesions, diarrhea, and behavioral abnormalities reverse themselves within days to weeks. Hair and body growth return to normal in a matter of months.

Dermatitis Herpetiformis

Dermatitis herpetiformis (DH) is characterized by involvement of extensor surfaces of the forearms, elbows, knees, and buttocks with grouped erythematous papules and vesicles. Biopsy reveals a blister at the basement membrane with the accumulation of neutrophils in dermal papillary tips. Perilesional skin demonstrates the pathognomonic deposition of granular IgA in dermal papillary tips.

Greater than 85% of patients with DH demonstrate some degree of small bowel atrophy on jejunal biopsy, which is identical to, but generally less severe than, ordinary gluten sensitive enteropathy (celiac disease). The attendant symptoms and signs of malabsorption are proportional to the severity of the gluten sensitive enteropathy.

DH is discussed in detail in Chapter 45. The present discussion will be limited to the association with malabsorption.

Pathogenesis

The association of DH with clinical malabsorption is on the basis of 2 pathogenetic mechanisms. First, greater than 85% of DH patients are HLA-B8DR3 positive. This genotype carries with it a high frequency of atrophic gastritis, achlorhydria, intrinsic factor deficiency, and resultant systemic deficiency of vitamin B_{12}. This clinical constellation of findings occurs in up to 20% of cases. Greater than 85% of DH patients have gluten sensitive enteropathy, which varies in severity from a mononuclear infiltrate in the lamina propria with minimal villous atrophy to complete flattening of the small intestinal mucosal cells. This abnormality may be patchy, requiring multiple biopsy specimens for documentation. Only about 15–20% of DH patients have symptomatic malabsorption, and these are the patients who represent the extreme of gluten sensitive enteropathy with severe mucosal flattening. The clinical signs of malabsorption in these severely affected patients are identical to those of celiac disease and are directly attributable to gluten sensitivity.

Classification

DH has become an incredibly homogeneous disease with several subgroups. This is attributable to the characteristic immunopathology of granular IgA deposition of perilesional skin, which is rapidly becoming a sine qua non for diagnosis. Previously, patients with linear IgA deposition along the basement membrane were included in the diagnosis of DH, but most investigators now consider this to be a separate disorder (see Chapter 45).

Symptoms of malabsorption, including steatorrhea and foul smelling stools, are present in a minority of patients. Many more complain of cramping, abdominal pain, and bloating after eating. Minimal symptoms may only be recognized by their cessation after institution of a gluten free diet.

The villous atrophy does not correlate with the severity of the skin disease and is not affected by dapsone therapy, which improves the skin disease. The bowel abnormality is caused by gluten; it improves with a gluten free diet, and it recurs with reinstitution of a regular diet.

Clinical findings of malabsorption, including weight loss, xerosis, alopecia, and steatorrhea, are present in only the most severe cases. Indeed, many patients with histologically significant small bowel atrophy appear well nourished and even obese.

Differential Diagnosis

The differential diagnosis of DH includes pemphigus, bullous pemphigoid, linear IgA disease, bacterial folliculitis, and eczematous processes. These are reviewed in detail in Chapter 45.

Patient Evaluation

Because virtually all patients with DH have gluten sensitive enteropathy, it can be questioned whether small bowel biopsy is even necessary. Although we do not perform this procedure routinely, it may be helpful to confirm the bowel abnormality and provide reassurance to the patient during long-term gluten free diet therapy that this diet is necessary. The real proof of gluten sensitive enteropathy comes with improvement of symptoms on gluten free diet therapy.

Ten to twenty per cent of patients have abnormal D-xylose absorption, but this finding adds little when the diagnosis of gluten sensitive enteropathy has already been made. Complete blood count is mandatory, and if anemia is seen (in the absence of dapsone-induced hemolysis), measurements of serum iron, folate, and vitamin B_{12} levels are indicated to rule out malabsorption as a cause of deficiency.

Low serum vitamin B_{12} levels necessitate a Schilling's test with and without intrinsic factor administration to differentiate between vitamin B_{12} malabsorption secondary to enteropathy and intrinsic factor deficiency associated with atrophic gastritis.

Treatment

Supplementation with vitamin B_{12}, folate, or iron is indicated, depending on results of the screening evaluation. The skin disease may be treated effectively with oral dapsone. Both the skin and the bowel disease respond to gluten restriction, but a minimum 6-month trial period should be undertaken before evaluating the effectiveness of therapy. See Chapter 45 for further details on treatment.

INFLAMMATORY BOWEL DISEASE

Inflammatory bowel disease is a general term for a group of idiopathic chronic in-

Table 28–4. SOME CUTANEOUS ASSOCIATIONS OF INFLAMMATORY BOWEL DISEASE

Specific Lesions
  Fissures and fistulae
  Metastatic Crohn's disease
  Mucosal lesions

Reactive Lesions
  Aphthous ulcers
  Pustular vasculitis (bowel-associated dermatosis-arthritis syndrome)
  Pyoderma gangrenosum
  Erythema nodosum
  Vasculitis
  Erythema multiforme
  Urticaria

Other Associations
  Epidermolysis bullosa acquisita
  Vitiligo
  Fingernail clubbing

Nutritional Deficiency–Associated Lesions

flammatory conditions that affect the bowel. The two major diseases are ulcerative colitis and Crohn's disease (i.e., regional enteritis and Crohn's disease of the colon). A number of non-intestinal signs and symptoms may occur in association with inflammatory bowel disease (Table 28–4). Many of the cutaneous associations of inflammatory bowel disease are discussed at length in other chapters. These conditions and others will be briefly reviewed here.

Patients with Crohn's disease may have associated perianal fistulae. These lesions are often presenting manifestations of the disease. They may histopathologically show granulomas highly suggestive of the diagnosis of Crohn's disease. Metastatic Crohn's disease is the name given to cutaneous granulomas that occur distant from the gastrointestinal tract in patients with Crohn's disease. Crohn's disease may be viewed directly in the oral mucosa. Cobblestoning and ulceration in the oral cavity appear to be identical to bowel lesions seen endoscopically. Patients with ulcerative colitis may have vegetating lesions of the oral cavity called pyostomatitis vegetans.

Oral aphthous ulcers have been well reported in association with Crohn's disease and ulcerative colitis. These lesions are not specific, as up to 20% of the normal population have aphthae. Malabsorption of iron, folic acid, and vitamin B_{12} may occur with inflammatory bowel disease. Correction of these deficiencies may result in improvement in associated aphthosis.

Cutaneous pustular vasculitis, like that seen in Behçet's disease, occurs in patients with inflammatory bowel disease (bowel-associated dermatosis-arthritis syndrome). This condition and its relationship to bowel bypass syndrome, the interpretation of aphthosis in the setting of enteropathic arthritis, and the issue of diagnosing Behçet's disease in a patient with bowel disease are all reviewed in Chapter 6.

Malabsorption has been reviewed earlier in this chapter. Many of the cutaneous changes seen in patients with inflammatory bowel disease are due to nutritional deficiencies secondary to malabsorption (see also Chapter 31, Nutritional Diseases).

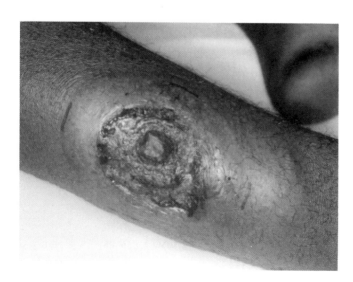

Figure 28–6. Pyoderma gangrenosum in a patient with chronic ulcerative colitis.

The incidence of pyoderma gangrenosum in patients with inflammatory bowel disease is probably less than 2%. However, up to one quarter of patients with pyoderma gangrenosum have inflammatory bowel disease (Fig. 28–6). Pyoderma gangrenosum is also reviewed in Chapters 4 and 9.

Erythema nodosum may occur in 1–5% of patients with inflammatory bowel disease. However, patients with erythema nodosum infrequently prove to have inflammatory bowel disease. They should still be questioned about signs and symptoms of bowel disease. Erythema nodosum is the subject of Chapter 42.

Additional reactive dermatoses discussed elsewhere in this text may occur in patients with inflammatory bowel disease. These reactive dermatoses include erythema multiforme (Chapter 41), urticaria (Chapter 7), necrotizing venulitis (i.e., leukocytoclastic vasculitis) and polyarteritis nodosa (Chapter 5), and epidermolysis bullosa acquisita (Chapter 45). Thrombophlebitis, digital clubbing, and vitiligo may also occur.

Suggested Readings

Beitler M, Eng A, Kilgour M, Lebwohl M: Association between acrochordons and colonic polyps. J Am Acad Dermatol 14:1042–1044, 1986.

Berde C, Willis DC, Sandberg EC: Pregnancy in women with pseudoxanthoma elasticum. Obstet Gynecol Surv 38:339–344, 1983.

Burgdorf W: Cutaneous manifestations of Crohn's disease. J Am Acad Dermatol 5:689–695, 1981.

Burt RW, Naylor EW, Emanuel L: Gardner's syndrome: Recent developments in research and management. Dig Dis Sci 12:945–959, 1980.

Clarkson JG, Altman RD: Angioid streaks. Surv Ophthalmol 26:235–246, 1982.

Eddy DD, Farber EM: Pseudoxanthoma elasticum. Internal manifestations: A report of cases and a statistical review of the literature. Arch Dermatol 86:729–739, 1962.

Pope FM: Historical evidence for the genetic heterogeneity of pseudoxanthoma elasticum. Br J Dermatol 92:493–509, 1975.

Prasad AS: Clinical manifestations of zinc deficiency. Ann Rev Nutr 5:341–363, 1985.

Reilly PJ, Nostrant TT: Clinical manifestations of hereditary hemorrhagic telangiectasia. Am J Gastroenterol 79:363–367, 1984.

Zone JJ, Petersen MJ: Dermatitis herpetiformis. In Thiers BH, Dobson R (eds): Pathogenesis of Skin Disease. New York, Churchill Livingstone, 1985, pp. 159–183.

29

Cutaneous Hepatology

KENNETH E. GREER

There are a number of cutaneous stigmata that are associated with liver disease, but none is specific. Even jaundice, classically associated with liver immaturity (neonatal jaundice) or failure, may occur with hemolysis and in the setting of perfectly normal hepatic function. The skin changes of liver disease may be related to primary diseases of the liver; to cutaneous diseases with associated liver abnormalities; and to a wide variety of disorders with changes in many organs, including the liver and the skin. There are also a number of drugs that are commonly used for the treatment of cutaneous disease but that may produce hepatic damage, such as methotrexate, ketoconazole, etretinate, and vitamin A. Finally, there are several drugs that produce hypersensitivity reactions characterized by fever, lymphadenopathy, hepatitis, and skin lesions. Drugs in this category include phenytoin, dapsone, and, rarely, allopurinol.

Classically, cutaneous manifestations have been associated with such primary liver diseases as alcoholic cirrhosis and hemochromatosis, but there are other disorders that produce similar changes, including Wilson's disease, viral hepatitis, primary biliary cirrhosis, and so forth. Porphyria cutanea tarda and erythropoietic protoporphyria, known primarily for their cutaneous manifestations, are associated with liver abnormalities, and the Gianotti-Crosti syndrome, neonatal hemangiomatosis, lichen planus, and pyoderma gangrenosum have been associated with hepatitis or with other forms of liver disease. Miscellaneous diseases affecting many organ systems, but with involvement of the liver and the skin, include syphilis, sarcoidosis, Gaucher's disease, polyarteritis nodosa, and cytophagic histiocytic panniculitis. Finally, with the increased incidence of liver transplantation, the skin becomes an important organ for the early recognition of the graft versus host reaction. Many of these disorders are discussed elsewhere in this text, and others occur too infrequently to be discussed in detail in this chapter.

Cutaneous symptoms, such as pruritus and jaundice, may be important evidence for considering the diagnosis of liver disease, especially in conjunction with such nonspecific symptoms as fatigue, anorexia, vomiting and weight loss, diminished libido, and right upper quadrant abdominal discomfort. In addition to the symptoms, certain physical findings, especially when considered collectively, suggest the diagnosis of liver disease. Cutaneous lesions are often prominent and include scleral icterus, spider telangiectasias, excoriations, xanthelasmas, changes in hair pattern, nail lesions, gynecomastia, and prominence of the cutaneous veins in the epigastrium.

CIRRHOSIS

Cirrhosis of the liver implies an irreversible alteration of liver architecture, consisting of hepatic fibrosis, areas of nodular regeneration, and a loss of a considerable number of hepatocytes. Although alcohol is the most common cause of cirrhosis (Laennec's cirrhosis) in the United States, cirrhosis can be caused by drugs and other toxins; infections (especially viral hepatitis); biliary obstruction (carcinoma of the pancreas or bile duct, gallstones, cystic fibrosis, etc.); metabolic diseases (hemochromatosis and Wilson's disease); chronic right-sided heart failure; and a group of miscellaneous diseases, such as sarcoidosis, primary biliary cirrhosis, and jejunoileal bypass. There are also a number of cases of cirrhosis that are idiopathic. Individuals with cirrhosis will usually present in one of two general ways: (1) evidence of acute hepatocellular necrosis with jaundice, nausea and vomiting, and tender hepatomegaly; (2) evidence of complications of cirrhosis, brought on primarily by the rise in intrahepatic vascular resistance and subsequent portal hypertension (ascites, splenomegaly, bleeding varices, and encephalopathy). Patients, not infrequently, will present with a mixed picture of the just mentioned two pathophysiologic pathways.

The dermatological stigmata of cirrhosis are well recognized and include changes in the skin, nails, and hair. Vascular lesions are common and include spider angiomas and other telangiectasias; palmar erythema; and dilated abdominal wall veins, which occur in patients with portal hypertension and represent the development of portal-systemic collaterals (Figs. 29–1 to 29–3). Spider angiomas occur in the large majority of patients with cirrhosis, but they are not pathognomonic of the disease, as they occur commonly in young children, pregnant

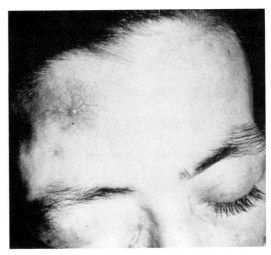

Figure 29–1. Spider angioma on the forehead.

women, and otherwise healthy adults. They are so named because of their central pulsatile arterial punctum with radiating branching vessels. They occur almost exclusively on the upper half of the body, especially on the face, neck, and upper trunk. The spider is formed by a coiled arteriole that spirals up to a central point and then branches out into thin-walled vessels that merge with normal capillaries. The pathogenesis of these unusual vascular malformations is unknown, but they do not appear to be related to portal hypertension, which is responsible for one of the most serious complications of cirrhosis, bleeding esophageal and gastric varices. Palmar erythema, manifested as a diffuse or splotchy erythema

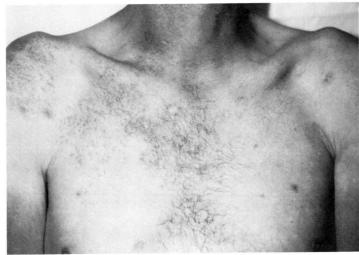

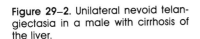
Figure 29–2. Unilateral nevoid telangiectasia in a male with cirrhosis of the liver.

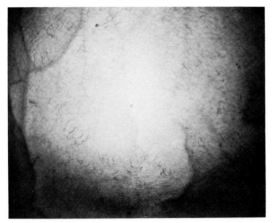

Figure 29–3. Dilated abdominal wall veins associated with cirrhosis and portal hypertension.

on the thenar and hypothenar eminences and tips of the fingers, frequently accompanies the development of the spider angiomas. Palmar erythema also occurs in healthy individuals as well as in association with non-hepatic diseases. There may be widespread appearance of thin, wiry telangiectasias in some patients, and, occasionally, the lesions appear in a unilateral distribution (Fig. 29–2).

Various forms of nail disease have been described in patients with cirrhosis, including the classic white nails of Terry. Terry's nails are characterized by a nailplate that is opaque white with the exception of the distal portion, which retains its normal pink color (Fig. 29–4). In addition, patients may develop transverse white bands (Muehrcke's nails), clubbed nails, or koilonychia (spoon-shaped nails), but none of these nail changes is specific for liver disease. Changes in body hair are common and are noted primarily in men. The axillary, pubic, and pectoral hair

is usually sparse, but thinning of all body hair is common also. There is often development of a female pubic hair pattern, coinciding with other evidence of feminization, including testicular softening and gynecomastia (Fig. 29–5).

There are a number of non-specific systemic symptoms associated with cirrhosis of the liver, especially weakness, anorexia, nausea, weight loss, and abdominal discomfort. Pruritus is less common in patients with cirrhosis than it is in patients with intrahepatic cholestasis, seen in such diseases as primary biliary cirrhosis, sclerosing cholangitis, or chronic extrahepatic biliary obstruction. The cirrhotic liver is usually small, firm, and nodular, and the spleen is often enlarged. Ascites may cause remarkable distention of the abdominal cavity. Owing to impaired hepatic function, prothrombin deficiency may develop, resulting in cutaneous purpura, epistaxis, and gingival bleeding. This deficiency also causes difficulty in controlling the bleeding from varices. The use of intramuscular vitamin K to help reverse the prothrombin deficiency has led to recent, but rare, reports of unusual annular erythematous reactions surrounding the injection site.

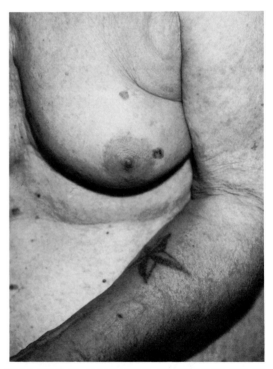

Figure 29–5. Gynecomastia in an adult male with cirrhosis of the liver.

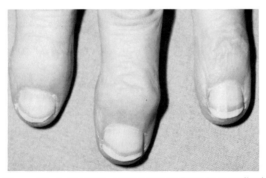

Figure 29–4. Opaque white nails of Terry in a patient with cirrhosis.

A view of the diagnosis, course, treatment, and prognosis of cirrhosis is beyond the scope of this chapter. There is, however, one additional point concerning cirrhosis that is especially important for dermatologists, and this is the inducement of the disease with methotrexate in the treatment of psoriasis. Methotrexate-induced cirrhosis appears to be related primarily to the total dosage of methotrexate therapy and is more likely to occur in patients who have been taking the drug for more than 5 or 10 years. Other parameters that may be important in increasing the likelihood of the development of cirrhosis in these patients include the age of the patient, obesity, presence of diabetes mellitus, and alcohol intake. There are well-established guidelines for liver biopsies, and, more recently, non-invasive scanning techniques have been used to follow liver function in patients on long-term methotrexate therapy.

PRIMARY BILIARY CIRRHOSIS

Primary biliary cirrhosis, a relatively uncommon form of cirrhosis occurring primarily in women between the ages of 40 and 60, deserves special recognition because the combination of pruritus, jaundice, hyperpigmentation, and xanthomas is specific for the disease. It is felt that the destruction of the small intrahepatic bile ducts, the primary defect in primary biliary cirrhosis, occurs on an immunologic basis. Abnormalities have been detected in both B and T cell function. Primary biliary cirrhosis may occur in patients with other autoimmune diseases, such as rheumatoid arthritis, thyroiditis, and the CREST* syndrome, and it may be familial. The first and often foremost symptom of primary biliary cirrhosis is pruritus, which is the presenting complaint in half the patients. Patients may have multiple excoriations, and it is not unusual to see a pattern of post-inflammatory hyperpigmentation in the so-called butterfly configuration on the back (Fig. 29–6). This pattern results from the fact that patients have difficulty reaching the skin of the upper central back but can readily scratch the periphery. The skin in the central area appears relatively normal, whereas the border is hyperpigmented and,

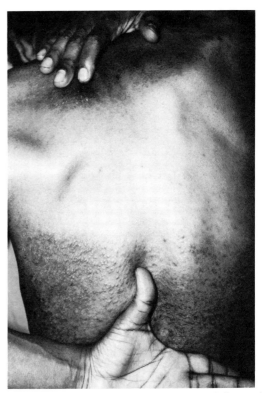

Figure 29–6. Post-inflammatory hyperpigmentation and lichenification from scratching, producing the "butterfly" configuration in a patient with primary biliary cirrhosis.

not infrequently, lichenified, producing the butterfly configuration. Patients also develop jaundice, hyperpigmentation, and xanthomas, which are due to the associated hyperlipidemia. The xanthomas may be very striking and include xanthelasma, planar xanthomas in palmar creases (Fig. 29–7; Plate VE) and in scars, tuberous xanthomas over the extensor aspects of joints and pressure areas, and, rarely, tendinous xanthomas. Late in the course of the disease, patients may develop osteomalacia (secondary to diminished absorption of vitamin D), portal hypertension, and hepatic failure.

HEMOCHROMATOSIS

Hemochromatosis, also known as bronze diabetes, is an autosomal recessive disease characterized by cutaneous hyperpigmentation, diabetes mellitus, and cirrhosis of the liver. There is a basic defect of iron metabolism in hemochromatosis, resulting in increased absorption of iron from the intestine and in deposition of this element in various

---

*Calcinosis, Raynaud's phenomenon, esophageal disease, sclerodactyly, and telangiectasia (see Chapter 3).

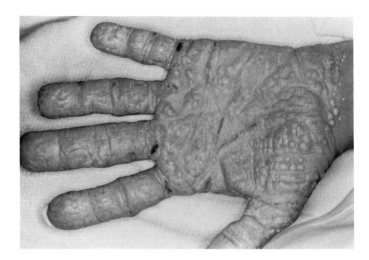

Figure 29–7. Multiple planar xanthomas in primary biliary cirrhosis (see also Plate V*E*).

tissues, especially the skin, liver, heart, pancreas, and endocrine organs. There are also secondary forms of hemochromatosis that may result from excessive oral intake of iron, from repeated transfusions in patients with refractory anemia, or from congenital transferrin deficiency. Unlike primary biliary cirrhosis, 90% of patients with hemochromatosis are male. The disease usually becomes clinically apparent between the ages of 40 and 60. The hyperpigmentation is generalized but accentuated in exposed areas. A small percentage of patients will develop pigmentation on oral mucous membranes and on the conjunctivae, which is not dissimilar to the pattern of pigmentation seen in Addison's disease. Hyperpigmentation is the presenting manifestation in one third of patients, and it is usually a distinctive metallic gray, although it may be brown. It results from an increase in melanin in the skin, presumably as a result of stimulation of the melanin producing system by the high iron stores. The skin also tends to be dry and scaly, and patients may develop other changes in the skin, hair, and nails identical to those seen with cirrhosis of the liver. There are extracutaneous features that are common as well, including diabetes mellitus, gonadal deficiency, heart disease, and a distinctive arthropathy with chondrocalcinosis. Unlike many other forms of cirrhosis, there is an effective form of therapy for some patients with hemochromatosis, namely, removal of iron stores by repeated phlebotomy.

WILSON'S DISEASE

Wilson's disease (hepatolenticular degeneration) is also a rare autosomal recessive

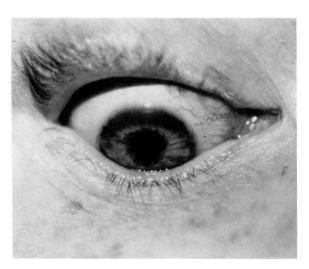

Figure 29–8. Pigmented band at the periphery of the cornea in Wilson's disease (Kayser-Fleischer ring).

disease associated with cirrhosis, but its clinical and pathologic manifestations result from excessive accumulation of copper in many tissues, especially the brain, liver, cornea, and kidneys. The triad of basal ganglia degeneration, cirrhosis of the liver, and a pathognomonic pigmentation of the corneal margins (Kayser-Fleischer ring) is characteristic of the disease. The Kayser-Fleischer ring is a golden brown or greenish-brown circle of pigment produced by the deposition of copper in Descemet's membrane at the periphery of the cornea (Fig. 29–8). This ocular finding can be important diagnostically, but the majority of patients present with either neurologic symptoms or hepatic insufficiency. The prognosis of Wilson's disease is often grave because of a delay in early diagnosis before irreparable damage has been done to the liver and nervous system. One other physical finding that might suggest the diagnosis of Wilson's disease is the presence of blue lunulae, although this azure color can be seen in normal individuals as well as in patients taking phenolphthalein or antimalarials. Wilson's disease is often treated with D-penicillamine, which is associated with many cutaneous problems, but in particular elastosis perforans serpiginosa may develop from this drug.

CUTANEOUS DISEASE ASSOCIATED WITH VIRAL HEPATITIS

Viral hepatitis is caused by several agents, and the clinical course varies from subclinical and inapparent infections to severe and fulminant disease with liver failure and death. There are viruses that preferentially attack the hepatocyte, especially hepatitis viruses A, B, and non-A–non-B; however, there are other viruses that are commonly associated with acute hepatitis, including the Epstein-Barr virus (infectious mononucleosis), cytomegalovirus, rubella, herpes simplex, and yellow fever.

The hepatitis virus that is most frequently associated with dermatological syndromes is hepatitis B virus, the causative organism of serum or long incubation hepatitis. Over 200,000 people in the United States develop hepatitis B infection annually, and 250 die of acute disease, 4000 die of hepatitis B–induced cirrhosis, and approximately 800 die of associated liver cancer. Hepatitis B is spread primarily via parenteral routes, either by overt inoculation (transfusion, infection with a contaminated needle, etc.) or by intimate personal contact, including contact between sexual partners and between affected patients and health professionals. Consequently, infection with hepatitis B occurs with an increased frequency among certain groups of people, not uncommonly in dentists and dental technicians, nurses, physicians, and medical laboratory technicians and personnel who are exposed to contaminated blood and blood products. This is extremely important because, unlike most other causes of viral hepatitis, hepatitis B infection may be chronic, either in association with demonstrable liver disease or in otherwise seemingly healthy carriers. This fact has led to increased emphasis for physicians and other health professionals to wear surgical gloves when they are exposed to possibly contaminated body fluids. This would include the use of protective gloves for minor office procedures. There has also been increased emphasis for health care personnel to receive immunization with the hepatitis B virus vaccine.

There are several dermatological syndromes that have been associated with hepatitis B infection, including a serum sickness–like prodrome, essential mixed cryoglobulinemia, papular acrodermatitis of childhood (Gianotti-Crosti syndrome), and polyarteritis nodosa. The cutaneous manifestations of the serum sickness–like prodrome include urticarial lesions, angioedema, erythema multiforme, or erythema nodosum–like lesions. Palpable purpura (vasculitis), erythrocyanosis, and Raynaud's phenomenon may be seen in patients with essential mixed cryoglobulinemia. A papular dermatitis on the face and limbs is seen in papular acrodermatitis of childhood, usually in association with lymphadenopathy and acute anicteric hepatitis (Fig. 29–9). There have been reports of this relatively uncommon disorder, which is seen primarily in children under 6 years of age, occurring in association with viruses other than hepatitis B. The high incidence of polyarteritis nodosa (PAN) and hepatitis B virus infection has been questioned, but it has been reported that up to 50% of PAN cases have evidence of infection with this virus. This multisystem disorder may have dermatological manifestations, especially nodules, livedo reticularis, and ulceration, most com-

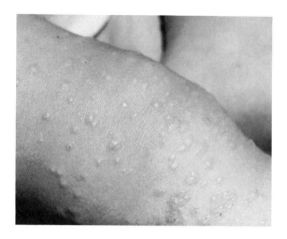

Figure 29–9. Multiple, 2–3 mm rounded papules on the knee in a 3-year-old male with papular acrodermatitis of childhood.

monly on the lower extremities. The nodules develop along the course of arteries, are frequently painful, and may ulcerate.

Suggested Readings

Cartwright GE, et al: Hereditary hemochromatosis. N Engl J Med *301*:175–179, 1979.

Food and Drug Administration: Safety of hepatitis B vaccine confirmed. FDA Drug Bull *15*:14–15, 1985.

Garden JM, Ostrow JD, Roenigk HH Jr: Pruritus in hepatic cholestasis. Arch Dermatol *121*:1415–1420, 1985.

McElgunn P: Dermatologic manifestations of hepatitis B infection. J Am Acad Derm *8*:539–548, 1983.

Ockner RK: Acute viral hepatitis. *In* Wyngaarden JB, Smith LH (eds): Cecil Textbook of Medicine, 16th ed. Philadelphia, WB Saunders Co., 1982, pp. 778–785.

Reynolds FS, Lee WM: Hepatotoxicity after long-term methotrexate therapy. South Med J *79*:536–539, 1986.

Sherlock S: Primary biliary cirrhosis. *In* Wright R, et al (eds): Liver and Biliary Diseases. Philadelphia, WB Saunders Co., 1979, pp. 715–734.

Strickland GT, Leu ML: Wilson's disease. Clinical and laboratory manifestations in 40 patients. Medicine (Baltimore) *54*:113–137, 1973.

Tomecki KJ, Cataloro CJ: Dapsone hypersensitivity: The sulfone syndrome revisited. Arch Dermatol *117*:38–39, 1981.

Weiss VC, West DP, Ackerman R, et al: Hepatotoxic reactions in a patient treated with etretinate. Arch Dermatol *120*:104–106, 1984.

30

Pancreatic Diseases

KENNETH E. GREER

The cutaneous manifestations of pancreatic disease are related to both the exocrine and endocrine functions of this gland as well as to pancreatic carcinoma. Until 20 years ago, the majority of reports were of patients who had cutaneous changes relating to acute or chronic pancreatitis and, only rarely, to metastatic nodules from carcinoma of the pancreas. Since 1966, most reports in the dermatological literature have dealt with patients who have the glucagonoma syndrome with its cutaneous manifestation, known as necrolytic migratory erythema. However, the skin lesions resulting from disorders of the pancreas are variable and include hemorrhage, panniculitis, thrombophlebitis, metastatic nodules, and necrolytic migratory erythema, which includes lesions of both skin and mucous membranes (Table 30–1).

The exocrine pancreas secretes large quantities of enzymes in response to duodenal secretin and cholecystokinin-pancreozymin. The enzymes are grouped into those that digest starch (amylase), fat (lipase), and protein (trypsin and other proteolytic enzymes).

Table 30–1. NON-DIABETIC CUTANEOUS
MANIFESTATIONS OF PANCREATIC DISEASE

Cutaneous changes related to pancreatitis
  Cutaneous hemorrhage (Cullen's and Turner's signs)
  Panniculitis
Cutaneous changes related to pancreatic endocrine
    tumors
  Glucagonoma syndrome
  Other islet cell tumors
Cutaneous changes related to pancreatic carcinoma
  Metastatic nodules—especially to umbilicus
  Panniculitis
  Migratory thrombophlebitis

Pancreatitis is presumably related to autodigestion by proteolytic enzymes, but there are a host of etiologic factors responsible for this process, and, although none are specific, there are several cutaneous lesions related to pancreatitis. Endocrine tissue accounts for less than 1% of the weight of the gland, and it is composed of small islets that release either insulin from beta-cells or glucagon from alpha-cells. There are a number of cutaneous lesions associated with abnormal beta-cell function and the resulting diabetes mellitus (see Chapter 22), and the cutaneous lesions of the glucagonoma syndrome are now well recognized. Cutaneous manifestations of other pancreatic tumors include specific metastatic nodules, in addition to nonspecific signs and symptoms related to pancreatic carcinoma or pancreatic endocrine tumors, excluding glucagonomas.

CUTANEOUS LESIONS ASSOCIATED WITH PANCREATITIS

Pancreatitis is classified as acute or chronic, based upon whether or not the patient recovers after an acute episode or continues to have pain or evidence of insufficient exocrine or endocrine pancreatic secretion. Cutaneous disease is most often associated with acute pancreatitis, which has many causes, such as alcohol ingestion, diabetes, infections (including mumps and hepatitis), biliary tract disease (gallstones primarily), trauma, and drugs (thiazide diuretics, azathioprine, sulfonamides, and estrogens, among others). Abdominal pain and tenderness, nausea, vomiting, fever, and hypotension are common clinical findings in

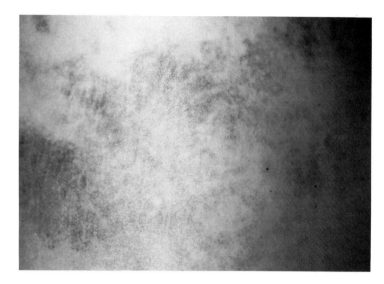

Figure 30–1. Purpura of left flank (Turner's sign) in a patient with acute hemorrhagic pancreatitis.

patients with acute pancreatitis, and the diagnosis can be established with the finding of an elevation of a single laboratory parameter, the serum amylase. There are 2 main types of skin lesions that may be seen in patients with acute pancreatitis: purpura and panniculitis. The first account of what was considered to be a specific cutaneous manifestation of acute hemorrhagic pancreatitis was recorded by Grey Turner in 1919. He reported a bluish patch of discoloration around the umbilicus in a patient suffering from pancreatitis. Initially believed to be due to fat necrosis, Turner's sign is, in reality, an ecchymosis arising from the subcutaneous extravasation of peritoneal hemorrhagic fluid (Fig. 30–1). This sign may be observed in as many as 5% of the cases of acute pancreatitis and may be seen occasionally in patients with other causes of hemorrhage into the peritoneum. Hemorrhagic discoloration of the flank (Fig. 30–2), described by Cullen in 1918 in association with ectopic pregnancy, may also occur in patients with acute pancreatitis as well as with other disorders causing retroperitoneal bleeding. Abdominal and truncal livedo reticularis has been reported in association with pancreatitis also.

Panniculitis is associated with both pancreatitis and pancreatic carcinoma and has been described as subcutaneous or nodular fat necrosis. It is thought to arise primarily from the action of enzymes (predominantly lipase) that are released into the circulation from the damaged pancreas, producing breakdown of subcutaneous fat. The result-

ing inflammatory subcutaneous nodules or plaques, 1–5 cm in diameter, occur especially on the lower legs, but also on the arms, buttocks, or trunk (Figs. 30–3 and 30–4). The lesions are frequently painful and, only in severe cases, spontaneously rupture, discharging a viscous, sterile material containing free and esterified cholesterol, neutral fats, soaps, and free fatty acids. In mild cases, the plaques involute within 2–3 weeks, leaving depressed hyperpigmented scars, but new crops tend to occur. Patients with extensive panniculitis are often febrile and have associated joint disease (synovitis, especially of small joints), abdominal pain, and vomiting. Panniculitis associated with pancreatitis usually occurs in patients in

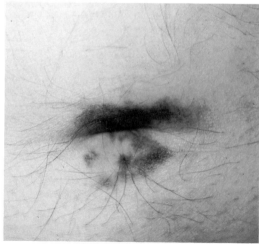

Figure 30–2. Periumbilical purpura (Cullen's sign) associated with acute hemorrhagic pancreatitis.

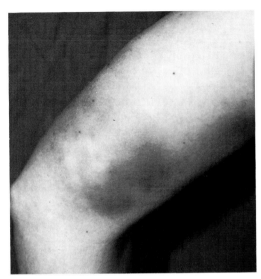

Figure 30–3. Large erythematous indurated area of posterior arm as a result of panniculitis.

their middle thirties or forties, whereas patients with cancer are usually significantly older and, in addition, are more likely to have blood eosinophilia and only slightly elevated or, occasionally, normal levels of serum amylase and lipase. The clinical differential diagnosis of pancreatic panniculitis includes erythema nodosum, Weber-Christian disease, nodular vasculitis, periarteritis nodosa, and lupus profundus.

Histologically, panniculitis associated with pancreatic disease is believed to be distinctive. These pathognomonic changes include foci of fat necrosis with "ghost-like"

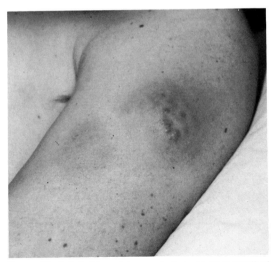

Figure 30–4. Painful nodules and plaques as a result of subcutaneous fat necrosis.

anucleate cells with thick "shadowy" walls and a surrounding inflammatory infiltrate of neutrophils, eosinophils, lymphocytes, histiocytes, and foreign body giant cells. Hemorrhage and secondary calcification are not uncommon, but vasculitis is not a part of pancreatic panniculitis. Therapy is supportive and is primarily treatment of the underlying pancreatic disease. The diagnosis of this disorder is important, owing to the fact that the underlying pancreatic disease may be carcinoma.

CUTANEOUS CHANGES RELATED TO PANCREATIC ENDOCRINE TUMORS

The majority of reports of cutaneous disease produced by non-diabetic pancreatic endocrine disorders have dealt with the glucagonoma syndrome. There are, however, pancreatic tumors that can synthesize a variety of hormones other than glucagon and insulin and that produce or are associated with cutaneous signs or symptoms. The tumors are usually benign and the hormones secreted by the tumors include gastrin (Zollinger-Ellison syndrome), somatostatin (somatostatinomas), ACTH (Cushing's syndrome), and prostaglandin and serotonin (pancreatic carcinoids). Patients with the carcinoid syndrome have typical flushing episodes. Patients or family members of patients with the Zollinger-Ellison syndrome have been reported to have an increased incidence of multiple lipomas. Patients with Cushing's syndrome as a result of ACTH secreting pancreatic islet cell tumors usually have less severe clinical manifestations than patients with Cushing's syndrome that is due to other causes, but the cutaneous changes, which are well known, may be very prominent. Other hormone secreting tumors may produce diarrhea, weight loss, and anemia, which may affect the skin indirectly and non-specifically.

The cutaneous eruption of the glucagonoma syndrome is known as necrolytic migratory erythema and, in the majority of cases, is a distinctive cutaneous marker of a tumor of pancreatic alpha-cells. The syndrome was first described by Becker and colleagues in 1942, was associated with carcinoma of the pancreas by McGovran in 1966, and was titled the glucagonoma syndrome by Maltinson and coworkers in 1974. Wilkinson named the distinctive skin changes "necrolytic migratory erythema" in 1971. Glucagonomas, which are usually malignant, occur more frequently without the typical cutaneous manifestations of the full syndrome. In addition, there have been rare reports of necrolytic migratory erythema occurring in patients without a pancreatic tumor or elevated levels of plasma glucagon. The majority of patients with the glucagonoma syndrome have insidious onset of symptoms that usually begin 1½–2 years before the diagnosis is made. By the time of diagnosis, however, the majority of patients have been found to have glucagonoma with metastases to the liver and regional lymph nodes. The disease has a predilection for middle-aged persons and has been reported more frequently in females.

There is considerable similarity of patients with the glucagonoma syndrome. In addition to the skin eruption necrolytic migratory erythema, patients frequently have stomatitis or glossitis, glucose intolerance, normochromic anemia (which may be profound and require repeated transfusions), weight loss, and diarrhea. Recurrent venous thrombosis, also a feature of non–endocrine secreting tumors of the pancreas, and depression have been reported to be associated with the glucagonoma syndrome. Fasting plasma glucagon levels (normally 50–200 pg/ml) are elevated in almost all patients and may be 5–10 times the normal level. Decreased blood amino acid levels are common also. The most distinctive feature of the syndrome is the cutaneous eruption, which usually occurs cyclically and has a characteristic distribution. The rash is frequently widespread but is most prominent in perioral and intertriginous areas, especially the perineum. The distal extremities and lower abdomen are common sites of involvement as well. Superficial necrosis of the epidermis produces an erosive and occasionally vesiculobullous dermatitis with crusting and eventual shedding of the skin. The base of the lesions is usually remarkably erythematous, and the borders are frequently annular or serpiginous. The active inflammatory process appears to cycle every 7–14 days. The differential diagnosis of well-developed skin lesions includes pemphigus, bullous pemphigoid, acrodermatitis enteropathica, essential fatty acid deficiency, and pellagra. However, the eruption frequently begins very insidiously and may mimic numerous cutaneous disorders, including eczema, contact dermatitis, configurate erythemas, moniliasis, psoriasis, and staphylococcal pyoderma. In addition, there are a number of reports of patients with glucagomas in whom there has been no mention of a skin eruption.

Histologically, biopsy specimens of early skin lesions may be very helpful in establishing the diagnosis of the glucagonoma syndrome. Marked spongiosis, frank necrolysis of the upper epidermis, and accumulation of neutrophils in the epidermis are characteristic. Occasionally clefting and intraepidermal bullae are seen, but acantholysis does not occur. The mild inflammatory infiltrate in the dermis is composed primarily of mononuclear cells and is predominantly perivascular. These same changes have been described in patients with pellagra and acrodermatitis enteropathica. The pathogenesis of the skin eruption is unknown, but there have been reports of improvement of the cutaneous process after the intravenous administration of amino acids.

Once the possibility of the diagnosis of glucagonoma syndrome has been raised (based usually on the skin lesions and elevated plasma glucagon levels), the search should be made for a pancreatic tumor. In addition, consideration should be given to other endocrine neoplasias in these patients and other family members, as familial glucagonoma has been reported in a family with multiple endocrine neoplasias. Resection of the tumor before metastatic spread has occurred is the goal, but partial removal of large tumors or metastases may result in significant clinical improvement. There are a number of chemotherapeutic agents that have been used with some success to treat patients with metastatic glucagonomas.

CUTANEOUS CHANGES RELATED TO NON–HORMONE SECRETING PANCREATIC CARCINOMA

Carcinoma of the pancreas is the fourth most common cancer causing death in the United States, accounting for over 20,000 deaths per year. The high mortality rate is largely due to the fact that over 85% of the tumors have metastasized at the time of diagnosis. Over 90% of the carcinomas are adenocarcinomas, with 65% involving the head of the pancreas, 30% involving both the body and tail, and 5% involving the tail alone. The classic symptoms of pancreatic

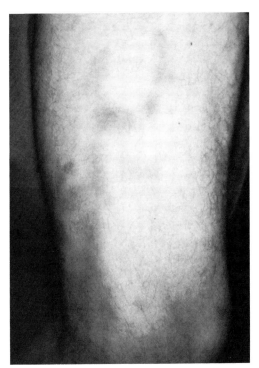

Figure 30–5. Multiple erythematous linear cords caused by superficial migratory thrombophlebitis.

thrombophlebitis of both superficial and deep veins is uncommon as well (Fig. 30–5). The association of this form of superficial phlebitis with carcinoma is attributed to Trousseau and was described in 1865. Interestingly, the presenting manifestation of the gastric cancer that led to Trousseau's death was venous thrombosis. Carcinoma of the pancreas accounts for approximately 30% of the tumors associated with thrombophlebitis, and it is second in this only to carcinoma of the lung. Classically, the phlebitis occurs in short segments of superficial veins and is distributed on the trunk and neck as well as on the extremities. Involvement of the veins of the upper extremities is not uncommon, a very unusual location in thrombosis unassociated with a malignant condition. The phlebitis is often resistant to anticoagulant therapy and may lead to a life-threatening embolic phenomenon. The inflammatory changes may resolve in a few weeks spontaneously, only to recur in the same or distant veins. The pathogenesis is unknown.

carcinoma are weight loss, abdominal pain, anorexia, and jaundice. The 3 most common cutaneous manifestations of non–hormone secreting pancreatic adenocarcinomas are metastatic skin nodules; migratory thrombophlebitis; and panniculitis, specifically subcutaneous or nodular fat necrosis. Panniculitis occurs most frequently with pancreatitis but has also been described in patients with adenocarcinoma of the pancreas and, rarely, with pancreas divisum, a congenital pancreatic ductal abnormality. Cutaneous metastases, especially to the umbilicus, are not common from pancreatic carcinoma, but approximately 10% of umbilical metastases (Sister Mary Joseph's nodule) occur from pancreatic tumors. Migratory

Suggested Readings

Huges PS, Aspisarnthanarax P, Mullins JF: Subcutaneous fat necrosis associated with pancreatic disease. Arch Dermatol *111*:506–510, 1975.

Nusbacher J: Migratory venous thrombosis and cancer. NY State J Med *64*:2166, 1964.

Parker CM, Hanke CW, Madura JA, et al: Glucagonoma syndrome: Case report and literature review. J Dermatol Surg Oncol *10*:884–889, 1984.

Powel F, Cooper A, Massa A, et al: Sister Mary Joseph's nodule: A clinical and histologic study. J Am Acad Dermatol *10*:610–615, 1984.

Sibrack LA, Gouterman IH: Cutaneous manifestations of pancreatic disease. Cutis *21*:763–768, 1978.

Sigmund WJ, Shelley WB: Cutaneous manifestations of acute pancreatitis with special reference to livedo reticularis. N Engl J Med *251*:851, 1954.

Vandersteen PR, Scheithauer BW: Glucagonoma syndrome. A clinicopathologic, immunocytochemical, and ultrastructural study. J Am Acad Dermatol *12*:1032–1039, 1985.

31

Nutritional Disease

JOSEPH L. JORIZZO

PROTEIN DISORDERS

Starvation in young children with protein-energy malnutrition is termed marasmus. Marasmus, unlike kwashiorkor, is not associated with edema or dermatological changes. Kwashiorkor is a form of protein-energy malnutrition that occurs in the setting of preserved subcutaneous fat. These patients compensate for an inadequate intake of protein by eating excesses of starches and sugars. The problem of starving children manifests itself primarily in impoverished areas of the world and is a major economic, moral, social, and political problem. In the United States, protein-energy malnutrition is more commonly seen in settings associated with abnormal protein absorption, increased protein loss, or diseases that produce generalized wasting. Examples would be short bowel syndrome, protein losing enteropathies, metastatic cancer, or chronic renal failure. Another set of causes is related to reduced protein-energy intake as a result of fad diets or psychiatric diseases such as anorexia nervosa.

Kwashiorkor is characterized classically by the recently weaned child who develops a peeling, "enamel paint" dermatosis, hyperpigmentation, edema, and depigmented bands in the hair (flag sign). Patients also have hepatosplenomegaly, muscle wasting, psychologic and behavioral changes, and diarrhea. Paradoxically, the appetite is reduced, which is not a feature of marasmus.

The initially erythematous cutaneous lesions become hyperpigmented and have a dry, cracked appearance (Fig. 31–1). The hair becomes thin, brittle, and hypopigmented, and it does not grow significantly.

The flag sign results from a demarcation by hypopigmentation of areas of hair produced during periods of the most severe protein-energy malnutrition. The nails also become thin.

Laboratory abnormalities include anemia, hypoalbuminemia, hypoglycemia, and hypolipidemia. Cardiac output and renal blood flow are often reduced. Cellular immunity is impaired, and complement components and secretory IgA levels are reduced.

The mortality rate in kwashiorkor exceeds 30%. Complications include parasitosis, sepsis, and tuberculosis. Ultimate body height and scholastic aptitude are also reduced.

Treatment is complicated by patient intolerance of fats and other foods as a result of reduced lipases. Vitamin supplementation that includes trace metals is critical, owing to the frequency of multiple simultaneous deficiencies. High protein diet supplements made with soybean protein or cow's milk are available. Parenteral hyperalimentation, if performed, must be accompanied by careful cardiocirculatory monitoring, owing to decreased cardiac reserve in these patients.

VITAMIN AND MINERAL DISORDERS

Vitamin A. Vitamin A and its precursor, beta-carotene, are present in the normal diet. The absorbed vitamin circulates as retinol, bound to specific retinol binding protein (pre-albumin on electrophoresis), and is stored in the liver. Vitamin A is an extremely important molecule that has crucial functions in vision, carbohydrate metabolism, glycoprotein synthesis, and the maintenance of epithelial surfaces. This last effect on

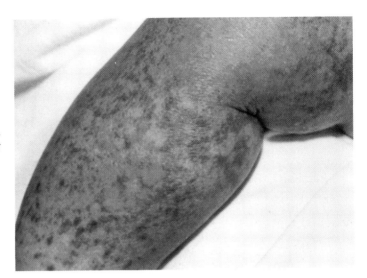

Figure 31-1. Edematous and slightly erythematous skin is present in this patient with malnutrition.

epithelial surfaces has prompted the search for safer derivatives of vitamin A to treat dermatological disorders of keratinization. Isotretinoin (Accutane) and etretinate (Tegison) are the currently available derivatives.

Vitamin A is stored in the liver, and acute and chronic toxicity is possible from excessive ingestion. Acute toxicity results in cutaneous exfoliation, increased intracranial pressure, and even death. Chronic toxicity includes the following changes: alopecia, generalized scaling, liver fibrosis, intracranial hypertension, remolding of bone, hypoplastic bone marrow, and other systemic toxicities.

Ocular signs of vitamin A deficiency include xerosis of the conjunctiva and cornea, and keratomalacia. Night blindness is often a presenting complaint. In some patients on oral retinoid therapy, competition for the vitamin A receptors in the eye may result in decreased night vision. Cutaneous lesions result from hyperkeratinization and epidermal hyperplasia. Although follicular hyperkeratosis, termed phrynoderma, was originally described as a classic cutaneous marker for vitamin A deficiency, the changes of phrynoderma are not seen in nutritional deprivation experiments. The most frequent cutaneous finding is extreme xerosis. Vitamin A deficiency may occur in the setting of inadequate dietary intake or with fat malabsorption secondary to diseases that affect the gastrointestinal tract.

Vitamin B$_1$ (Thiamine). Thiamine is a vitamin that is concentrated in the outer layer of seeds, grains, and peas and is present in yeast and in certain animal tissues. This vitamin is important in carbohydrate metabolism and in decarboxylation of keto acids. Deficiency of this important vitamin is associated with several well known syndromes, including beriberi, Wernicke's encephalopathy, and Korsakoff's syndrome. Although dietary deficiency (e.g., diet of exclusively polished rice) is a cause of thiamine deficiency in Asia, malabsorption of thiamine as a result of the folate deficiency of alcoholism is the principal cause in the United States. Dry beriberi leads to peripheral neuritis–induced muscle wasting. Wet beriberi is characterized by generalized edema that is due to cardiac enlargement and cardiac failure. The edema and a burning, red tongue are the mucocutaneous finding of beriberi.

Vitamin B$_2$ (Riboflavin). Animal protein and some vegetables are good sources of riboflavin, which is an important coenzyme in many oxidation-reduction reactions in the body. Deficiency of riboflavin is associated with corneal vascularization, interstitial keratitis and other ocular changes, inflammation of the lips, flattened lingual papillae, and a seborrheic dermatitis–like eruption and a scrotal dermatitis. These changes are termed oro-oculo-genital syndrome.

Vitamin B$_6$ (Pyridoxine). Vitamin B$_6$ is present in meats, dairy products, eggs, and whole grains. It functions as a coenzyme in various metabolic reactions involving proteins, carbohydrates, and lipids. The most common settings for deficiency are alcoholism; infantile deficiency as a result of use of processed foods; and an increase in the minimal daily requirement induced by drugs such as isoniazid, hydralazine, and D-penicillamine.

Excess vitamin B$_6$ is associated with a sensory neuropathy and deficiency with a dermatological syndrome with combined features like those of pellagra and essential fatty acid deficiency. Glossitis and a seborrheic dermatitis–like eruption are also features of pyridoxine deficiency.

Vitamin B$_{12}$ (Cobalamin). Cobalamin, with folic acid, is involved in deoxyribonucleic acid synthesis. Symmetrical hyperpigmentation of the extremities is a dermatological feature of cobalamin deficiency.

Niacin. Nicotinamide, a niacin derivative, is a crucial component of coenzyme I and coenzyme II, which are important in oxidation-reduction reactions in the body. Niacin can be produced in the body via conversion from tryptophan. Dietary deficiency of niacin or tryptophan can produce the niacin deficiency syndrome known as pellagra. Pellagra may occur as a result of deficiency in chronic alcoholism or food faddism or from alterations in tryptophan metabolism in carcinoid syndrome, Hartnup's disease, and with isoniazid therapy for tuberculosis.

Pellagra is characterized clinically by the "three Ds": dermatitis, diarrhea, and dementia. Severe diarrhea is the usual initial manifestation of pellagra. The initial dermatosis is an erythematous eruption in a sun-exposed distribution. The eruption then becomes bullous and later is characterized by a hyperpigmented, "peeling paint" appearance. The skin becomes progressively harder, darker, and drier. The skin, on the chest and face especially, shows a sebaceous gland prominence called "goose skin." Casal's necklace is a band of dermatosis around the neck. There frequently is an associated oro-oculo-genital syndrome, as is seen in riboflavin deficiency, with severe genital dermatitis. Neuropsychiatric disease may be irreversible if allowed to persist for too long without treatment.

Biotin. Biotin is synthesized by intestinal bacteria and is an important coenzyme in many carboxylation reactions. Patients who eat raw eggs may become biotin deficient as a result of biotin-avidin binding (i.e., avidin is present in uncooked egg white). A scaly eczematous eruption, alopecia, lethargy, and hypotonia have been attributed to biotin deficiency.

Pantothenic Acid. This vitamin forms part of coenzyme A, which is involved in acetylation metabolic reactions. Neuromuscular signs and symptoms, diarrhea and vomiting, and possibly the "burning feet" syndrome seen in World War II prisoners are manifestations of deficiency of this vitamin.

Folic Acid. Folic acid is important for thymidine (a building block of deoxyribonucleic acid) synthesis. Deficiency may be dietary or a result of malabsorption. Megaloblastic anemia is a reflection of a megaloblastosis of all cells. Glossitis is a mucocutaneous feature. Peripheral neuropathy may occur.

Vitamin C. Vitamin C (ascorbic acid) is available in citrus fruits, tomatoes, and green vegetables. It is required for proper collagen production. The disease state associated with deficiency of vitamin C is scurvy. Vitamin C deficiency in the United States may

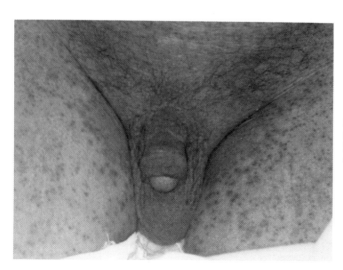

Figure 31–2. Vitamin C deficiency. Seborrheic distribution with purpuric lesions are present in this man with scurvy that is due to excessive alcohol intake.

occur in association with alcohol abuse or in food faddists. Follicular hyperkeratosis with "corkscrew hair" is an early cutaneous feature of scurvy (Fig. 31–2). These lesions become hemorrhagic as a result of poor connective tissue support in immediate hemostasis. Gingivitis may be severe. Peripheral edema, slow wound healing, and depressed mental activity are later features of scurvy.

Vitamin D. Vitamin D derivatives are formed by ultraviolet light effects on the epidermis. Precursors are absorbed from the bowel and are found in milk, egg yolk, and fish liver oils. The vitamin and its derivatives are crucial for calcium regulation. Rickets, with its resultant bone and cartilage abnormalities, results from deficiency of vitamin D. Metastatic calcification of skin may occur with vitamin D excess.

Vitamin E (Tocopherol). Vitamin E deficiency may be associated with shortened erythrocyte survival and possibly with a seborrheic dermatitis–like eruption.

Vitamin K. Vitamin K is present in many plants and is produced by intestinal bacteria. It is necessary for the synthesis of prothrombin by the liver. Ecchymoses are the findings in vitamin K deficiency. Vitamin K is a fat soluble vitamin (like vitamins A, D, and E) and can be malabsorbed. Coumarin derivatives are competitive antagonists of vitamin K.

Zinc. Zinc is an essential mineral that is required for growth and differentiation. It is involved in the metabolism of proteins, carbohydrates, lipids, and nucleic acids.

Acrodermatitis enteropathica was for years a perplexing dermatosis characterized by a "peely paint" cutaneous eruption in the groin, acral, and perioral area; by alopecia; by severe diarrhea; and by growth retardation and mental status changes. The condition is inherited as an autosomal recessive trait. Acrodermatitis enteropathica, which is potentially fatal, was shown in the mid-1970s to result from an inherited abnormality in gastrointestinal zinc transport. Pharmacologic doses of oral zinc result in a disappearance of all clinical signs and symptoms in these patients.

A clinicopathologically identical syndrome has been described as acquired zinc deficiency in patients on total parenteral nutrition that does not contain zinc (Fig. 31–3). Abnormalities of neutrophil chemotaxis have been reported in patients with zinc deficiency. These abnormalities are reversi-

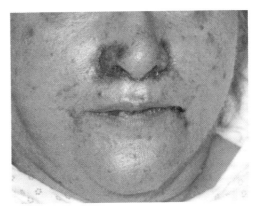

Figure 31–3. Zinc deficiency in a patient with hyperalimentation following surgery. Note the seborrheic distribution.

ble with correction of the zinc deficiency state. Other factors involved in inflammation are also modulated by zinc.

Copper. Copper is another essential mineral. Menkes kinky hair syndrome is a rare X-linked disorder that may result from an inherited defect in intercellular copper transport. The hair changes are pili torti, and a seborrheic dermatitis–like cutaneous eruption occurs. Patients experience progressive neurologic disease and early death. There is no effective treatment.

An infantile nutritional copper deficiency syndrome has been described. These infants have anemia, bone changes, psychomotor retardation, and defective pigmentation of skin and of hair.

Iron. Hemochromatosis, with iron overloading, is associated with hyperpigmentation (i.e., bronze diabetes), cirrhosis, and diabetes mellitus. Koilonychia (spoon nails) has been associated with iron deficiency.

Suggested Readings

Ellis CN, Vanderveen EE, Rasmussen JE: Scurvy: A case caused by peculiar dietary habits. Arch Dermatol 120:1212–1214, 1984.

James WPT: Kwashiorkor and marasmus: Old concepts and new developments. Proc R Soc Med 70:611–619, 1977.

Logan WS: Vitamin A and keratinization. Arch Dermatol 105:748–753, 1972.

Norris D: Zinc and cutaneous inflammation. Arch Dermatol 121:985–989, 1985.

Stratigos JD, Katsambas A: Pellagra: A still existing disease. Br J Dermatol 96:99–106, 1977.

Williams MC, Packman S, Cowan MJ: Alopecia and periorificial dermatitis in biotin-responsive multiple carboxylase deficiency. J Am Acad Dermatol 9:97–103, 1983.

VI

CUTANEOUS INFECTIOUS DISEASES

32

Viral Diseases

NEAL PENNEYS

A panoply of skin changes can be associated with systemic viral disease. Recognition of the primary lesion can immediately narrow the list of diagnostic possibilities of the cause of the exanthem. Viral exanthems will be considered in groups, depending on their primary lesion in the skin.

SYSTEMIC VIRAL DISEASES ASSOCIATED PRIMARILY WITH A MACULAR RASH

Rubella

Rubella, or German measles, is a common viral infection that primarily affects children and young adults. The prodrome, which lasts 1–2 days, is followed by a pink-red eruption that begins on the face and spreads to the neck, trunk, and extremities. Characteristic tender lymphadenopathy is found in the posterior occipital and nuchal regions. As the rash resolves, there may be fine scaling. Rubella infection of the fetus leads to a syndrome characterized by a number of findings, primarily affecting a variety of internal organ systems. In the skin, there may be a morbilliform rash similar to that seen in adults. An unusual manifestation that leads to a characteristic skin finding is bone marrow infection that leads to widespread bleeding in the skin, resulting in the "blueberry muffin baby."

Patient Evaluation. In adults, the diagnosis is usually made on clinical grounds. In children, virus may be grown from various sites. A variety of antibodies can be detected against rubella, and serologic testing can be obtained to confirm infection with the virus. An increase in titer of several dilutions is necessary to confirm diagnosis. Rubella must be differentiated from other infections, particularly rubeola and scarlet fever. The characteristic tender lymphadenopathy coupled with the rash and the mild nature of the infection usually serves to differentiate rubella from rubeola (which also has Koplik's spots) and scarlet fever (which characteristically has circumoral pallor, strawberry tongue, and Pastia's sign).

Therapy. Rubella is usually a self-limited disease with no serious sequelae. Treatment is supportive. When infection occurs in a pregnant woman in her first trimester, a therapeutic abortion is recommended.

Measles (Rubeola)

Measles is produced by infection with a paramyxovirus. After a 7–14 day period of incubation, a prodrome of conjunctivitis, upper respiratory symptoms, and coryza develops. Several days later the rash appears and lasts for several days. The most characteristic mucocutaneous finding associated with measles is the Koplik spot, a red spot with a blue-white center that occurs most commonly on the buccal mucosa. The cutaneous expression of this viral disease begins as a macular eruption on the forehead and ears and subsequently spreads downward to involve other body areas. The eruption usually resolves in the same sequence, with mild desquamation.

Histopathology. In the skin, the predominant histopathologic change is the presence of an inflammatory infiltrate in the dermis. Epidermal giant cells may be present, as they are in Koplik's spots. Rarely, intranuclear

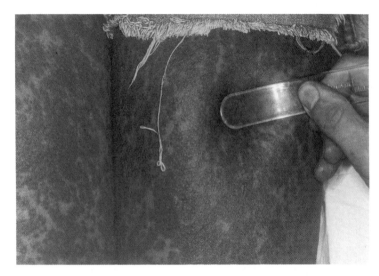

Figure 32–1. Ampicillin rash in a patient with infectious mononucleosis.

inclusion bodies may be noted in keratinocytes.

Patient Evaluation. Many serologic tests are available to identify antibodies specific for measles virus. The clinical presentation is so typical as to be diagnostic in itself. In patients who have received incomplete immunization for measles virus but who are exposed to measles and develop clinical infection, the rash and clinical picture may be atypical. In these cases, a history of exposure and immunization usually lead to the diagnosis of atypical measles infection.

Therapy. Treatment is supportive.

Infectious Mononucleosis

Infectious mononucleosis follows infection with the Epstein-Barr virus. Infection with this virus is widespread. It usually occurs in childhood and is largely asymptomatic. There is a well-described association of infection by this virus with the subsequent development of nasopharyngeal carcinoma and Burkitt's lymphoma.

Clinical Findings. A typical case of infectious mononucleosis begins with sore throat, fever, and lymphadenopathy. A number of cutaneous manifestations may be present in association with Epstein-Barr virus infection, and they include palatal petechiae, urticaria, macular and petechial eruptions, and erythema multiforme. When hepatic involvement is severe, jaundice may be present. A diffuse maculopapular eruption may develop in patients with infectious mono-

nucleosis who are treated with ampicillin (Fig. 32–1).

Patient Evaluation. Patients with infectious mononucleosis characteristically have a lymphocytosis. Atypical lymphocytes may be observed in the peripheral smear. Neutropenia and thrombocytopenia may also be present. Heterophile antibodies are present in about 90% of patients. Epstein-Barr virus–specific antibodies also appear during the course of the illness, and the virus can be cultured from the oropharynx or from lymphocytes. In typical cases, the diagnosis can be made on clinical grounds with serologic confirmation. A similar syndrome can be produced by infection with cytomegalovirus, which is heterophile antibody–negative. Viral hepatitis and toxoplasmosis can be separated by hepatitis-specific and toxoplasmosis-specific serologies, respectively.

Therapy. Therapy is for the most part supportive.

Cytomegalovirus

Cytomegalovirus belongs to the herpesvirus group and is a double-stranded DNA virus. Studies of antibodies to cytomegalovirus indicate that infection by this virus is ubiquitous and is often inapparent.

Clinical Findings. In congenital cytomegalovirus infection, the most common cutaneous manifestation is a petechial rash. In adults, cytomegalovirus infection can produce a syndrome similar to that of mononucleosis induced by Epstein-Barr virus.

The rash observed in adults may resemble rubella or may be non-specific in pattern. In patients who are immunosuppressed, cytomegalovirus has been known to produce hemorrhagic macular lesions and ulcerations.

Histopathology. Skin biopsy may show neutrophilic vasculitis. Characteristic intranuclear inclusion bodies may be seen in endothelial cells.

Patient Evaluation. The diagnosis of cytomegalovirus infection can be confirmed by growth of the virus or by demonstration of a rise in serologic titer.

Therapy. At the present time, treatment is primarily supportive.

Viral Hepatitis Infection

Acute viral hepatitis is a common and potentially dangerous infectious disease associated with a number of viral agents. There seems to be no association between the pattern of cutaneous eruption and a specific viral agent. Cutaneous manifestations of viral hepatitis are discussed in Chapter 29.

SYSTEMIC VIRAL DISEASES ASSOCIATED WITH A VESICULAR RASH

Hand-Foot-Mouth Disease

A variety of enteroviruses of the Coxsackie group (particularly coxsackievirus A16) have been associated with this syndrome. Children and young adults are most frequently infected. After a brief incubation period, a mild prodrome of malaise, fever, and abdominal discomfort develops. This is followed by the development of tender oral lesions found on the tongue and palate. Skin lesions develop simultaneously and are found primarily on the hands and feet. The lesions are well-circumscribed red papules with a vesicular center. The process resolves by slow desquamation.

Histopathology. There is an intraepidermal vesicle. Marked intracellular edema affects keratinocytes, and a dense inflammatory infiltrate occurs in the papillary dermis.

Patient Evaluation. Most of the exanthems produced by enterovirus are central and are therefore easily distinguished from those of hand-foot-mouth disease, which are acral. The eruption of hand-foot-mouth disease

may superficially resemble that of herpes simplex infection. Herpetic infection may be rapidly excluded by failure to demonstrate herpetic cytopathic changes in smears taken from the blister (Tzanck's preparation).

Therapy. This disease is self-limited. Treatment is supportive.

Herpes Simplex

Herpes simplex virus is a member of the herpesvirus family, which contains the varicella-zoster virus, cytomegalovirus, and Epstein-Barr virus.

Clinical Findings. Herpes simplex infection produces a characteristic recurrent vesicular eruption in healthy individuals (Fig. 32–2). Unusual morphologic presentations can herald and be associated with serious systemic disease. Neonatal disseminated herpetic infection is usually acquired by passage of the fetus through an actively infected birth canal. In this instance, vesicular lesions may be widespread on the skin and may be associated with spread to internal organs and to the central nervous system. In patients with acquired immune deficiency syndrome (AIDS), herpetic lesions are frequently indolent and present with a wide spectrum of morphologies. Chronic herpetic lesions may resemble ulcers, vegetations, blisters, and non-specific abrasions and may be on the skin and mucous membranes. Cutaneous disseminated herpes simplex infection can occur superimposed upon exten-

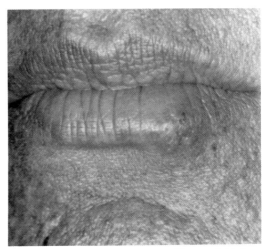

Figure 32–2. Typical appearance of herpes labialis on the lower lip in a patient with recurrent herpes simplex infection.

sive dermatitic processes such as atopic dermatitis and is known as Kaposi's varicelliform eruption.

Histopathology. Skin specimens show characteristic viral cytopathic changes, including epidermal giant cells and enlargement of nuclei with slate-gray tinctorial change. A variable inflammatory infiltrate occurs in the dermis.

Patient Evaluation. Tzanck's preparations (removal of blister roof, scraping of blister base, and staining of the material) reveal viral cytopathic changes typical of herpesvirus infection. Viral cultures will show growth of herpes simplex virus. Skin biopsy will also demonstrate characteristic features. In patients with AIDS or who have iatrogenic immunosuppression, it is important to suspect chronic herpetic infections, particularly in perianal, oral, and genital regions, even though the lesions may not be vesicular. In some patients, herpetic infections must be differentiated from other viral diseases such as hand-foot-mouth disease and from other vesicular processes such as contact dermatitis.

Therapy. Herpes simplex infection in normal individuals is self-limited and requires only local care. In patients with recurrent symptomatic herpes simplex infection, oral acyclovir may be used for long-term, low dose suppression because this agent has been reported to reduce the recurrence rate; however, there does not appear to be a long-term benefit. Topical acyclovir is only of use in shortening the course of the primary herpetic infection. In immunosuppressed individuals, topical acyclovir may be of use in suppressing some of the local changes induced by chronic infection. Extensive infection in these individuals demands systemic treatment with acyclovir, by either oral or intravenous routes.

Varicella

Varicella (chicken pox) is produced by a virus in the herpesvirus group. In healthy individuals, varicella is characterized by a minimal prodrome and by the onset of a vesicular rash about 2 weeks after exposure. The primary lesion evolves rapidly into a clear vesicle surrounded by a red flare (likened to a dew drop on a rose petal) (Fig. 32–3). The lesions develop over a period of several days, and thus at any one time there

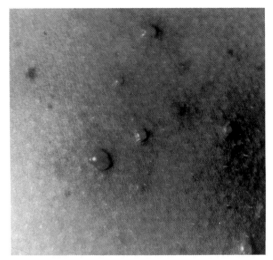

Figure 32–3. Small, vesicular lesions surrounded by a slight erythematous hue, representative of acute varicella.

are lesions in many stages. Healing with scarring is not uncommon, probably because of the associated pruritus. The greatest density of lesions is found centrally, and recurrent crops can occur. In children, varicella is usually a self-limited disease; in adults, varicella can be a serious systemic disease associated with primary varicella pneumonia. In immunosuppressed individuals, varicella infection may be associated with extensive pneumonia, involvement of the liver or central nervous system, and extensive internal dissemination. Extensive hemorrhagic skin lesions may also be present in these cases.

Histopathology. Skin biopsy reveals an intraepidermal vesicle containing epidermal giant cells and intranuclear changes typical of herpesvirus infection. There may be less inflammatory infiltrate than that seen in herpes simplex infection.

Patient Evaluation. Tzanck's preparation reveals characteristic herpesvirus-induced changes. If necessary, viral culture can be performed to confirm the diagnosis. Skin biopsy will reveal the changes described previously. Other viral vesicular diseases such as disseminated herpes simplex infection, dissemination in herpes zoster, and hand-foot-mouth disease must be considered. In adults, careful evaluation for pulmonary involvement is important.

Therapy. In healthy children and adults, varicella is a self-limited disease and therapy is supportive. In immunosuppressed patients or patients with severe pulmonary involvement, oral or intravenous acyclovir may be administered to help control the process.

Herpes Zoster

Herpes zoster is produced by the same virus that causes varicella (the varicella-zoster virus). In this case, the infection represents a reactivation of the patient's viral infection.

Clinical Findings. Most commonly, herpes zoster is associated with a painful prodrome in the involved dermatome (Fig. 32–4). When unusual dermatomes are involved, ordinary symptoms such as pleuritic pain, pain mimicking cardiac disease or gallbladder disease, and renal colic may occur. The eruption of herpes zoster is unilateral and evolves from urticarial red plaques to intense grouped vesicles and finally to ulcerations. Occasionally, herpes zoster will be associated primarily with urticarial lesions and few vesicles. Herpes zoster is acutely painful, and in certain individuals the pain may persist and will produce post-herpetic neuralgia. The frequency of post-herpetic neuralgia increases with age.

Patient Evaluation. The diagnosis is often obvious because of the dermatomal distribution and the prodromal symptoms. Viral cytopathic changes can be demonstrated in Tzanck's preparations and in tissue sections. Viral culture can be used to confirm the diagnosis. In disseminated forms of herpes zoster infections, there may be a problem separating this entity from varicella. However, accentuation of the eruption in a dermatome leads to the correct diagnosis.

Therapy. In healthy individuals, herpes zoster infection is self-limiting over several weeks. Local therapy and oral analgesics are usually sufficient. In patients over the age of 60, it has been shown that the administration of systemic corticosteroids within the first 7 days of the eruption decreases the risk of post-herpetic neuralgia. Corticosteroids, usually prednisone, are given orally over a 10–15 day course, starting with 60 mg per day. In disseminated disease, possibly with associated immunosuppression, oral or intravenous acyclovir can be administered to control the eruption. Acyclovir has not been shown to alter the incidence or severity of pain, either acutely or when occurring as post-herpetic neuralgia. The recent release of capsaicin, used topically, may be helpful for post-zoster neuralgia.

Systemic viral infection may produce an array of secondary lesions and alterations in the skin. Perhaps the most dramatic changes are those associated with infection by viruses of the human lymphotropic virus group.

HTLV-I INFECTION

HTLV-I infection is associated with human adult T cell lymphoma-leukemia syndrome.

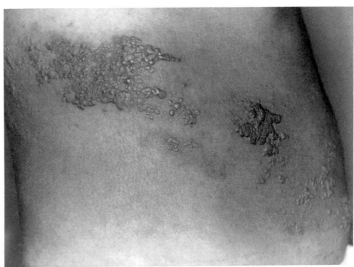

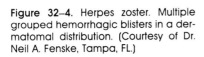

Figure 32–4. Herpes zoster. Multiple grouped hemorrhagic blisters in a dermatomal distribution. (Courtesy of Dr. Neil A. Fenske, Tampa, FL.)

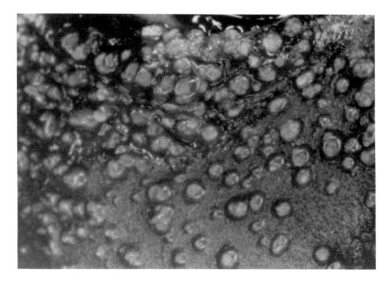

Figure 32–5. Multiple papules of molluscum contagiosum are present on the lower eyelid in this Haitian male with acquired immune deficiency syndrome.

HTLV-II INFECTION

HTLV-II has been isolated from sporadic cases of hairy cell leukemia. Infection with this virus has not been associated with significant cutaneous lesions.

HUMAN IMMUNODEFICIENCY VIRUS (HIV, FORMERLY HTLV-III)

Several lines of research have linked the retrovirus HIV to the pathogenesis of AIDS (acquired immune deficiency syndrome). HIV infects mature T cells, especially those of the helper-inducer phenotype, resulting in destruction of these cells and immunosuppression of the host. HIV differs from HTLV-I and II on morphologic, immunologic, and genetic grounds. The virus has a high degree of genetic polymorphism.

Clinical Findings. This infection is more commonly found in hemophiliacs, drug addicts who share contaminated syringes, individuals from Haiti, homosexual men, and individuals sexually exposed to a homosexual or bisexual male. There are no specific skin findings associated with the initial infection. Patients may have systemic symptoms at the time of infection. Cutaneous changes associated with AIDS almost invariably are related to the effects of immunosuppression or to the presence of neoplastic disease, usually in the form of Kaposi's sarcoma (see also Chapter 19). The most banal of cutaneous infections may present in

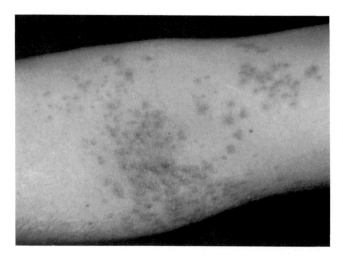

Figure 32–6. Chronic herpes simplex infection in a drug addict.

chronic, atypical, or florid forms in patients with AIDS (see also Chapters 33 and 34). The most frequently noted superficial infections include chronic herpetic infection, widespread and giant molluscum contagiosum (Fig. 32–5), extensive papillomavirus infection, chronic oral candidiasis, and disseminated herpes zoster or simplex infection (Figs. 32–6 and 32–7). Disseminated fungal disease, particularly cryptococcosis and histoplasmosis, can present with cutaneous lesions as the initial sign of infection. Unusual mycobacterial diseases, including hematogenous spread of tuberculosis as well as *Mycobacterium intracellularis* infection, have been reported in the skin. Patients with AIDS frequently have Kaposi's sarcoma. When this entity presents in the skin, it may be subtle and not have the characteristic features expected in Kaposi's sarcoma as seen in elderly individuals. Lesions can vary in color from pink to dark brown and purple. The skin lesions are usually macular, and there may be extensive involvement of the mucous membranes.

Histopathology. There is no specific histopathologic pattern associated with infection by this retrovirus. The pathologic pattern will reflect the secondary process, that of chronic infection; that of neoplasia, such as Kaposi's sarcoma; or that of a number of processes known to be associated with AIDS, such as seborrheic dermatitis.

Patient Evaluation. A number of serologic tests exist to document exposure to the retrovirus HIV. Positive ELISA screens should be confirmed by Western blot studies that demonstrate antibodies against specific viral products. Lymphopenia is frequently present with inversion of the T helper to T suppressor cell ratio (i.e., reduced T helper cells). Evaluation of the secondary skin lesions that are associated with HIV will depend on the type of lesions and might include KOH preparations, Tzanck's smears, fungal and viral cultures, and skin biopsy. Unusual persistent extensive superficial infections should alert the physician to the possibility of underlying HIV infection.

Therapy. A variety of experimental antiviral agents are being tested in the treatment of AIDS; however, as of this time there is no effective treatment for HIV infection. Specific treatment is directed at suppression of secondary infection, supportive care, and treatment of neoplasia. Cautionary measures such as "safe sex," the use of condoms, public education, and screening of blood products may help prevent the spread of AIDS.

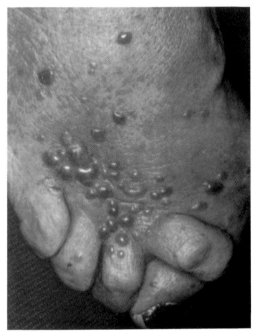

Figure 32–7. The vesicular lesions on the dorsum of the foot represent disseminated herpes zoster in a patient with chronic lymphocytic leukemia.

Suggested Readings

Broder S, Gallo R: A pathogenic retrovirus (HTLV-III) linked to AIDS. N Engl J Med *322*:1292–1297, 1984.

Bunn PA Jr, Schechter GP, Jaffe E, et al: Clinical source of retrovirus-associated adult T-cell lymphoma in the United States. N Engl J Med *309*:257–264, 1983.

Corey L, Spear PG: Infections with herpes simplex viruses. N Engl J Med *314*:686–691, 1986.

Friedman-Kien AE, Laubenstein LJ, Rubenstein P, et al: Disseminated Kaposi's sarcoma in homosexual men. Ann Intern Med *96*:693–700, 1982.

Klein RS, Harris CA, Small CB, et al: Oral candidiasis in high risk patients as the initial manifestation of the acquired immunodeficiency syndrome. N Engl J Med *311*:354–358, 1984.

Miller GD: Hand-foot-and-mouth disease. J Am Med Assn *203*:827–830, 1968.

Nahmias AJ, Roziman B: Infection with herpes-simplex virus 1 and 2. N Engl J Med *289*:667–674, 781–789, 1973.

Penneys NS, Hicks B: Unusual cutaneous lesions associated with acquired immunodeficiency syndrome. J Amer Acad Dermatol *13*:845–852, 1985.

33

Cutaneous Fungal Infections

NEAL PENNEYS

Systemic fungal infections that can present with skin lesions include sporotrichosis, blastomycosis, coccidioidomycosis, histoplasmosis, paracoccidioidomycosis, cryptococcosis, phycomycosis (mucormycosis discussed in this chapter), candidiasis, and aspergillosis.

SPOROTRICHOSIS

Sporotrichosis, caused by *Sporothrix schenckii*, follows direct inoculation of the organism into the skin. The organism is a dimorphic fungus, and yeast-like forms are found in tissue. *S. schenckii* has been isolated from soil, living plants, and organic debris.

Clinical Findings. The pattern of disease is very distinctive, with lymphatic spread usually following the initial chancriform lesion (Fig. 33–1). This infection is frequently found in persons who have contact with thorny plants such as roses or sphagnum moss, either through occupational exposure or through gardening. Usually, there is a puncture wound produced by a thorn or foreign body that allows penetration of the spores. One to 12 weeks following the injury, a small papule forms, which eventually enlarges to produce a chancriform nodule, frequently ulcerated. At a variable time, dissemination through regional lymphangitic occurs, producing the characteristic clinical picture (Fig. 33–2). The individual lesions may wax and wane for prolonged periods of time. Dissemination to other body regions is

most unusual and occurs primarily in the immunosuppressed patient. Pulmonary sporotrichosis and arthritic sporotrichosis have been reported to occur in the absence of cutaneous infection and probably represent infection following inhalation of spores.

Histopathology. The clinical diagnosis of sporotrichosis can be supported by skin biopsy findings. Within the dermis, there are stellate microabscesses composed of neutrophils surrounded by plasma cells and histiocytes. Periodic acid–Schiff (PAS) stains may demonstrate the organism in many instances.

Patient Evaluation. Sporotrichosis is a process that is often limited to the inoculation site with regional lymphatic spread. Following biopsy, tissue should also be obtained for culture to confirm the diagnosis. If there are signs of dissemination, appropriate diagnostic studies should be obtained to confirm dissemination. The extent of the differential diagnosis will vary, depending on the site and extent of the infection. Sporotrichosis may be difficult to recognize when lesions occur in unusual locations, such as on the face or on the trunk. In these sites with the absence of the characteristic lymphatic pattern, the process may resemble a non-specific inflammatory plaque and the infectious nature of the lesion may not be recognized. When patients are seen early in the development of the process, a solitary chancriform lesion may be the sole clinical finding. The causes of chancriform lesions include blastomycosis, histoplasmosis, coccidioidomycosis, *Nocardia asteroides* and

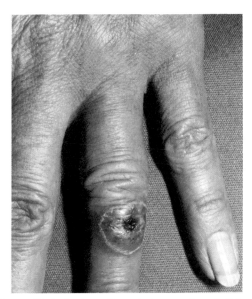

Figure 33–1. A chancriform lesion on the digit in a patient with sporotrichosis.

Nocardia brasiliensis, and *Mycobacterium marinum.* Once extension along a lymphatic has occurred, the most likely other possibilities are infection by *M. marinum, Leishmania brasiliensis,* and *N. brasiliensis.* The diagnosis is confirmed by growth of the fungus with demonstration of its dimorphism.

Treatment. The treatment of choice is an increasing dosage schedule of orally administered solution of supersaturated potassium iodide (SSKI). For persons of average adult weight, the standard initial dosage is 5–10 drops three times a day; the dosage is slowly increased to 30 drops three times daily for an extended length of time, until the lesions have completely resolved. Acneiform lesions and stuffy nose may be side-effects of

this treatment. If necessary, localized heat may have a beneficial effect. Oral ketoconazole may also have a beneficial therapeutic effect; however, recurrences after this treatment are common. Systemic therapy with amphotericin B is effective in systemic sporotrichosis.

BLASTOMYCOSIS (NORTH AMERICAN BLASTOMYCOSIS)

Blastomycosis, caused by *Blastomyces dermatitidis,* usually affects the skin secondarily through hematogenous spread following an asymptomatic pulmonary infection. The organism is a dimorphic fungus that is yeast-like in tissue. The disease occurs most frequently in the midwestern United States. Dissemination of the infection usually follows a primary pulmonary focus.

Clinical Findings. The characteristic skin lesion is an expanding circinate or arcuate plaque, and this is the most common extrapulmonary manifestation. The initial skin lesion is a papule that expands, may ulcerate, and develops a thickened, verrucous scale (Fig. 33–3 and 33–4). As the lesion expands, there is a tendency for flattening within the center of the lesion with the loss of scale and scar formation. The expanding border retains its hyperkeratotic, verrucous appearance, and it is occasionally studded with small, draining sinuses. A spectrum of skin lesions of blastomycosis occurs, including plaques, ulcers, abscesses, and nodules. Other organs, such as genitourinary tract, central nervous system, and joints, may be involved in disseminated disease.

Histopathology. To maximize the chance of finding organisms in tissue sections, skin biopsy should be obtained from a clinically

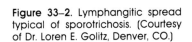

Figure 33–2. Lymphangitic spread typical of sporotrichosis. (Courtesy of Dr. Loren E. Golitz, Denver, CO.)

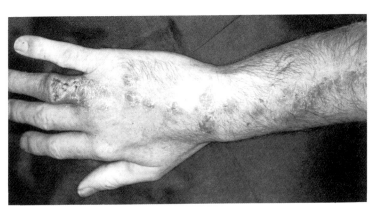

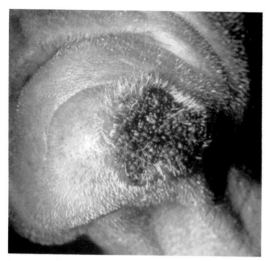

Figure 33–3. Verrucous plaque on the chin in a patient with North American blastomycosis (see also Plate V*F*).

in the lungs or in the genitourinary tract. The organism can be identified directly in secretions (KOH preparation), or material can be placed on Sabouraud's or enriched agar and the organisms grown at both 30° C and 37° C. Complement fixation tests for blastomycosis are not reliable.

Therapy. The presence of cutaneous blastomycosis indicates disseminated disease. Amphotericin B is the appropriate treatment of this disease. Secondary agents used to manage blastomycosis include imidazole derivatives such as oral ketoconazole and 2-hydroxystilbamidine. These agents produce results less predictable than those obtained with amphotericin B. Prior to therapy with an imidazole, a spinal tap to exclude CNS disease is necessary, since these agents do not cross the blood-brain barrier.

active region. There is irregular epidermal hyperplasia, beneath which there is a polymorphous infiltrate. Organisms are most often found within giant cells. Facilitation of the search for organisms occurs with the use of special stains such as PAS or methenamine silver.

Patient Evaluation. Differential diagnoses include squamous cell carcinoma, metastatic carcinoma, other disseminated fungal infections, tuberculosis verrucosis cutis, sarcoidosis, and halogenoderma. Because the skin is most often involved as a site of secondary dissemination, attempts should be made to define the primary focus, which is usually

COCCIDIOIDOMYCOSIS

This systemic fungal disease is found primarily in residents or visitors to the southwestern United States, in particular the San Joaquin Valley. The disease is produced by inhalation of the spores of *Coccidioides immitis*. In tissue, the fungus forms spores with a thick wall (the spherule) that reproduce by endosporulation. Following inhalation, a primary pulmonary infection develops and is associated with conversion to skin test positivity.

Clinical Findings. A number of non-specific cutaneous reactions occur in association with this infection, including erythema multiforme, erythema nodosum, and nonspecific cutaneous rashes. When this disease disseminates, a number of signs and symptoms develop, including weight loss, fever, and adenopathy. Dissemination to the skin produces a variable clinical picture, which includes papules, pustules, plaques, nodules, and abscesses (Fig. 33–5). Ulceration, which may persist indefinitely, can occur. The ulceration is usually found in the acral areas. A second pattern of cutaneous dissemination is a verrucous plaque found most commonly on the face and scalp. Erythema nodosum developing in a patient who has traveled through an endemic area should alert the physician to the possibility of coccidioidomycosis.

Histopathology. The histologic picture of coccidioidomycosis is similar to that noted in blastomycosis, with epidermal hyperpla-

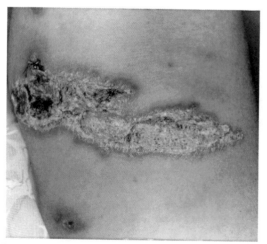

Figure 33–4. Verrucous, irregular plaque on the arm of a patient with blastomycosis.

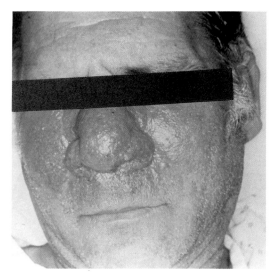

Figure 33–5. Erythematous, cellulitic-appearing rash on the malar skin as well as on the nose in a man with coccidioidomycosis (see also Plate V*G*).

sia, a polymorphous infiltrate with giant cells, and occasional fungal organisms.

Patient Evaluation. Excluding rare primary inoculation lesions, skin infection represents dissemination. The organism can be demonstrated directly in infected tissue fluids. *C. immitis* should be grown on standard media containing cyclohexamide to inhibit saprophytic fungi. Infection is confirmed by the demonstration of dimorphic growth and by the demonstration of complement fixation antibodies that develop at varying times after initial infection.

Treatment. Amphotericin B is the treatment of choice. Ketoconazole also has therapeutic efficacy against this fungus.

HISTOPLASMOSIS

Histoplasmosis is primarily a pulmonary infection caused by the organism *Histoplasma capsulatum*. This fungus is a dimorphic fungus that has a yeast form in tissue. This infection is most commonly seen in residents of the central United States, where skin test positivity is common among healthy young adults. Infection follows inhalation of spores, which are most commonly found in contaminated soil.

Clinical Findings. Skin lesions are very common in histoplasmosis. They usually reflect dissemination in an immunosuppressed patient. Disseminated histoplasmo-

sis with skin lesions has been reported in patients with the acquired immune deficiency syndrome (AIDS). The skin lesions are usually non-descript papules or small ulcers. Oropharyngeal and nasal ulcers are common and are of diagnostic significance; however, other signs and symptoms may be non-specific.

Histopathology. Skin biopsy reveals perivascular inflammation containing lymphocytes, plasma cells, and histiocytes in the dermis. The organism is best demonstrated with methenamine silver stains.

Patient Evaluation. Confirmation of the diagnosis is by dimorphic growth of the organism in culture. Demonstration of a rising complement fixation antibody titer is also important. Skin lesions are almost invaribly a sign of dissemination, and the other affected sites should be defined.

Treatment. The appropriate therapy is with intravenous amphotericin B. Ketoconazole may also be used but is less effective.

PARACOCCIDIOIDOMYCOSIS

Paracoccidioidomycosis, or South American blastomycosis, is a severe and progressive ailment that occurs rarely in the United States and reflects exposure to the organism by a visit to an endemic area, including Mexico, Central America, and South America. The organism, *Paracoccidioides brasiliensis*, has not been cultured.

Clinical Findings. The primary site of infection is usually pulmonary. However, symptoms may reflect infection in sites such as the reticuloendothelial system. The most common signs and symptoms include difficulty in swallowing, mucosal ulcerations, lymphadenopathy, shortness of breath, and facial skin lesions. The skin lesions are mucocutaneous and include red ulcerations of the oral cavity as well as of other mucosal surfaces. Other skin lesions include nonspecific papules, and nodules, some of which may be verrucous and vegetative. Dissemination of the disease may occur years after the initial infection.

Histopathology. Skin biopsy reveals granulomatous changes with an associated polymorphous infiltrate similar to that of blastomycosis. PAS and methenamine silver stains can be used to demonstrate the fungus.

Patient Evaluation. Mucocutaneous involvement indicates dissemination. Patients should be evaluated for internal organ involvement, including the lungs, lymph nodes, and adrenal glands. Confirmation of the diagnosis is by direct demonstration of the organism by a simple KOH preparation from sputum or from skin and mucosal tissue. Attempts at culture should be made, using Sabouraud-dextrose media at room temperature. Serologic studies may also be helpful in confirming the diagnosis and evaluating the effectiveness of therapy.

Treatment. Sulfonamides are the treatment of choice for this disease. Amphotericin B and imidazole derivatives may also be used.

CRYPTOCOCCOSIS

Cryptococcosis is a systemic infection caused by the fungus *Cryptococcus neoformans*. The fungus is a yeast that reproduces by budding. Evidence indicates that the organism is acquired following inhalation. There is increased incidence of infection in patients who are immunosuppressed (e.g., as a manifestation of AIDS, from corticosteroid or cytotoxic therapy in association with lymphoma, or with sarcoidosis).

Clinical Findings. Central nervous system manifestations are the most common severe and the most common initial presentation. Pulmonary, bone, and other sites may also be involved. Skin lesions are not uncommon in cryptococcosis and may be solitary papules, some with central dells or pustules, nodules, cellulitic lesions, or ulcers. The face and scalp are the most common locations for skin lesions. The morphologic characteristics of the skin lesions are not specific, but they may resemble those of molluscum contagiosum, basal cell carcinoma, and a variety of other skin lesions.

Histopathology. In tissue, the organism can be identified by its positivity with Mayer's mucicarmine, which stains the yeast's capsule red but does not stain other fungi with similar morphologic characteristics.

Patient Evaluation. Because involvement of the skin is most often a result of dissemination, affected internal foci must be identified, particularly the central nervous system. The presence of disseminated cryptococcal infection may reflect endogenous immunosuppression, such as that noted in AIDS.

Treatment. The treatment of choice for cryptococcosis is systemic amphotericin B in combination with flucytosine.

MUCORMYCOSIS

Mucormycosis refers to infections produced by the members of the order Mucorales. These infections occur primarily in patients who have uncontrolled diabetes mellitus, allogeneic organ transplants, or hematologic malignancies.

Clinical Findings. A variety of clinical presentations are known. Rhinocerebral mucormycosis is characterized by the relatively acute development of orbital or facial edema associated with a variety of local symptoms and signs. Ulcerative lesions can be found on the hard palate and on the nasal mucosa. Lesions on the palate represent direct extension from infection in the sinus. In disseminated mucormycosis, skin lesions are nondiagnostic morphologically but can resemble those seen in ecthyma gangrenosum.

Histopathology. In tissue, there are large, non-septate hyphae surrounded by polymorphous inflammation. The organisms are better seen with PAS and methenamine silver stains. These organisms produce a tremendous necrosis of blood vessel walls with massive tissue necrosis.

Patient Evaluation. If primary inoculation mucormycosis of wound infections is excluded, the most common form in the skin is rhinocerebral mucormycosis. The differential diagnosis of mucormycosis includes aspergillosis of the nasal cavity and *Pseudomonas aeruginosa* infection. The diagnosis may be confirmed by direct observation of hyphal forms in tissue scrapings from affected areas. Studies to exclude underlying diabetes mellitus should be performed. Radiographic examination, including computer-assisted tomography, can be used to define sinus and bone involvement. Specimens for culture should be inoculated onto Sabouraud's glucose agar and incubated at 37° C and at 30° C.

Treatment. Control of the associated systemic condition (e.g., diabetes mellitus) coupled with intravenous amphotericin B therapy is the usual approach to therapy.

CANDIDIASIS

Candida organisms are yeasts with a multitude of species, 8 of which are considered to be pathogenic in humans. *Candida* organisms are commensals of humans and are found routinely in the gastrointestinal tract and on the skin. Skin and mucosal lesions produced by infection with *Candida* species can indicate a profound alteration of the immunologic status of the individual and can thus be associated with a number of syndromes characterized by altered immune status.

Clinical Findings. One of the most well-recognized presentations of candidal infection is thrush, a painful infection of the tongue characterized by the presence of whitish plaques. Thrush may occur as a consequence of immunosuppression by systemic corticosteroid administration. Its presence is a reliable marker of AIDS-related complex (ARC) and indicates the likelihood of progression of that disease to AIDS. Candidal infection can affect all mucosal surfaces and produce similar lesions.

In patients who are immunosuppressed (usually as a consequence of chemotherapy), especially those with a central intravenous line, candidal septicemia can occur. Generally, candidal sepsis is associated with nonspecific skin lesions that are macular, papular, or pustular; or with vasculitis lesions that may progress to ulcerative lesions (Fig. 33–6).

Chronic mucocutaneous candidiasis is found in association with a heterogeneous group of disorders characterized by failure of T cell lymphocyte function. In a recessively inherited subgroup, endocrinopathy may be associated. Most forms of this disease have skin signs that are seen early in childhood, although a rare patient will develop symptoms in adulthood, often in association with thymoma and myositis. Candidal organisms can infect all cutaneous structures, ranging from an isolated fingernail to extensive tumorous growths (candidal granuloma) (Figs. 33–7 and 33–8).

Histopathology. In tissue, both spore and hyphal forms may be present in a varying amount of inflammatory infiltrate. The organisms are best demonstrated with either PAS or methenamine silver stains.

Patient Evaluation. There are a number of different clinical syndromes that can be associated with dissemination of *Candida* progressive to the skin. If patients are immunosuppressed and have suggestive lesions, candidal sepsis should be considered and blood cultures obtained. Furthermore, the

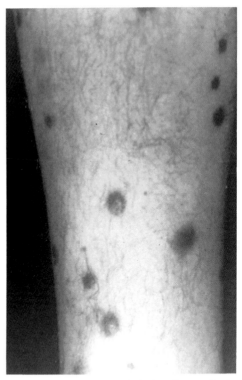

Figure 33–6. Multiple purpuric lesions in a patient with candidal sepsis.

organisms are easily grown on routine media. Chronic mucocutaneous candidal infection may indicate the presence of immunosuppression such as that seen in AIDS and in inherited forms of chronic mucocutaneous candidiasis. In the inherited forms, testing for endocrinopathies such as insulin resistant diabetes mellitus, hypothyroidism, or hyperparathyroidism is necessary. Immunologic testing for assessment of cellular immune competence should be obtained, as well as serologic tests to exclude the presence of HIV infection.

Treatment. Candidal infections can be managed by either topical or systemic therapy, the mode of which depends on the location and the associated syndrome. Topical clotrimazole is an example of one such anticandidal agent. Oral candidiasis can be managed with oral nystatin suspension, clotrimazole troches, gentian violet solutions, and dilute hydrogen peroxide solutions. When there is an associated immune defect, topical therapy is frequently ineffective. In these cases, systemic ketoconazole or amphotericin B may be required. Candidal sepsis is treated with intravenous amphotericin B.

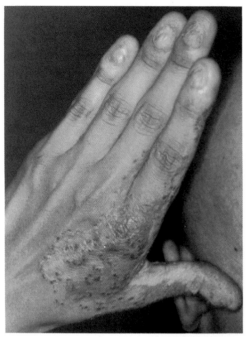

Figure 33–7. This male with alopecia areata and insulin-resistant diabetes has candidal granulomas on the hand as well as dystrophic nail changes representative of chronic mucocutaneous candidiasis.

ASPERGILLOSIS

Aspergillus is an ubiquitous fungus that can produce disease in immunosuppressed patients. Skin lesions occur rarely by direct inoculation or by hematogenous spread, usually from pulmonary foci.

Clinical Findings. The skin lesions are not diagnostic and range from papules to vasculitic lesions to ulcerations.

Histopathology. In tissue, non-septate hyphae are seen surrounded by a mixed cell infiltrate. PAS and methenamine silver stains can be used to demonstrate the organisms.

Patient Evaluation. Both primary and disseminated aspergillosis occur primarily in immunocompromised individuals. Usually, these persons have associated severe blood dyscrasias and are receiving chemotherapy. Organisms are easily grown in culture.

Treatment. Systemic amphotericin B is the treatment of choice.

GENERAL COMMENT ON THERAPY

Throughout this chapter, we have referred to the use of amphotericin B and ketoconazole for deep fungal infections. With either agent there is a significant incidence of side-effects. Amphotericin B has major toxicity to the kidney, and if given enough drug almost all patients will lose some renal function. It also must be given intravenously, and is started at a low dosage (1 mg per day) and raised to as high as 16–32 mg per day. Ketoconazole was initially believed to be free of major systemic toxicity, but it has been associated with an idiosyncratic hepatotoxicity that on occasion has resulted in death. In addition, it has "steroid"-like activity, and anaphylactic reactions have occurred, even with the first dose.

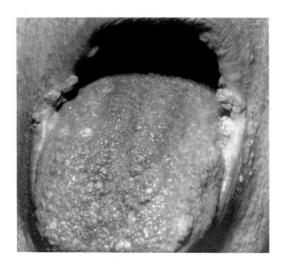

Figure 33–8. Mucosal surface involvement with chronic mucocutaneous candidiasis.

Suggested Readings

Bodey GP, Luna M: Skin lesions associated with disseminated candidiasis. J Am Med Assn 229:1466–1468, 1974.

Borton LK, Wintroub BU: Disseminated cryptococcosis presenting as herpetiform lesions in a homosexual man with acquired immunodeficiency syndrome. J Am Acad Dermatol 10:387–390, 1984.

Curtis AC, Grekin JN: Histoplasmosis. J Am Med Assn 134:1217–1224, 1947.

Grossman ME, Silvers DN, Walther RR: Cutaneous manifestations of disseminated candidiasis. J Am Acad Dermatol 2:111–116, 1980.

Hammond DR, Winkelmann RK: Cutaneous phycomycosis. Arch Dermatol 115:990–992, 1979.

Harrell ER, Curtis AC: North American blastomycosis. Am J Med 27:750–766, 1959.

Londero AT, Ramos CD: Paracoccidioidomycosis. Am J Med 52:771–775, 1972.

Mayoral F, Penneys NS: Disseminated histoplasmosis presenting as a transepidermal elimination disorder in an AIDS victim. J Am Acad Dermatol 13:842–844, 1985.

Meyer RD, Kaplan MH, Ong M, et al: Cutaneous lesions in disseminated mucormycosis. J Am Med Assn 225:737–738, 1973.

Prystowsky SD, Vogelstein B, Ettinger DS, et al: Invasive aspergillosis. N Engl J Med 295:655–658, 1976.

Rico MJ, Penneys NS: Cutaneous cryptococcosis resembling molluscum contagiosum in a patient with AIDS. Arch Dermatol 121:901–902, 1985.

Schwartz RA, Lamberts RJ: Isolated nodular cutaneous coccidioidomycosis. J Am Acad Dermatol 4:38–46, 1981.

Segal RJ, Jacobs PH: Sporotrichosis. Int J Dermatol 18:639–644, 1979.

Young RC, Bennett JE, Vogel CL, et al: Aspergillosis: The spectrum of the disease in 98 patients. Medicine 49:147–173, 1970.

34

Bacterial Diseases

NEAL PENNEYS

Systemic bacterial diseases involve the skin by dissemination via the blood stream and lymphatics, by direct extension to the skin, and by the production of characteristic toxic or hypersensitivity eruptions in the skin. Many of the eruptions associated with systemic bacterial diseases are sufficiently recognizable to assist in the rapid diagnosis of the underlying process. Antibiotic therapy is used for most of these disorders. As new antibiotics are developed, the recommendations for therapy change. As this is not a reference text, to avoid outdating in many cases we will not specify the antibiotic of choice nor its dose or route of administration.

CHARACTERISTIC ERUPTIONS ASSOCIATED WITH STREPTOCOCCAL DISEASES

Scarlet Fever

Certain strains of group A streptococci elaborate an erythrogenic toxin that produces a chracteristic rash. Scarlet fever usually occurs only once, because specific antibodies are synthesized as a response to the toxin and these antibodies protect against recurrence of the rash (although not against recurrent streptococcal infection).

Clinical Findings. Scarlet fever primarily affects children and rarely adults. The incubation period varies from 2 to 4 days and is followed by fever, nausea, vomiting, headache, and abdominal pain. The streptococcal infection is most often in the oropharynx (but may be rarely in other locations), and initial signs and symptoms relate to the local effects of the infection. The pharynx is red and edematous, and exudates can be present on the tonsils. Tender lymphadenopathy may be present below the jaw. The tongue may be coated with swollen, red papillae. The rash is macular and spreads from the neck to the trunk and finally to the extremities. Palms and soles are spared. The cheeks are red, and there is circumoral pallor. There is accentuation of the rash in all skin folds; in the antecubital fossae, this results in a linear quality known as Pastia's sign. The intensity of the rash varies, and it is not characteristic in mild cases. At its maximum, the rash is scarlet (hence the name). Occasionally the eruption is purpuric. After 4–5 days, the rash fades and there is desquamation (Fig. 34–1). The scaling process begins on the face, spreads to the trunk, and finally involves the extremities. Peeling on the distal extremities may be in large sheets.

Patient Evaluation. Confirmation of the diagnosis is by throat culture that reveals group A streptococci and by increases in serum levels of antistreptolysin O (ASO, now known as streptozyme) titer. Other bacterial processes must be considered in the initial evaluation. Perhaps the most confusing is the staphylococcal scalded skin syndrome (SSSS), which is produced by infection with group II phage type 71 *Staphylococcus aureus*. Generally, the cutaneous eruption in SSSS is bullous, and this separates it from scarlet fever. The skin eruptions associated with a number of viral diseases may resemble the eruption of scarlet fever; however, exudative pharyngitis is usually absent. Infectious mononucleosis may mimic scarlet fever; however, this entity can be separated by appropriate serologic tests.

262

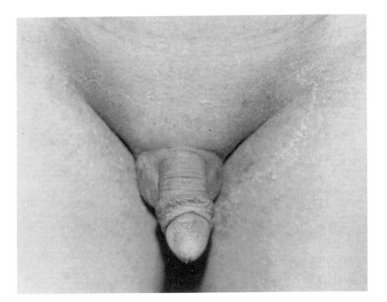

Figure 34–1. Faint, erythematous rash with desquamation in a patient with scarlet fever. (Courtesy of Dr. Lorey Golitz, Denver, CO.)

Therapy. Penicillin is the therapy of choice. It may be given intramuscularly or orally. In penicillin-sensitive individuals, erythromycin may be used.

Rheumatic Fever

Rheumatic fever is characterized by an inflammatory process primarily involving the heart, joints, skin, and central nervous system. The disorder is acute, febrile, and largely self-limited. All cases of rheumatic fever follow an upper respiratory tract infection with certain group A strains of streptococcus. The temporal relationship between streptococcal pharyngitis and the appearance of rheumatic fever is variable. Rheumatic fever does not follow cutaneous streptococcal infections. The mechanism by which the disease occurs is not known.

Clinical Findings. Acute rheumatic fever is found primarily in children aged 6–15. In the United States, the peak incidence varies, occurring in March and April in the Northeast and in the fall in the Southeast. The most important manifestations include carditis, polyarthritis, chorea, subcutaneous nodules, and erythema marginatum. The latent period between the onset of preceding streptococcal pharyngitis and the onset of acute rheumatic fever is approximately 19 days. The skin manifestations are two: (1) subcutaneous nodules, and (2) erythema marginatum. Subcutaneous nodules are firm and painless and vary in size up to 2.0 cm. The nodules are usually found over extensor surfaces and over the tendons. Common sites are over the elbows, knees, wrists, ankles, Achilles tendon, occiput, and vertebrae. The number will vary, and the lesions can persist for 1–2 weeks. Subcutaneous nodules are associated with severe carditis. Erythema marginatum is a macular, evanescent rash that usually is found on the trunk and proximal extremities. The eruption forms serpiginous patterns and rapidly advances. The rash remains for a variable period of time but may persist for an indefinite period.

Histopathology. Skin biopsy of erythema marginatum shows neutrophils, some degenerated, and focal hemorrhage in the dermis. Skin biopsy of subcutaneous nodules reveals infiltration of fibrohistiocytic cells in a pattern similar to that seen in granuloma annulare or in early rheumatoid nodule.

Patient Evaluation. The diagnosis of acute rheumatic fever rests on the recognition of the diverse manifestations of the disease, since there is no specific diagnostic test for this disorder. Differential diagnosis includes rheumatoid arthritis, juvenile rheumatoid arthritis, systemic lupus erythematosus, serum sickness, rubella, infectious endocarditis, viral syndromes with myocarditis, and Henoch-Schönlein purpura. Most experts believe that the presence of 2 major criteria or 1 major and 2 minor criteria (as defined by Jones) support with a high degree of probability the diagnosis of acute rheumatic fever. The absence of serologic evidence of an antecedent streptococcal infection (such as positive antistreptolysin O titer, positive anti-DNAase B or positive antihyaluronidase titers) is strong evidence against the presence of acute rheumatic fever.

Treatment. The mainstays of treatment are bed rest, systemic corticosteroids, and nonsteroidal anti-inflammatory agents. Prophylaxis such as with penicillin is necessary to prevent recurrent disease.

Erysipelas

Erysipelas is a cellulitic infection following infection with group A streptococci.

Clinical Findings. The infection in adults usually is found in the vicinity of a wound or ulceration. It may also affect the facial skin, presumably following some minor trauma. The skin lesion is edematous, well-demarcated, and dusky red and may have prominent vesicles and bullae at the advancing edge. The patient may have toxemia and a high fever. Recurrent erysipelas has been associated with the development of lymphedema as a result of the accompanying lymphangitis.

Histopathology. Skin biopsy reveals marked edema and a perivascular and diffuse, primarily acute, infiltrate. Intraepidermal vesicle formation may be present.

Patient Evaluation. Although not common, this infection has a characteristic clinical appearance. Attempts to culture organisms from tissue aspirates usually fail. Erysipelas must be separated from other cutaneous infections that have acute presentations. Streptococcal cellulitis is a similar process; however, the skin lesions are not as well-defined and the process is not as acute. Systemic toxicity is frequently less.

Treatment. Penicillin given intravenously is the antibiotic of choice. The patient usually requires 10–14 days of antibiotic therapy. In penicillin-sensitive individuals, another antibiotic effective against streptococci may be used, such as erythromycin.

Lymphangitis

Lymphangitis is usually an infection by group A streptococci with involvement of lymphatic channels.

Clinical Findings. Usually there is a portal of entry, frequently on an extremity. From this cutaneous entry point, red streaks extend cephalad toward regional lymph nodes, which may be tender. Skin lesions may be very painful. The disease has a characteristic clinical appearance. Patients may show signs of significant toxicity. Attempts to culture organisms from skin lesions are usually fruitless. As in erysipelas, penicillin is effective therapy.

ERUPTIONS ASSOCIATED WITH STAPHYLOCOCCAL INFECTION

Staphylococcal Scalded Skin Syndrome (SSSS)

Strains of group II *Staphylococcus* produce this disease, with most organisms belonging to phage type 71. These strains, frequently found on the skin and in the nasopharynx in affected individuals, elaborate an exotoxin that produces the superficial blistering. Injection of the toxin into neonatal mice results in similar pathologic changes with exfoliation.

Clinical Findings. SSSS primarily affects children and infants. Adults, particularly those with renal failure, may also develop SSSS. The first sign is perioral redness; erythema then extends to involve all cutaneous surfaces. As the disease evolves, crusts and thin-roofed bullae develop (Fig. 34–2; Plate II A). If bullae rupture, extensive denudation will be present. Frequently, Nikolsky's sign (formation of an intraepidermal separation by torsion on normal-appearing skin) will be positive. The condition resolves by desquamation and re-epithelialization.

Histopathology. SSSS has a characteristic histologic picture in which there is a superficial split in the uppermost layers of the epidermis, forming a superficial blister. There is little inflammatory infiltrate. Rapid diagnosis can be made by examining frozen sections taken from a lesion.

Patient Evaluation. Diagnosis is primarily made on clinical grounds, confirmed by skin biopsy. Growth of *Staphylococcus* phage type 71 in culture confirms the diagnosis.

Therapy. Administration of appropriate antibiotics, usually a penicillinase-resistant penicillin intravenously, combined with intravenous fluids is the indicated treatment for this syndrome.

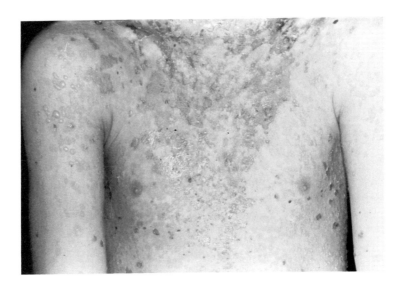

Figure 34–2. Crusted and vesiculated skin in a patient with staphylococcal scalded skin syndrome (see also Plate VIA).

Toxic Shock Syndrome

The development of the toxic shock syndrome has been convincingly linked to the presence of varieties of *Staphylococcus aureus* that produce exotoxin C.

Clinical Findings. The patient characteristically affected by this syndrome is a young woman who uses tampons and who develops signs and symptoms during a menstrual period. During menses, there is the acute development of fever, vomiting, myalgias, and diarrhea. Severe hypotension may develop with associated hypovolemic shock. These patients may have a diffuse erythematous eruption. The most characteristic cutaneous finding, however, is edema, redness, and eventual desquamation of the skin of the palms and soles (Fig. 34–3; Plate VI B). Erosions may affect mucous membranes. The mortality rate is approximately 3 per cent. The fact that this syndrome affects primarily menstruating females who use certain tampons suggests that these tampons have a permissive effect on the development of the syndrome.

Patient Evaluation. The patient must be evaluated for other causes of hypotension and shock. Usually, the history of menstruation and the use of tampons points the way to a correct diagnosis. Cultures from blood and other sites should be performed if there is doubt concerning the source of infection.

Therapy. As with SSSS, the therapy for this process includes an appropriate antibiotic, usually penicillinase-resistant peni-

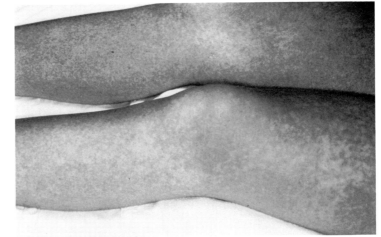

Figure 34–3. Erythematous lesions representative of toxic shock syndrome (see also Plate VIIB).

cillin coverage, coupled with fluid replacement.

BACTEREMIAS

Skin lesions are not unusual in patients who have bacteremia. A spectrum of lesions may be present that support a clinical diagnosis of sepsis. These include subconjunctival hemorrhage, acral petechiae, hemorrhagic macules, papules, vesicles, ulcerated papules, and larger lesions. Certain skin lesions favor the presence of specific organisms and can provide diagnostic clues to the nature of the bacteremia before culture results are available. The following organisms produce skin lesions that are suggestive of their presence.

Pseudomonas aeruginosa Infection

Ecthyma gangrenosum is the most well-recognized skin lesion of bacteremia produced by *P. aeruginosa*. These lesions start as small vesicles that progress to hemorrhagic ulcerations. The central portion of the lesion has a black eschar, and there is a surrounding red-purple rim (Fig. 34–4). The lesions are usually sparse and may be found on any body surface and on mucous membranes. *Pseudomonas* sepsis may also produce a wide variety of non-diagnostic skin lesions ranging from isolated hemorrhagic vesicles to large areas of ulceration known as gangrenous cellulitis.

Patient Evaluation. Examination of the skin lesion under Wood's light may reveal green fluorescence, which supports the diagnosis of *Pseudomonas* infection. Cultures should be obtained from the skin lesion and from blood to confirm the clinical diagnosis.

Therapy. Appropriate antibiotic therapy and fluid support must be administered. Local therapy, such as with tap water compresses, may be useful in helping to loosen the eschar.

Gonococcal Septicemia

Gonococcal bacteremia is found in a small percentage of persons who are infected by *Neisseria gonorrhoeae*. Women are much more commonly affected than men, and dissemination may occur from a number of primary sites, including the urinary tract, rectum, and oropharynx.

Clinical Findings. The most common symptoms are migratory polyarthralgia or arthritis and a discrete acral skin eruption. The morphology of the skin lesions varies from petechiae to papules or pustules on a hemorrhagic base (Fig. 34–5). The skin lesions are frequently tender. The patients have accompanying malaise and a high, spiking fever.

Histopathology. Skin biopsy reveals an acute inflammatory vasculitic process characterized by the presence of neutrophils, vascular damage, small vessel thrombi, and a variable degree of epidermal changes. The

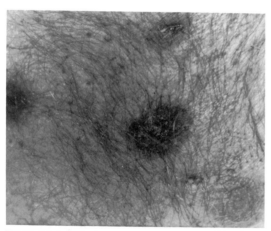

Figure 34–4. Ecthyma gangrenosum caused by *Pseudomonas*.

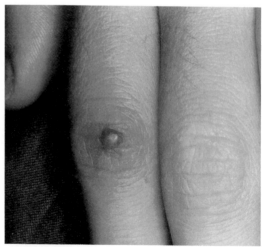

Figure 34–5. Pustular necrotic lesion representative of disseminated gonorrheal infection. (Courtesy of Dr. Neil A. Fenske, Tampa, FL.)

changes are not specific but are compatible with a septic process. Organisms are generally difficult to demonstrate in tissue with routine methods.

Patient Evaluation. Other causes of sepsis with arthritis must be excluded. The diagnosis is confirmed by a positive blood culture, a positive culture from the site of primary infection, and/or a positive smear from the site of initial infection. Gonococcus is rarely able to be cultured from the skin lesions or the joints.

Therapy. Appropriate antibiotic therapy is required, as is bed rest and other supportive care.

Meningococcal Septicemia

A variety of clinical syndromes are associated with meningococcal sepsis. Cutaneous lesions are varied and include petechial lesions, exanthem-like eruptions that resemble those seen in viral syndromes, papules, and hemorrhagic vesicles and pustules. In acute syndromes, the pattern of the eruption may resemble that seen in disseminated intravascular coagulopathy with large areas of confluent purpura. Skin lesions in chronic meningococcemia resemble those seen in gonococcemia and are characterized by crops of papules and vesiculopustules.

Histopathology. Skin biopsies reveal changes similar to those seen in septic events. In chronic lesions, the pathologic changes are similar to those seen in gonococcal sepsis. In acute lesions, there is a polymorphous infiltrate coupled with extravasation of erythrocytes and variable degrees of epidermal change.

Patient Evaluation. Confirmation of the diagnosis is by culture of the organism. Depending on the presentation, a variety of other septic processes need to be excluded. Appropriate evaluation will vary, depending on the associated systemic signs and symptoms.

Therapy and Prognosis. Acute meningitis with septicemia is often fatal; therefore, a rapid initiation of antibiotic therapy coupled with fluid support is indicated. Chronic meningococcemia is more subtle and less frequently associated with a fatal outcome. Once it is diagnosed, antibiotics are necessary.

Enteric Fever

Typhoid fever, produced by *Salmonella typhi,* is the most common enteric fever. Initial symptoms of typhoid fever are headache, fever, and diarrhea. The characteristic skin lesion of typhoid fever is the rose spot, a small red macule that is found in less than 50 per cent of patients with typhoid fever about 1 week after the onset of symptoms. The lesions usually occur on the abdomen, are slightly palpable, and are transient. Rose spots may also be found with other forms of enteric fever produced by *Salmonella* species. Confirmation of the diagnosis is made by blood culture. Serologic tests for typhoid fever are frequently negative early in the course of the disease but may be of help at a later point. Many infectious processes need to be considered, including Rocky Mountain spotted fever, infection by other *Salmonella* species, malaria, and viral exanthems. Chloramphenicol is the antibiotic of choice.

Cellulitis Produced by *Haemophilus influenzae*

Most commonly seen in children on the face and neck, cellulitis produced by *H. influenzae* rarely occurs in adults. This lesion is an infiltrated edematous red plaque associated with a primary focus of infection, usually in the upper respiratory tract or oropharynx. Other forms of cellulitis may be similar, so that the diagnosis must be confirmed by culture. Appropriate antibiotic administration is the treatment of choice.

Skin Lesions Associated with Bacterial Infections of the Endocardium

The well-known skin lesions of bacterial endocarditis are Osler's nodes, Janeway's lesions, and subungual splinter hemorrhages. Osler's nodes are small, transient, red, tender papules on the volar surfaces of the fingers and toes that are found in a minority of patients with subacute bacterial endocarditis. Janeway's lesions are non-tender, red macules on the palms and soles. Besides splinter hemorrhages, widespread petechial skin lesions are characteristic of bacterial infection of the endocardium.

Histopathology. Osler's nodes are reported to contain a polymorphous inflammatory infiltrate with dermal edema and varying degrees of vasculitis. Descriptions of Janeway's lesion include the formation of dermal abscess as well as polymorphous inflammation. Patients with these lesions should be assayed for the presence of subacute bacterial endocarditis. Tissue aspirates from these skin lesions have been used to isolate organisms; however, blood cultures are a more direct means of determining the presence of sepsis. Appropriate cardiac evaluation should also be performed.

Therapy. Therapy is directed at the cardiac lesions, the treatment of which will result in the resolution of skin lesions. Usually long-term (more than 6 weeks) intravenous antibiotic therapy is needed.

NON-VENEREAL SPIROCHETAL DISEASE

Lyme Disease

Lyme disease is caused by infection with the spirochete *Borrelia burgdorferi.* Infection is transmitted by *Ixodes dammini* or a related ixodid tick. Although the illness has been widely observed, it is most frequently found in the northeastern United States, the northern Midwest, and the Far West.

Clinical Findings. The illness is associated with a characteristic skin eruption known as erythema chronicum migrans. This eruption begins as a central papule from which an expanding red, slightly palpable circular and arcuate eruption develops, associated with central clearing (Fig. 34–6). The gyrate erythema can become quite large. Color variations are noted as the lesion advances and ages. The affected area may be warm. Other skin lesions that may appear with Lyme disease include urticaria and conjunctivitis. Systemic findings, including arthritis, cardiac involvement, and central nervous system findings, develop.

Histopathology. Biopsies taken from erythema chronicum migrans show variability with dermal edema and a heavy mononuclear infiltrate around superficial vessels. Spirochetes may be demonstrated with tissue silver stains.

Patient Evaluation. Serologic tests may be helpful in confirming the diagnosis, and the spirochete can occasionally be demonstrated in skin biopsies taken from lesions of erythema chronicum migrans. Appropriate consultation should be obtained, depending on the systemic signs and symptoms that accompany the rash.

Therapy. Antibiotic management with tetracycline is the treatment of choice.

MYCOBACTERIAL DISEASES

Cutaneous Mycobacterial Disease Produced by *Mycobacterium tuberculosis*

Although tuberculosis is primarily a disease of internal organs, mostly the lungs, there are a number of well-described skin

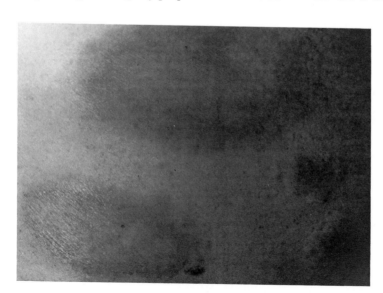

Figure 34–6. Erythematous annular lesions of erythema chronicum migrans.

lesions associated with infection by *M. tuberculosis*.

Clinical Findings. *M. tuberculosis* may be inoculated directly into the skin of a person who has never had tuberculosis; in this situation, the primary lesion is usually a verrucous papule that may be crusted or eroded (Prosector's chancre). The primary lesion is small but may enlarge. This lesion plus the affected regional lymph nodes forms the primary complex following skin inoculation. The diagnosis can be supported and confirmed by skin biopsy and culture.

Inoculation of *M. tuberculosis* into the skin of a person who has previously been infected by this organism results in a lesion known as tuberculosis verrucosa cutis. The lesion is acral and asymptomatic, and it slowly expands in a radial fashion. The surface is warty and is covered by keratinous debris. This form of tuberculosis must be separated from other hyperkeratotic verrucous processes such as blastomycosis, chromomycosis, and other chancriform lesions.

Another skin lesion that can be found in patients with previous exposure to *M. tuberculosis* is lupus vulgaris. This asymptomatic lesion, found primarily on the head and neck, slowly expands and can eventually form a large plaque with surface features that range from atrophy to hyperkeratosis (Fig. 34–7). Over a long period, this lesion may produce significant scarring as well as distortion and destruction of underlying structures. Lupus vulgaris must be differentiated from sarcoidosis, discoid lupus erythematosus, and a variety of chronic bacterial and fungal diseases. A large percentage of patients with lupus vulgaris have underlying tuberculosis in other organs. A late sequela of lupus vulgaris is the development of squamous cell carcinoma within the lesion.

The skin may be secondarily involved by spread of *M. tuberculosis*. Scrofuloderma is produced by direct extension of tuberculosis to the skin from an underlying structure (usually involved lymph nodes, but also from bone and joints). The most commonly involved area is the head and neck. A second pattern of secondary extension to the skin is the formation of metastatic tuberculous abscesses from hematogenous spread. However, acute miliary tuberculosis of the skin is found almost exclusively in children who are gravely ill. A third manifestation of sec-

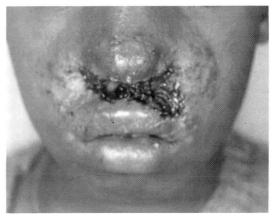

Figure 34–7. Crusted plaques in a malar distribution also involving the nose and the mustache area in a patient with cutaneous tuberculosis (lupus vulgaris).

ondary cutaneous involvement is orificial tuberculosis; these lesions are found on mucous membranes and periorificial skin and represent spread from an internal focus. This is a rare manifestation of *M. tuberculosis* infection and indicates widespread disease. Pulmonary disease generally precedes oral involvement; intestinal disease precedes perianal involvement; and genitourinary disease precedes genital involvement.

There are a number of skin lesions known as tuberculids. Originally these skin lesions were thought to represent true involvement of the skin by *M. tuberculosis*. It is now apparent that the pathogenesis of these lesions is poorly understood and that their relationship to active infection is unclear. These lesions include lichen scrofulosorum (a lichenoid eruption found on the trunk, primarily in children), papulonecrotic tuberculid (symmetrical crops of papules with central necrosis that heal with a scar), and erythema induratum of Bazin (a chronic, tender, nodular, and ulcerating process of the posterior legs in women).

Histopathology. Cutaneous tuberculosis produces variable changes, depending on the type and age of the lesion. Primary lesions initially contain a neutrophilic infiltrate. As the lesion ages, epithelioid cells and giant cells may be present and caseation necrosis becomes a feature. Tuberculous organisms can be identified by acid-fast stain. Similar histologic changes occur with hematogenous spread of tuberculosis to the skin. In tuberculosis verrucosa cutis, there is prominent epidermal hyperplasia coupled with an acute inflammatory infiltrate. Organisms can be demonstrated with acid-fast stains. In lupus vulgaris, early granulomas are found with a variable inflammatory infiltrate. Variable epidermal alterations are present. In scrofuloderma, there is an abscess composed of necrotic material surrounded by an inflammatory reaction. Acid-fast–positive organisms are generally present.

Patient Evaluation. Patients with cutaneous tuberculosis should be evaluated for underlying or disseminated disease. Material should be collected for culture to confirm the diagnosis. Skin testing can be performed to support the clinical diagnosis.

Therapy. A variety of anti-tuberculous agents are available, including isoniazid, rifampin, and ethambutol. The recommendation for the exact combination and length of treatment changes periodically.

Leprosy

Leprosy is a chronic granulomatous disease caused by *Mycobacterium leprae*, an acid-fast–positive bacterium rod found primarily within histiocytes. Despite historical beliefs, the disease is not highly communicable. The method of transmission is not clearly defined but probably involves direct contact or fomites. Skin lesions represent a panoply of findings that indicate the type of host response induced by the infection. Leprosy affects the relatively cool areas of the skin; thus, lesions are most apt to occur on exposed surfaces such as earlobes.

Clinical Findings. The earliest skin lesions of leprosy occur as indeterminate leprosy, which is characterized by ill-defined macules. As the disease advances to one of the more clearly defined stages, these early lesions may fade.

Patients with tuberculoid leprosy have active cellular immunity to *M. leprae* and have a strongly positive lepromin test (cutaneous response to standardized extracts of infected tissue). Skin lesions may be single or multiple. The lesions are variable in size, clearly defined, and frequently hypopigmented (Fig. 34–8; Plate *VI C*). Within these lesions, there are sensory alterations such as loss of touch discrimination and thermal sensation that are secondary to nerve infiltration and damage. Another characteristic finding of tuberculoid leprosy is nerve enlargement, partic-

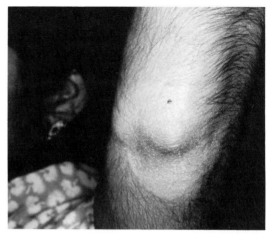

Figure 34–8. Hypopigmented anesthetic skin in an Indian physician with tuberculoid leprosy (see also Plate VI C).

ularly affecting the ulnar and greater auricular nerves, but also involving other superficial nerves (Fig. 34–9). Enlargement may be to the point at which these nerves are grossly visible on general physical examination.

In patients with a reduced cellular immune response to *M. leprae*, the pattern of skin disease changes and evolves into lesions that are typical of lepromatous leprosy. Lepromatous leprosy represents an immune state in which there is anergy and a negative lepromin reaction. Skin lesions are pleomorphic and range from macules to nodules, plaques, and diffuse infiltrative lesions (Fig. 34–10). Patients can develop the leonine facies, in which there is diffuse facial thickening associated with loss of eyebrows and eyelashes. Lesions are usually widespread and multiple. A rare form of lepromatous leprosy is the diffuse leprosy of Lucio. This form is characterized by a diffuse skin infiltrate by *M. leprae* with few localized stigmata of leprosy.

Borderline, or dimorphous, leprosy can present a spectrum of skin lesions ranging from those similar to polar tuberculoid leprosy (in borderline tuberculoid leprosy) to those similar to polar lepromatous leprosy (in borderline lepromatous leprosy). The lepromin reaction is variable. Skin lesions in a given patient can vary from one extreme to the other as the unstable immune response to the organism alters. If there is a shift to the tuberculoid pole, the patient may have a reversal reaction in which skin lesions may redden and become tender and nerves may become tender and enlarged. If

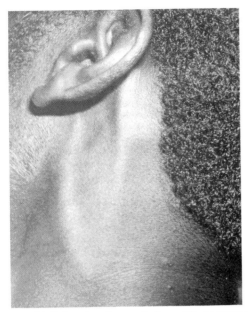

Figure 34-9. Prominent nerve in lipomatous leprosy.

there is a shift toward the lepromatous pole, the patient may experience a downgrading reaction heralded by widespread lesions of erythema nodosum leprosum (painful, red nodules that clinically mimic those of erythema nodosum) accompanied by fever and other constitutional symptoms. Downgrading reactions are frequently chronic and may be disabling.

Histopathology. Skin biopsy will reveal a spectrum of findings, depending on the type of disease. Specimens from indeterminate leprosy are not diagnostic and contain a minimal inflammtory infiltrate. Tissue sections from tuberculoid leprosy reveal well-

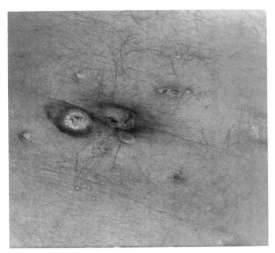

Figure 34-10. Multiple nodules present in lipomatous leprosy.

formed granulomas, perineural inflammation, and rare organisms demonstrable with Fite's stain. Tissue from skin lesions of lepromatous leprosy reveals a perivascular and diffuse infiltrate of histiocytes, and numerous organisms can be found with Fite's stain. Borderline lesions vary between changes noted in polar tuberculoid leprosy and those seen in polar lepromatous leprosy.

Patient Evaluation. Slit smear (a small superficial skin incision with expression of tissue fluid that is stained with acid-fast or Fite's stain) can be used to confirm the diagnosis from borderline tuberculoid to lepromatous leprosy (cases in which ample quantities of organisms are present in tissue). Appropriate neurologic, otolaryngologic, ophthalmologic, and surgical evaluation should be performed, depending on the symptoms and signs exhibited by the patient. The differential diagnosis of leprosy is truly legion and again varies with the clinical presentation. For example, leonine facies may be a manifestation of lepromatous leprosy; however, leonine facies can also be seen secondary to leukemic and lymphomatous infiltration of the skin. Skin biopsy dramatically reduces the list of diagnostic possibilities.

Therapy. Therapy involves the use of 2 principal drugs, dapsone and rifampin. Therapy depends on the stage of the disease. For patients who have indeterminate, polar tuberculoid, or borderline tuberculoid leprosy, the concurrent administration of rifampin, 600 mg once monthly, and oral dapsone, 100 mg daily for 6 months, is the regimen of choice. For patients with multibacillary forms of leprosy, a similar regimen with the addition of clofazimine, 50 mg per day, is used, and treatment must be continued for at least 2 years. Of course, there are many variations in the treatment of this complex disease. Patients must be followed for prolonged periods of time. Response of patients to therapy may be monitored by repeated skin biopsies and slit smears.

Atypical Mycobacterial Infections

Skin involvement in healthy individuals by atypical mycobacteria is primarily caused by *Mycobacterium marinum* (a member of Runyon's group I, photochromogens). This organism is found in aquatic environments and is usually inoculated into the skin following an abrasion. Thus, the lesion occurs

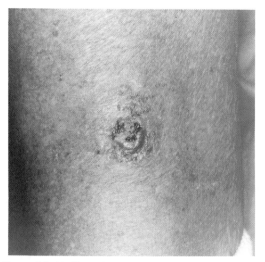

Figure 34-11. Ulcerated nodular lesion representative of atypical mycobacterial infection (swimming pool granuloma).

primarily in persons exposed to fish tanks, boats, stagnant pools, and so forth. Lesions for the most part occur on the hands and the arms.

The primary lesion of M. marinum infection is chancriform, hyperkeratotic, and occasionally ulcerative (Fig. 34–11). Secondary lesions may spread in a sporotrichoid fashion along the regional lymphatic vessels. The disease is self-limited and usually resolves in 1–2 years.

A rare skin lesion is Buruli's ulceration, an extensive ulcerative process that results from infection with Mycobacterium ulcerans. Most of these lesions are solitary and are on the lower extremities. This diagnosis should be considered if the patient has traveled to an endemic area (Uganda, Mexico, Australia) and has a large, ulcerative skin lesion.

Lastly, Mycobacterium intracellularis rarely can produce non-specific skin lesions following dissemination in patients who have the acquired immune deficiency syndrome (AIDS).

Histopathology. Skin biopsy of a swimming pool granuloma lesion (M. marinum) reveals granulomatous dermatitis with overlying epidermal hyperplasia. Occasional Langerhans giant cells can be found within the infiltrate. Acid-fast stains will demonstrate organisms in some cases, usually in early lesions. Failure to demonstrate acid-fast organisms does not exclude the diagnosis of atypical mycobacteriosis. Skin biopsy of Buruli's ulcer reveals cutaneous ulceration with necrosis and a sparse infiltrate.

Acid-fast stains will demonstrate organisms in the ulceration. Biopsy of skin lesions of M. intracellularis reveals granulomatous dermatitis with myriads of acid-fast organisms within the cytoplasm of histiocytes.

Patient Evaluation. A disease similar to swimming pool granuloma is rarely produced by the photochromogen Mycobacterium kansasii. Confirmation of the diagnosis is by culture on special media. Confirmation of infection by M. ulcerans and M. intracellularis is by culture under appropriate conditions.

Therapy. A variety of treatments can be used for M. marinum infection, including the local application of heat; local excision; and oral therapy with minocycline, tetracycline, or antituberculous drugs such as rifampin.

Suggested Readings

Catanzaro FJ, Stetson CA, Morris AJ, et al: The role of the streptococcus in the pathogenesis of rheumatic fever. Am J Med 17:749–752, 1954.

Dalldorf FG, Jennette JC: Fatal meningococcal septicemia. Arch Pathol 101:6–9, 1977.

Dorff GJ, Geimer NF, Rosenthal DR, et al: Pseudomonas septicemia: Illustrated evolution of its skin lesions. Arch Intern Med 128:591–595, 1971.

Elias PM, Fritsch P, Epstein EH Jr: Staphylococcal scalded skin syndrome: Clinical features, pathogenesis, and recent microbiological and biochemical developments. Arch Dermatol 113:207–211, 1977.

Goette DK, Jacobson KW, Doty RD: Primary inoculation tuberculosis of the skin. Arch Dermatol 114:567–569, 1978.

Goihman-Yahr M: Leprosy, an overview. Int J Dermatol 423:430, 1982.

Gott RE, Carter DM, Sall T: Cutaneous infection caused by atypical mycobacteria. Arch Dermatol 95:259–268, 1967.

Kerr A, Tan JS: Biopsies of the Janeway lesion of infective endocarditis. J Cutan Pathol 6:124–129, 1979.

Masi AT, Eisenstein BI: Disseminated gonococcal infection (DGI) and gonococcal arthritis (GCA): II, Clinical manifestations, diagnosis, complications, treatment and prevention. Semin Arthritis Rheum 10:173–186, 1981.

Melish ME, Glasgow LA: The staphylococcal scalded skin syndrome: Development of an experimental model. N Engl J Med 282:1114–1117, 1970.

Penneys NS, Hicks B: Unusual cutaneous lesions associated with acquired immunodeficiency syndrome. J Am Acad Dermatol 13:845–852, 1985.

Schlievert PM, Shands KN, Dan BB, et al: Identification and characterization of an exotoxin from Staphylococcus aureus associated with toxic shock syndrome. J Infect Dis 143:509–514, 1981.

Wannamaker LW: Differences between streptococcal infections of the throat and of the skin. N Engl J Med 282:23–27, 1970.

35

Venereal Disease with Disseminated Cutaneous Manifestations

NEAL PENNEYS

Venereal diseases are an important area of internal disease in which cutaneous lesions are guides to appropriate diagnosis. AIDS, gonorrhea, herpes simplex, and Reiter's syndrome are discussed in Chapters 32, 34, 32, and 6, respectively. Discussion of warts, molluscum contagiosum, scabies, and pediculosis is beyond the scope of this text, but can be found in recent review articles or dermatological textbooks.

SYPHILIS

Transmission of syphilis is most often through sexual contact. The causative agent is the spirochete *Treponema pallidum*. The pattern of disease varies, and cutaneous signs are multiform, numerous, and will vary depending on the duration of the infection. At the portal of entry, a chancre develops approximately 7–21 days after infection. The chancre may be asymptomatic and last from 1 to 5 weeks. Chancres begin as papules and evolve into firm, superficial nodules that ulcerate and are covered by a crust. The most typical locations for these lesions are in the genital area, although chancres can be in perianal, oral, and other locations. Usually regional lymphadenopathy is present.

Progression to secondary syphilis occurs at a variable time after infection, usually 8 weeks to 6 months after development of the chancre. In some cases, the chancre may still be present. Secondary syphilis is characterized by a wide variety of lesions that may be flat, palpable, nodular, ulcerative, or follicular. Macular lesions are most common, and they are usually non-pruritic and widespread (Fig. 35–1). Involvement of the palms and soles by secondary lesions is characteristic (Fig. 35–2). Individual lesions can masquerade as almost any dermatosis. Lesions can resemble psoriasis, acne, fungal disease, and ulcerative processes. When these lesions are on mucous membranes, they are named condylomata lata (Fig. 35–3). Secondary syphilis is often associated with systemic symptoms, including malaise, headache, and myalgias. Liver, bone marrow, kidney, and other organs may be involved in secondary syphilis. Lesions of secondary syphilis will disappear, and latent syphilis can develop and will persist indefinitely unless there is treatment or disease progression.

When syphilis is acquired *in utero*, the pattern and variety of subsequent skin lesions vary considerably from those noted previously, depending on the age of the patient and the persistence of the infection. Neonatal syphilis may be of serious import to the infant. It is characterized by a variety

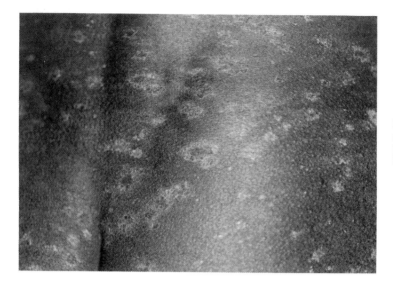

Figure 35–1. Multiple scaly plaques similar to pityriasis rosea are present in this patient with secondary syphilis.

of secondary signs, including abdominal distention, edema, and hepatosplenomegaly. Unlike syphilis in adults, the skin lesions may be vesicular. Fissures of the angles of the mouth and surrounding the anus are present in a majority of patients. Syphilitic rhinitis may also be present and is charac-

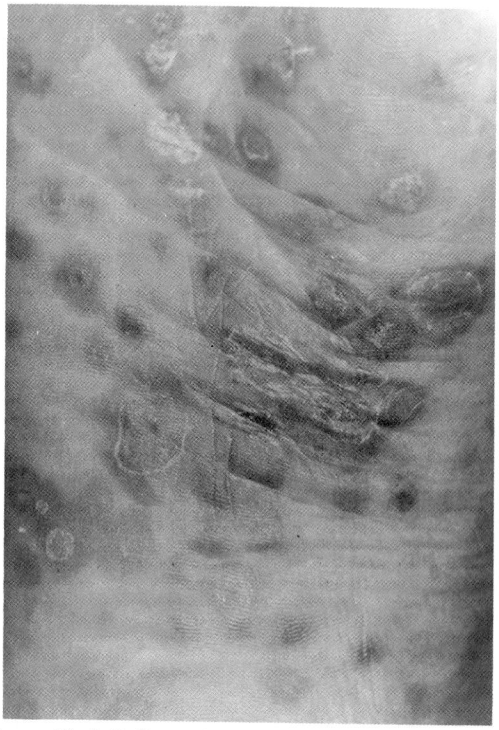

Figure 35–2. Erythematous plaques are present on the sole of this individual with secondary syphilis.

terized by an associated bloody mucinous secretion known as snuffles. Multiple other organ systems may be affected in this form of the disease. Neonatal syphilis should be considered a potentially fatal condition. The course of syphilis after infancy is slowly progressive, and a variety of skin lesions may be associated with progression of the disease. Hutchinson's triad is considered typical of late pre-natal syphilis. The triad includes interstitial keratitis, eighth cranial nerve deafness, and Hutchinson's teeth (an abnormality of the upper central incisors). Other sequelae of late pre-natal syphilis are rhagades (linear scars radiating from the nose, eyes, mouth, and chin); Higouménakis sign (unilateral enlargement of the clavicle); frontal bossing (of Parrot); saber shin deformity; and a high, arched palate.

Histopathology. Syphilis is associated with an array of histologic findings, which depend on the stage of the disease. Early lesions are characterized by endothelial swelling coupled with a polymorphous infiltrate containing plasma cells. Lesions of secondary syphilis may have a variety of histologic appearances, ranging from interface dermatitis to granulomatous dermatitis; the presence of plasma cells coupled with these other features should suggest the possibility of secondary syphilis. Characteristically, gummatous lesions of tertiary lues contain areas of tissue necrosis coupled with a polymorphous infiltrate that frequently contains plasma cells. In early lesions of syphilis, spirochetes may be identified in tissue using silver stains.

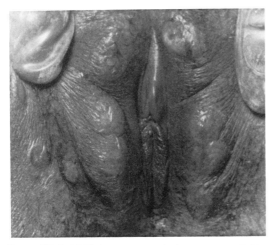

Figure 35–3. Multiple verrucous lesions representative of secondary syphilis (condylomata lata).

Patient Evaluation. Primary syphilis should be diagnosed by darkfield microscopy with serologic follow-up. The sensitivity of the Venereal Disease Research Laboratory (VDRL) test is high in secondary and early latent syphilis but is reduced in primary and late syphilis and in cerebrospinal fluid studies. Asymptomatic persons, including pregnant women, and asymptomatic contacts of persons with syphilis should be screened with the VDRL test with confirmation of a positive result by a more specific treponemal test (FTA-ABS). Quantitative VDRL determinations should be obtained at 3, 6, and 12 months after treatment, to assess adequacy of the treatment regimen for both early and late latent syphilis. VDRL determinations in spinal fluid should be restricted to persons who are seropositive and who have a high risk for the development of neurosyphilis. Because syphilis is a disease with protean manifestations, a complex differential list of other dermatological diseases must be considered and excluded. Because of the ease and reliability of serologic tests for syphilis, it is often important to exclude syphilis by performing serologic follow-up.

Therapy. Treatment for early stages of syphilis is the administration of 2.4 million units of benzathine penicillin G by intramuscular injection or 600,000 units of procaine penicillin G daily by intramuscular injection for 8 days. Latent or indeterminate syphilis is treated by the intramuscular administration of 2.4 million units of benzathine penicillin G weekly for 3 weeks. For patients allergic to penicillin, tetracycline hydrochloride, 500 mg four times a day by

mouth for 15 days (or for 30 days for late syphilis), is considered adequate. However, careful patient follow-up for adequacy of treatment is mandatory.

CHANCROID

Chancroid is a sexually transmitted disease caused by infection by the organism *Haemophilus ducreyi*, a gram-negative, nonmotile baccilus. Chancroid is characterized by multiple papules and small ulcerations, primarily in the genital region, that develop about 2–5 days after infection. Cutaneous ulcers are irregular in shape, are soft, and have slightly undermined borders (Fig. 35–4). Lesions often bleed and may be quite painful. Lesions are found most frequently on the prepuce, corona, and shaft of the penis and on the labia, clitoris, fourchette, and vestibule. The cervix and vagina may also be involved. Extragenital lesions are very unusual. Chancroid is associated with painful lymphadenopathy (i.e., the bubo). Systemic symptoms such as headache and fever may be present.

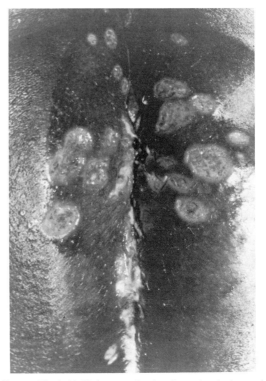

Figure 35–4. Multiple, punched-out, erosive lesions of chancroid.

Patient Evaluation. The diagnosis of chancroid is most often based on clinical findings and on the exclusion of other infections such as syphilis, herpes simplex, lymphogranuloma venereum, and granuloma inguinale by darkfield examination, serologic testing, viral culture, and skin biopsy. Gram stains of infected tissue reveal large numbers of gram-negative coccobacilli, which may be arranged in "school of fish" patterns. Cultures should be obtained, and an attempt should be made to grow the organism on special media.

Treatment. Erythromycin, 500 mg four times a day, or trimethoprim-sulfamethoxazole, 160/800 mg twice a day, are the antibiotic regimens of choice for chancroid.

GRANULOMA INGUINALE

Granuloma inguinale is a venereal disease that is most prevalent among poorer socioeconomic groups. The infection is most common in Asia, the West Indies, and South America. In the United States, blacks are infected more frequently than whites. The causative organism is *Donovania granulomatis*, a short, plump bacillus that is gramnegative and heavily encapsulated. The organisms are usually found intracellularly in the cytoplasm of macrophages. The incubation period for this disease has not been established but it is probably on the order of several weeks.

Clinical Findings. The lesions usually be-

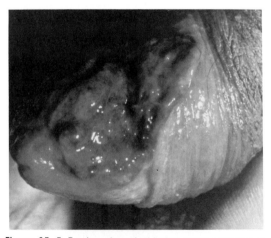

Figure 35–5. Erosive ulcerated lesion representative of granuloma inguinale infection.

gin as asymptomatic, small papules that enlarge and become superficially eroded (Fig. 35–5). Individual lesions may become quite large. The lesions are found most commonly in the perineal, perianal, and vaginal areas. Rarely, lesions are found on other body sites.

Histology. The lesion may be focally ulcerated. In the dermis, there is a dense infiltrate composed predominantly of plasma cells and histiocytes. Scattered, small collections of neutrophils are also present. With Giemsa's stain, the organism may be seen within the cytoplasm of histiocytes as small inclusion bodies surrounded by a non-staining capsule.

Patient Evaluation. Granuloma inguinale must be differentiated from other ulceronodular lesions, including squamous cell carcinoma; cutaneous fungal disease; bacterial infections, including tuberculosis; and other granulomatous skin lesions. Confirmation of the diagnosis is by the demonstration of Donovan bodies (bipolar structures with unstained capsules in the cytoplasm of histiocytes) in crush preparations of tissue taken from the clinical lesion. Syphilis should be excluded by appropriate serologic tests.

Therapy. Tetracycline, 500 mg four times a day, or trimethoprim-sulfamethoxazole, 2 tablets every 12 hours, is considered effective treatment. Medication should be continued until the lesions have resolved.

LYMPHOGRANULOMA VENEREUM

Lymphogranuloma venereum is an infection produced by microorganisms belonging to the *Chlamydia trachomatis* group that is usually transmitted in association with sexual intercourse. The primary lesion is a transitory papule that is usually not recognized. Inguinal lymphadenitis develops after initial infection, most commonly in males. Lymphadenopathy may be either unilateral or bilateral and is frequently tender. Coalescence of lymph nodes above and below Poupart's ligament produces the groove sign. Eventually, lymphadenopathy will resolve, although rupture and drainage to the surface may occur with fistula formation. Chronic infection leads to local forms of elephantiasis, chronic ulcerations, and fistulae. Lymphogranuloma venereum may be associated with severe rectal symptoms, including pain, tenesmus, and discharge. Late sequelae of rectal involvement include stricture, elephantiasis, and ulceration. Non-specific cutaneous manifestations that have been recorded with lymphogranuloma venereum include urticaria, non-specific eruptions, erythema multiforme, and photosensitivity.

Patient Evaluation. At the present time, the diagnosis is best suspected by clinical impression and confirmed by an increase in titer of the complement fixation test. Other venereal disease can be excluded by serologic means, viral cultures, and skin biopsy findings.

Therapy. Fluctuant buboes should be aspirated prior to their rupture. Tetracycline, 500 mg four times a day for at least 14 days, is the recommended treatment.

GONORRHEA AND REITER'S SYNDROME

Gonorrhea and Reiter's syndrome are discussed in Chapters 34 and 6, respectively.

Suggested Readings

Becker LE: Lymphogranuloma venereum. Int J Dermatol 15:26–33, 1976.

Chapel TA: The variability of syphilitic chancres. Sex Transm Dis 5:68–73, 1978.

Chapel TA: The signs and symptoms of secondary syphilis. Sex Transm Dis 7:161–169, 1980.

Davis CM: Granuloma inguinale. J Am Med Assn 211:632–636, 1970.

Dodson RF, Fritz GS, Hubler WR Jr, et al: Donovanosis: A morphologic study. J Invest Dermatol 62:611–614, 1974.

Fiumara NJ: Reinfection with primary, secondary, and latent syphilis. Sex Transm Dis 6:243–249, 1979.

Gaisin A, Heaton CL: Chancroid: Alias the soft chancre. Int J Dermol 14:188–197, 1975.

Hammond GW, Slutchuk M, Scatliff J, et al: Epidemiologic, clinical, laboratory and therapeutic features of an urban outbreak of chancroid in North America. Rev Infect Dis 2:867–874, 1980.

Jeerapaet P, Ackerman AB: Histologic patterns of secondary syphilis. Arch Dermatol 107:373–377, 1973.

Margolis RJ, Hood AF: Chancroid: Diagnosis and treatment. J Am Acad Dermatol 6:493–499, 1982.

Rockwell DH, Yobs AR, Moore MB: The Tuskegee study of untreated syphilis; the 30th year of observation. Arch Intern Med 114:792–796, 1964.

Schachter J: Chlamydial infections. N Engl J Med 298:428–435, 1978.

36

Cutaneous Signs of Protozoan Disease

NEAL PENNEYS

The parasitic diseases such as the helminth diseases are of critical importance in many areas of the world. However, a review of these conditions is beyond the scope of this text. Scabies and pediculosis are very important dermatological diseases; however, they are not "skin" signs of systemic disease. This chapter will focus very briefly on an overview of leishmaniasis and amebiasis.

LEISHMANIASIS

Leishmania is a genus of dimorphic protozoa that are found within the cells of the reticuloendothelial system as amastigotes in the mammalian host. The disease leishmaniasis is transmitted by the sandfly.

Clinical Findings. The most common forms of leishmaniasis (cutaneous leishmaniasis of the Old World, or Oriental sore; cutaneous leishmaniasis of the New World) are localized cutaneous lesions produced by *L. tropica* and *L. braziliensis*, and *L. mexicana*, respectively (Fig. 36–1). Lesions may occur along draining lymphatics (i.e., sporotrichoid spread). Infection by *L. donovani* produces visceral leishmaniasis, which in turn can be associated with characteristic skin changes. The primary inoculation site in visceral leishmaniasis is usually inapparent. The clinical manifestations vary but usually include the insidious onset of abdominal discomfort, fever, weakness, and pallor. Organomegaly develops, and the spleen may become dramatically enlarged. Many cutaneous signs develop, which are not specific and include dryness, pallor, petechiae, ecchymoses, jaundice, and alopecia. A characteristic change is a darkening of the skin of the hands, feet, abdomen, and face, a change that gave rise to the Indian name "kala-azar," or black fever. If patients survive the acute phase of the disease, a variable number of individuals will develop a post–kala-azar dermal leishmaniasis. These skin lesions may appear up to 2 years following treatment of the acute phase. Lesions range from hypopigmented macules to large nodules that resemble those seen in leprosy.

Leishmaniasis is associated with a number of cutaneous manifestations, including primary cutaneous inoculation lesions and sec-

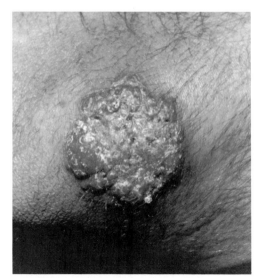

Figure 36–1. Nodular lesion representative of cutaneous leishmaniasis.

ondary skin lesions in visceral leishmaniasis. There are a number of non-specific cutaneous changes associated with visceral disease, including pallor, darkening of the skin, petechiae, and alopecia.

Histopathology. In acute lesions, there is a dermal infiltrate composed of macrophages containing intracellular *Leishmania* organisms. Organisms are best seen with Giemsa's stain. In chronic lesions, there is a granulomatous infiltrate and organisms are rarely found. In biopsies from skin lesions of kala-azar, a granulomatous infiltrate is present and organisms are usually demonstrable in tissue sections.

Patient Evaluation. Appropriate cultures on special media and serologic testing will facilitate diagnosis of the acute phase. Skin biopsy will reveal the organism in specific cutaneous lesions.

Therapy. The drugs of choice are pentavalent antimonials. For localized cutaneous leishmaniasis, a variety of local treatments, including cryotherapy and surgical excision, have been described.

AMEBIASIS

Amebae are spherical organisms that exist in 2 forms: a motile form called a trophozoite, and a non-motile, encysted form that is found when conditions are not favorable for the single cell protozoan. *Entamoeba histolytica* is the most common member of the *Amoeba* group to be pathogenic in humans.

Clinical Findings. Amebiasis is primarily an intestinal disease, but it may also present as cutaneous amebiasis. Usually, intestinal amebiasis is present concomitantly with cutaneous amebiasis (the skin being involved by direct extension from an internal viscus). Consequently, cutaneous amebiasis is most frequently seen in the groin and perineal regions but also can be found on the face, abdomen, and buttocks, and around colostomy sites. The typical skin lesion is a rapidly enlarging ulcer with a necrotic slough covered by exudate. Disseminated amebiasis with subcutaneous abscesses has been observed in the acquired immune deficiency syndrome (AIDS).

Patient Evaluation. Confirmation of the diagnosis depends on the demonstration of the trophozoite in fresh sample material from the ulcer bed.

Therapy. Treatment is by an assortment of medications, depending on the site of involvement, since some medications may be active for luminal disease whereas others are necessary for tissue involvement. Treatment of cutaneous amebiasis includes topical ulcer care as well as systemic medications.

Suggested Readings

Adams EB, MacLeod IN: Invasive amebiasis. I. Amebic liver abscess and its complications. Medicine 56:325, 1977.

Kerdel-Vegal F: American leishmaniasis. Int J Dermatol 121:291, 1982.

Marsden PD, Nonata RR: Mucocutaneous leishmaniasis—a review of clinical aspects. Rev Soc Bras Med Trop 9:309, 1975.

Most H, Lavietes PH: Kala-azar in American military personnel. Report of 30 cases. Medicine 26:221, 1947.

37

Rickettsial Diseases

NEAL PENNEYS

The family of microbes Rickettsiaceae is composed of obligate intracellular organisms transmitted to humans by a variety of arthropods. The microbes are small coccobacilli-like organisms that produce a spectrum of cutaneous eruptions that greatly facilitate diagnosis of infection. The general characteristics of the rickettsial diseases, including Weil-Felix reactions, are presented in Table 37–1.

ROCKY MOUNTAIN SPOTTED FEVER

The most frequent rickettsial infection in the United States is Rocky Mountain spotted fever. The disease, caused by *Rickettsia rickettsii*, ranges in severity from an asymptomatic form to a potentially life-threatening disease. The incidence of the disease correlates with increased tick activity and with exposure to the tick vectors, *Dermacentor andersoni* and *Dermacentor variabilis*. This generally occurs in the spring and summer months. Originally, the disease was confined to the western United States; however, now more than one half of all cases are reported from the southeastern region of the United States. A history of tick exposure can be obtained in a majority of patients.

Clinical Findings. The highest incidence of disease is in children 5–9 years of age. The incubation period will vary but averages 8 days. The illness begins with chills, myalgias, and headache. Muscle tenderness may be present, along with photophobia and conjunctivitis. The characteristic rash appears 4 days after the onset of symptoms and is macular and initially pink. It begins acrally, affecting the palms, soles (Fig. 37–1), wrists,

and arms; it then proceeds centrally. At a variable time after the appearance of the rash, extravasation of erythrocytes occurs and the eruption becomes rose-colored and non-blanchable. Rarely, ulceration occurs, usually in distal locations.

Histopathology. Skin biopsy reveals necrotizing vasculitis with a perivascular, focally dense inflammatory infiltrate and focal extravasation of erythrocytes. Using Giemsa's stain, the organism can occasionally be demonstrated in tissue sections associated with endothelium. Organisms can also be identified rapidly in skin biopsy specimens by immunofluorescence microscopic examination.

Patient Evaluation. Rocky Mountain spotted fever must be separated from other serious infectious diseases. A history of tick bite supports this diagnosis. Because of severe headache, viral and bacterial meningitis has to be excluded. Meningococcemia produces a delicate, discrete rash that varies from macular to slightly papular and that occasionally is petechial in character. Also, the association of disseminated intravascular coagulopathy with meningococcemia may be confused with Rocky Mountain spotted fever. Viral diseases, such as measles, that may be confused with Rocky Mountain spotted fever can be excluded based on differing patterns of skin eruption, self-limiting behavior, and appropriate history suggesting viral exposure. Other related rickettsiae produce milder forms of disease similar to Rocky Mountain spotted fever, but these conditions (listed in Table 37–1) are generally milder and are not frequently found in the United States. Of note is the primary lesion in this group, a necrotic ulcer at the

Table 37–1. GENERAL CHARACTERISTICS OF THE RICKETTSIAL DISEASES

Disease	Organism	Vector	Predominant Area	Weil-Felix Reaction		
				OX-19	OX-2	OX-K
Rocky Mountain spotted fever	R. rickettsii	Tick	United States	+	+	−
North Asian tick typhus	R. siberica	Tick	Eastern Asia	+	+	−
Queensland tick typhus	R. australis	Tick	Australia	+	+	−
Boutonneuse fever (and others)	R. conorii	Tick	Africa, India, southern France	+	+	−
Rickettsialpox	R. akari	Mite	United States, widespread	−	−	−
Murine typhus	R. typhi	Flea	Widespread	+	Variable	−
Q fever	C. burnettii	—	Widespread	−	−	−
Epidemic typhus	R. prowazekii	Body louse	Widespread	+	Variable	−
Scrub typhus	R. tsutsugamushi	Mite	Asia, Australia	−	−	+

site of tick attachment, the tache noire. Confirmation of cause depends on serologic techniques, including the agglutination by serum of various strains of *Proteus* organisms (Weil-Felix reaction) and by complement fixation tests.

Treatment. Treatment of the spotted fever group is with appropriate supportive therapy and with tetracycline or chloramphenicol. Dosages vary from 50 to 100 mg/kg/day. Because of lower inherent toxicity, tetracycline is the preferred drug. In endemic areas, a low threshold for the treatment with oral tetracycline in patients with acral exanthems and a systemic toxic illness is warranted.

RICKETTSIALPOX

Rickettsialpox is a mild, non-fatal febrile process caused by infection with *R. akari*. It

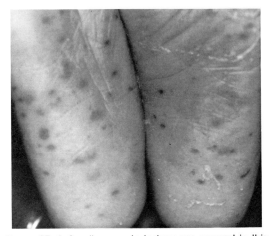

Figure 37–1. Small, purpuric lesions are present in this patient with Rocky Mountain spotted fever.

is transmitted by a mouse mite and occurs primarily in urban areas of the United States. As with Rocky Mountain spotted fever, the onset is sudden and is characterized by chills, fever, headache, and sweating. The initial lesion is a papule, frequently vesicular, that precedes the generalized eruption by 4–7 days. The papule ulcerates and forms an eschar. The eruption becomes generalized and involves the palms and soles and occasionally the oral mucosa. The eruption resolves by crusting and healing without scar formation.

Patient Evaluation. The rash resembles varicella in its early stages; however, varicella occurs most commonly in children and becomes diffusely vesicular, whereas rickettsialpox does not. Other rickettsial diseases associated with eschar formation should be excluded, including scrub typhus, boutonneuse fever, and Siberian and Queensland tick typhus. The Weil-Felix test is negative after infection by *R. akari*. However, specific complement fixing antibodies are present.

Therapy. Tetracycline is the favored form of treatment. The dosage is similar to that used for Rocky Mountain spotted fever.

ENDEMIC (MURINE) TYPHUS

Endemic (murine) typhus is an infectious process that follows exposure to a rat flea and is caused by *R. typhi*. This disease occurs in individuals who have exposure to rats, either as an occupational hazard or through living conditions. Endemic typhus occurs primarily in the southern United States. The infection begins acutely with headache, fever, and myalgias. The rash, present in the majority of patients, develops from the third to the fifth day of symptoms and is macular. The eruption is truncal in distribution; it may be evanescent or may persist throughout the infection. Confirmation of infection is through serologic means. The Weil-Felix reaction to *Proteus* OX-19 is positive during the second week of infection. The reaction to OX-2 may be positive, but OX-K remains non-reactive. Specific complement fixing antibodies can be obtained. Therapy is the administration of tetracycline or chloramphenicol.

Q FEVER

Q fever is caused by infection with the obligate intracellular rickettsial organism *Coxiella burnetii*. This organism is widely distributed and can produce an infection in domestic livestock. Human infections result from contact with infected sheep, goats, or cattle with infected placentas, milk, hides, or straw. Although most human infection is probably subclinical, the most common presentation is as primary Q fever, a severe influenza-like syndrome characterized by acute onset of headache, fever, chills, and myalgia and often accompanied by pneumonitis and hepatitis. Q fever is *not* associated with a characteristic skin eruption, although a faint erythematous skin rash of the trunk has been reported. Uncommonly, Q fever is an indolent infection and is characterized by low grade fever, sweats, weight loss, abdominal pain, and hepatitis.

EPIDEMIC TYPHUS

The causative agent of this disease is *R. prowazekii*, an organism closely related to *R. typhi*, the agent that produces murine typhus. This disease is louse-borne and is transmitted from one person to another by this vector. This infection is most frequently seen in association with famine and with poor living conditions. The infection has an abrupt onset, with intense headache, chills, fever, and myalgias. A rash may be present beginning 4–5 days after onset of systemic symptoms. It is usually found in the axillary folds and on the trunk. The rash is initially macular, discrete, and pink, but it progresses and becomes purpuric and confluent. It tends to spread peripherally and involve all body surfaces, excluding the face, palms, and soles. The progress of the eruption separates this disease from Rocky Mountain spotted fever. Occasionally, the rash is transitory. Epidemic typhus must be differentiated from bacterial diseases, including meningococcemia, typhoid fever, meningitis, and leptospirosis; and from certain viral diseases, primarily measles and infectious mononucleosis. The Weil-Felix reaction is identical to that of endemic typhus; however, specific complement fixing antibodies do develop after infection. Either tetracycline or chloramphenicol is considered effective therapy.

SCRUB TYPHUS

Scrub typhus, caused by *R. tsutsugamushi*, is found primarily in the Orient, but occasionally imported cases have been identified in the United States. The vector is the larval stage of the trombiculid mite. Following the bite of an infected mite, a papule forms that eventually ulcerates and forms an eschar. Approximately 10–12 days after the bite, fever, headache, and myalgias develop concomitantly with tender lymph nodes in the region of the eschar. Symptoms vary widely in severity. An eruption develops on the trunk about 5 days after onset of symptoms and gradually spreads to the limbs. In a study of 87 patients with this disease in Viet Nam, only 30 affected individuals had a rash but 85% had lymphadenopathy. The symptoms and rash are not specific and can be confused with those of other viral illnesses, particularly infectious mononucleosis; as well as with those of a variety of bacterial diseases, including leptospirosis, typhoid fever, and brucellosis. Confirmation of the diagnosis is by serologic testing. Antibodies to *Proteus* OX-K are present in sera from 50% of patients by the second week of illness. Patients with leptospirosis can have cross-reactions, giving a positive Weil-Felix reaction. Treatment is by appropriate supportive measures and with tetracycline or chloramphenicol. Doxycycline has also been reported to be effective in this disease.

Suggested Readings

Berman SJ, Kundin WD: Scrub typhus in South Vietnam, a study of 87 cases. Ann Intern Med 79:26–30, 1973.

Brettman LR, Lewin S, Holzman RS, et al: Rickettsial pox: Report of an outbreak and a contemporary review. Medicine 60:363–373, 1981.

Brown GW, Robinson DM, Huxsoll DL, et al: Scrub typhus: A common cause of illness in indigenous populations. Trans Royal Soc Trop Med Hyg 70:444–450, 1976.

Duma RJ, Sonenshine DE, Bozeman FM, et al: Epidemic typhus in the United States associated with flying squirrels. J Am Med Assn 245:2318–2320, 1981.

Kaplowitz LG, Lange JV, Fischer JJ, et al: Correlation of rickettsial titers, circulating endotoxin, and clinical features of Rocky Mountain spotted fever. Arch Intern Med 143:1149–1153, 1983.

McDade JE, Shephard CC, Redus MA, et al: Evidence of Rickettsia prowazekii infections in the United States. Am J Trop Med Hyg 29:277–283, 1980.

Torres J, et al: Rocky Mountain spotted fever in the mid-South. Arch Intern Med 132:340–347, 1973.

Woodward TE, Pedersen CE Jr, Oster CN, et al: Prompt confirmation of Rocky Mountain spotted fever. Identification of rickettsiae in skin tissues. J Infect Dis 13:297–301, 1976.

VII

OTHER SYSTEMIC DISEASES WITH CUTANEOUS MANIFESTATIONS

38

Sarcoidosis

JEFFREY P. CALLEN

Sarcoidosis is a multisystem disorder of unknown etiology. It most commonly involves the lungs, lymph nodes, liver, spleen, skin, eyes, glandular tissue, and bone; however, it can involve any organ system in the body. There are no consistent laboratory findings that allow for the diagnosis of sarcoidosis. Thus, the diagnosis rests on the finding of a characteristic, although nonspecific, histopathologic finding. When this histologic appearance is present in multiple organ systems and when appropriate tests are performed to rule out other causes of sarcoidal granulomas, the diagnosis is confirmed.

The first reports of sarcoidosis date back to the descriptions of the classic skin lesions, which have been referred to as Mortimer's malady in reference to the first patient described by Sir Jonathan Hutchinson (also called Hutchinson's papillary psoriasis). Following these first reports, many other names have been attached to various manifestations of sarcoidosis, including those of Boeck and Besnier. The immunology of sarcoidosis is fascinating and has led to various theories of the pathogenesis of this disease. The course of sarcoidosis is highly variable. It ranges from an acute self-healing process to a chronic disease affecting exclusively the skin to a debilitating entity causing blindness or progressive respiratory insufficiency. Sarcoidosis, although associated with morbidity, rarely is a primary cause of death.

ETIOLOGY AND PATHOGENESIS

The etiology of sarcoidosis is unknown. It has been postulated that the disease may be due to one or more infectious agents, which in a genetically predisposed individual will cause a sarcoidal reaction to develop. The clinical manifestations depend upon host response as well as on a causative organism. Through the years multiple agents have been postulated to be involved, including fungi, viruses, bacteria, and foreign materials. Cases with coexistent "autoimmune" disease have been reported, suggesting that patients with various collagen vascular diseases may be more prone to the development of sarcoidosis. Genetic factors have been implicated by HLA testing.

Sarcoidosis is believed to be a lymphoproliferative disorder characterized by the depression of delayed type hypersensitivity, imbalance of OKT4–T8 cells (helper-inducer to suppressor-cytotoxic T cell ratio), hyperreactivity of B cells, and increased production of circulating immune complexes. It is believed that in the presence of appropriate antigen, circulating immune complexes are formed and serum inhibitors may be activated that affect T cell function, allowing increases in B cell activity. Prolonged antigenemia and macrophage stimulation may occur. With the development of the sarcoidal granuloma, enzyme secretion (in particular, angiotensin converting enzyme) may occur. Elevation of the angiotensin converting enzyme is probably an effect rather than a cause of disease. The precise reasons for the effects of antigens on these patients are not understood. However, the end result appears to be anergy to recall antigens such as purified protein derivative (PPD) and mumps, and an inability to sensitize an individual with sarcoidosis to an antigen such as dinitrochlorobenzene (DNCB). Elevated levels of gammaglobulin and non-specific elevation of antibody titers to various viruses and fungal elements also occur. The pathogenesis of sarcoidosis remains a mystery despite recent studies.

CLINICAL FEATURES

Cutaneous Manifestations

Cutaneous manifestations of sarcoidosis are either "specific" or "non-specific," based upon the histopathologic examination. Those skin lesions represented histopathologically by non-caseating granulomas are termed "specific" skin lesions of sarcoidosis. Those lesions that do not show non-caseating granulomas are termed "non-specific" lesions. The most common "non-specific" skin lesion is erythema nodosum. The "specific" skin lesions include papules, plaques, nodules, lesions in scars, and so forth.

As cited, the most common "non-specific" manifestation of sarcoidosis is erythema nodosum (see also Chapter 9). These lesions are firm, slightly erythematous, subcutaneous nodules, most commonly occurring on the anterior tibial surface. The lesions are often tender to palpation. Sarcoidosis is the cause of up to 25% of all cases of erythema nodosum. When erythema nodosum is associated with sarcoidosis, the symptom complex is usually characterized by asymptomatic bilateral hilar lymphadenopathy, uveitis, fever, and arthritis. This four-symptom complex is referred to as Löfgren's syndrome. It is an acute form of sarcoidosis that resolves without treatment in 90% or more of affected individuals. It is postulated that these patients have circulating immune complex disease causing erythema nodosum. Biopsies of the lung as well as the lymph nodes in these patients have revealed sarcoidal granulomas. Lung biopsy is not indicated in patients who have the typical tetrad. Other non-specific lesions of sarcoidosis are extremely rare but include pruritus, erythema multiforme, and an exfoliative erythroderma. The association between these skin findings and sarcoidosis may be coincidental.

"Specific" skin lesions of sarcoidosis occur in roughly 10–35% of patients with documented systemic sarcoidosis. The diagnosis of a cutaneous sarcoidal granuloma is

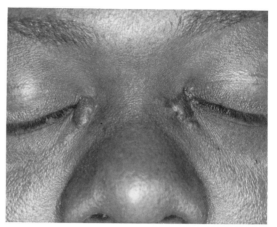

Figure 38–1. Small papular lesions are present at the inner canthus in this patient with sarcoidosis.

made by skin biopsy. The lesions, however, are not diagnostic clinically. Sarcoidosis can mimic many dermatoses, and should be included on many lists of differential diagnoses. The most common presentation of sarcoidosis is a papular lesion. Small papules, 3–6 mm in diameter, with little epidermal change are frequently noted on the head and neck in sarcoidosis (Fig. 38–1). In particular, the periorbital region seems more commonly involved. The papules may be flesh-colored, red, violaceous, or slightly hyperpigmented. In blacks, the papules may be hypopigmented. The papules will at times enlarge or coalesce to form either annular lesions or plaques (Fig. 38–2; Plate VI D).

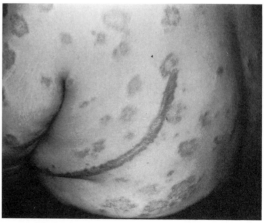

Figure 38–2. Multiple annular lesions are present in this female with sarcoidosis (see also Plate VI*D*).

Plaque-type lesions were first reported by Hutchinson and are known as Hutchinson's papillary psoriasis. They represent a deeper cutaneous infiltration of sarcoidal granulomas than is seen in the papular lesions. The plaques may be indurated and can involve any area of the body. When they involve the scalp, a scarring alopecia may result. Involvement on the face or neck with telangiectatic infiltrated lesions is termed angiolupoid sarcoidosis or lupus pernio. Patients with plaques of sarcoidosis on the face, particularly when around the nose and nostril openings (Fig. 38–3; Plate VI*E*), have an increased incidence of sarcoidosis of the upper respiratory tract (SURT) as well as pulmonary fibrosis. Patients with lupus pernio and angiolupoid sarcoidosis frequently have pulmonary manifestations that are persistent and progressive.

Subcutaneous nodular lesions were first described by Darier and Roussy. The subcutaneous lesions are often asymptomatic and frequently occur on the trunk and extremities. Tenderness of these lesions is extremely rare.

Sarcoidosis often occurs in scars (Fig. 38–4) or on areas of skin chronically damaged by infection, radiation, or mechanical trauma. Sometimes it becomes difficult to determine if these lesions are indeed cutaneous sarcoidosis or whether they are local sarcoidal reactions to a foreign substance. In the absence of systemic disease, a diagnosis of sarcoidosis cannot be made with confi-

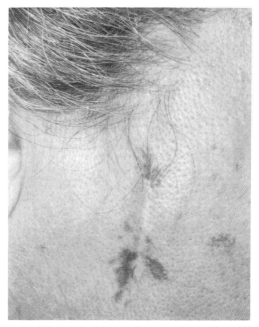

Figure 38–4. Sarcoid granulomas occurring in a scar.

dence, particularly when only one area of the body is involved. However, if multiple areas of the body including or excluding scars are involved with cutaneous sarcoidal granulomas, even in the absence of systemic disease, a diagnosis of sarcoidosis can be made.

There are multiple unusual forms of sarcoidosis. Erythroderma has been described in some patients. Ulcerations in sarcoid lesions are unusual, except in lupus pernio. Verrucous lesions have been described in a rare patient, but often the patients will have typical nodular cutaneous lesions elsewhere. Pustular lesions in a follicular pattern have been described. Ichthyosis-like lesions have been described in multiple patients with sarcoidosis. The lesions have the appearance of ichthyosis vulgaris, and an association of these lesions with systemic disease has been reported. On rare occasions, nail involvement can occur.

Intrathoracic Disease

Intrathoracic disease, including hilar adenopathy and pulmonary parenchymal disease, is the most common manifestation of systemic sarcoidosis. Pulmonary sarcoidosis has been staged, according to chest roentgen-

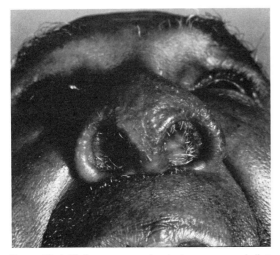

Figure 38–3. Violaceous, scarring lesions representative of lupus pernio are present in this patient with sarcoidosis of the upper respiratory tract (see also Plate VI*E*).

ographic findings, from 0 to III. Stage 0 disease consists of no changes seen on chest x-ray. Stage I disease consists of bilateral hilar adenopathy in the absence of parenchymal disease recognized by chest x-ray. Stage II disease consists of hilar adenopathy with the presence of pulmonary fibrosis. Stage III disease consists of extensive pulmonary fibrosis in the absence of hilar adenopathy. It is not infrequent that a diagnosis of sarcoidosis is made on routine chest x-ray in an entirely asymptomatic patient. Patients who have bilateral hilar adenopathy without the evidence of any symptoms do not need extensive systemic evaluation, and resolution of their disease may occur spontaneously. In all stages of pulmonary sarcoidosis, abnormalities may be found on careful testing with pulmonary function tests or bronchial alveolar lavage.

Bilateral hilar adenopathy is the earliest and most common intrathoracic manifestation of sarcoidosis. These patients are often asymptomatic, although erythema nodosum, uveitis, arthritis, and fever may accompany the hilar lymphadenopathy as previously mentioned. It is rare for these patients with stage I disease to develop progressive parenchymal disease. In most patients with bilateral hilar adenopathy with symptoms of Löfgren's syndrome or in those who are asymptomatic, biopsy is not necessary. However, in those patients who have either unilateral adenopathy or dyspnea only a small portion will have sarcoidosis, and in these patients lung biopsy and possibly mediastinal nodal biopsies are indicated. Stages II and III pulmonary sarcoidosis are associated with a much higher incidence of chronic, progressive disease, and resolution of the radiographic findings becomes less likely. Symptoms may be present or absent. However, abnormal pulmonary function testing correlates with greater disease seen on chest x-ray.

Ocular Manifestations

Sarcoidosis may affect any portion of the eye and occurs in between one fourth and one half of the patients with systemic sarcoidosis. Acute ocular sarcoidosis generally runs a course of 2 or less years, during which time active therapy may be needed. Chronic eye disease is less common. It appears that early aggressive intervention can prevent scarring and blindness.

The most common ocular manifestation of sarcoidosis is uveitis, which usually affects the anterior segment of the eye. Patients may be entirely asymptomatic, or they may present with a red eye, photophobia, or increased tearing. The diagnosis of anterior uveitis is made by slit lamp examination, which will reveal "mutton fat" keratotic precipitates in the anterior chamber. Less commonly, the posterior segment of the eye is involved and its appearance correlates well with chorioretinitis and with neurosarcoidosis. Uveitis must be aggressively treated to prevent adhesions with resulting glaucoma, cataract development, or blindness.

Another common ocular finding in patients with sarcoidosis is conjunctival involvement. This may or may not produce symptoms of ocular irritation. Conjunctival granulomas occur in about one third of patients with sarcoidosis. Conjunctival biopsies have been positive even when patients lack clinical evidence of conjunctival involvement.

Lymph Nodes

Sarcoidal granulomas commonly infiltrate the lymph nodes. The incidence of peripheral lymphadenopathy not involving the hilar nodes is roughly 30% in patients with systemic sarcoidosis. Lymphadenopathy has been associated with both acute and chronic disease patterns. The lymph node involvement is detected by palpation, is usually non-tender, and is often not noticed by the patient.

Splenic involvement in sarcoidosis is detected in approximately 10–25% of patients. It is manifested by splenomegaly, but functional abnormalities are quite rare.

Musculoskeletal Manifestations

Symptomatic muscle involvement in sarcoidosis is rare, although biopsy detection of a sarcoidal infiltrate is not uncommon. Clinical series of large numbers of patients with sarcoidosis have revealed that approximately 1% of patients have symptoms of muscle involvement. However, when pa-

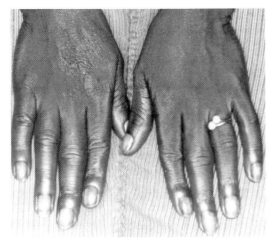

Figure 38–5. Sarcoid arthritis. This patient also had papular lesions of cutaneous sarcoidosis.

tients with sarcoidosis have random muscle biopsies, more than 50% will have histologic evidence of granulomatous disease.

Bone lesions occur in 10–15% of patients, usually correlating with chronic, progressive disease. The radiographic changes are cystic lesions that usually occur in the terminal phalanges of the hands. They may be accompanied by soft tissue swelling. Arthralgias are commonly experienced in acute sarcoidosis, particularly in patients with Löfgren's syndrome, and they may be accompanied by arthritis (Fig. 38–5). The wrists, knees, and ankles are the most commonly affected joints. Although chronic granulomatous arthritis has been reported, it is a rare complication of systemic sarcoidosis.

Neurosarcoidosis

Neurosarcoidosis affects 5–15% of patients with systemic sarcoidosis. Central nervous system involvement occurs in one half of the patients with neurosarcoidosis. The presence of neurosarcoidosis appears to correlate with the presence of posterior uveitis and of chronic cutaneous disease. The most common neurologic manifestations of sarcoidosis include optic nerve disease, facial nerve palsy, meningitis, and cerebral granulomas that can lead to encephalopathy and seizures. Uveoparotid fever (Heerfordt's syndrome) is a symptom complex of sarcoidosis consisting of uveitis, facial nerve palsy, fever, and parotid gland enlargement. This syndrome is also frequently associated with central nervous system involvement. The detection of neurosarcoidosis can be difficult, because the tissue is not readily available for microscopic evaluation. Evaluation of a patient with suspected neurosarcoidosis should include skull x-rays, brain scan, electroencephalogram, and a computed axial tomographic (CAT) scan of the head. Lumbar puncture can also be useful in patients with meningeal involvement.

Hepatic Sarcoidosis

Hepatic involvement in sarcoidosis is common. In a large study, hepatomegaly was detected in 20% of patients with sarcoidosis. Abnormal liver function tests are present in approximately one half of the patients with liver involvement. Liver biopsy is a useful procedure in establishing a diagnosis of sarcoidosis, although care must be taken to exclude other causes of granulomatous disease of the liver and the findings must be correlated with evidence of sarcoidal disease elsewhere in the body. Liver involvement rarely progresses to functional abnormalities or to cirrhosis.

Endocrine, Metabolic, and Laboratory Abnormalities

Endocrine glands may be infiltrated by sarcoidal granulomas. Functional abnormalities are not common, although pituitary or hypothalamic infiltration can cause diabetes insipidus or, on rare occasions, panhypopituitarism. An elevated prolactin level has been a useful indicator of hypothalamic sarcoidal involvement. Other endocrine organs, such as thyroid, parathyroid, adrenals, and pancreas, may be involved. However, functional impairment of these organs is very unusual.

Hypercalcemia occurs in a small percentage of patients with systemic sarcoidosis. The serum calcium elevation is often transient and seems to be very responsive to therapy with systemic corticosteroids. In occasional patients with widespread sarcoidosis, serum calcium elevation can be persistent and can lead to urinary tract stones, nephrocalcinosis, and even renal failure. Hypercalciuria is more common than hypercalcemia and may be used as a correlate with disease activity. The mechanism by which hypercalcemia is produced in sarcoidosis may be through overt production of 1,25-dihydroxyvitamin D by macrophages.

The serum angiotensin converting enzyme (SACE) level is raised in approximately 60% of patients with systemic sarcoidosis. SACE is produced by epithelioid cells and may reflect the granuloma load in the body. Thus, SACE has been useful in monitoring both disease activity and response to therapy in patients with pulmonary sarcoidosis. However, the diagnostic usefulness of the SACE is limited because "false" negative as well as "false" positive tests may occur. Other enzymes produced by sarcoidal granulomas include lysozymes and glucuronidase. These enzymes, however, have not been clinically useful in evaluating patients with systemic sarcoidosis.

Cardiac Disease

The true incidence of cardiac involvement in sarcoidosis is not known. However, autopsy studies suggest that it is common and frequently asymptomatic. Cardiac sarcoidosis can result in symptoms of congestive heart failure, arrhythmia, or conduction defects. Sudden death in sarcoid patients has been linked to cardiac involvement.

Other Clinical Manifestations of Sarcoidosis

Almost any area of the body can be affected by sarcoidosis. Granulomatous renal disease has been reported on several occasions. Gastric granulomas, bone marrow granulomas, spinal cord lesions, and gonadal granulomas have also been reported.

Relationship of Cutaneous Disease to Systemic Disease

Multiple studies have detailed the cutaneous disease in patients with sarcoidosis. Unfortunately, none of the studies have used the same methodology and many fail to define the skin lesions adequately. However, a few generalizations can still be made:

1. Patients with lupus pernio more frequently have sarcoidosis of the upper respiratory tract (SURT).
2. Patients with cutaneous involvement more frequently have systemic sarcoidosis that is chronic.
3. Patients with lupus pernio with SURT have more frequent bone involvement than do patients without this combination of problems.
4. Patients with cutaneous involvement may have more frequent splenomegaly and hepatomegaly.

It is not known whether or not patients who have cutaneous disease other than lupus pernio have any difference in prognosis from those patients who do not have cutaneous disease.

HISTOPATHOLOGY

Sarcoidosis is characterized by granulomas composed principally of epithelioid cells with an occasional giant cell and little or no caseation necrosis. Inclusion bodies are frequently observed, but these are not specific for sarcoidosis and may be seen in other granulomatous conditions. The granulomas may remain, seemingly unchanged for months or years; may resolve completely; or may undergo a fibrotic change.

Because non-caseating granulomas are not specific for sarcoidosis, other conditions must be vigorously ruled out before a diagnosis of sarcoidosis can be strongly considered. Thus, the diagnosis is one of exclusion. Special stains of the histopathologic specimens should include Fite's stain; stains for Microbacterium; and PAS stain, looking for fungal elements. In addition, examination for a foreign body reaction with at least polarized light should be undertaken. Various neoplasms should be excluded, particularly lymphomas, since there are occasional reports of sarcoidal reactions occurring in nodes adjacent to neoplastic change. Immunologic testing (e.g., T cell subset determination) of specimens has not been shown to be of diagnostic value.

DIAGNOSIS AND DIFFERENTIAL DIAGNOSIS

Sarcoidosis is diagnosed by a combination of clinical, radiologic, and laboratory findings in the presence of histologically confirmed non-caseating granulomas in tissue. The only exception to this is the diagnosis in patients with asymptomatic bilateral hilar lymphadenopathy or those patients who have Löfgren's syndrome. These two presentations are characteristic enough not to warrant further laboratory or other considerations. The differential diagnosis of cutaneous sarcoidosis is wide and varied and contains such common entities as granuloma annulare, cutaneous lupus erythematosus, and cutaneous infections with fungus or tuberculosis, among others. Histopathologically, the differential diagnosis involves the exclusion of other granulomatous disease. The differential diagnosis of pulmonary sarcoidosis and sarcoidosis in other organ systems is equally varied. Thus, it is necessary for the diagnosis to have appropriate clinical support as well as histopathologic and laboratory support. Techniques such as gallium-67 scan and bronchial alveolar lavage with cell counts may be helpful, particularly in following the patient for activity of disease.

Tissue diagnosis through biopsies of various sites remains the main procedure to establish the diagnosis of sarcoidosis. Care must be taken to exclude other causes of granuloma, such as infections or foreign bodies. A prime biopsy site is the skin, as it is an accessible and fairly "high yield" organ. Particular attention should be paid to changes in scars or to any papular, nodular, or plaque-type lesion of recent onset. In addition, conjunctival biopsy, even in the absence of conjunctival nodules, may be positive in up to one third of patients with sarcoidosis. Palpable lymph nodes may be biopsied when feasible. Lung biopsy via fiberoptic bronchoscope and bronchial alveolar lavage are helpful in establishing a diagnosis as well. Blind biopsy of the minor salivary glands on the lower lip has been said to be positive in up to 60% of patients with sarcoidosis. Liver biopsy is a high yield procedure; however, morbidity and mortality make it less useful than the previously mentioned techniques. Muscle biopsy may reveal sarcoidal granulomas in up to 50% of patients, particularly when a needle is used. Other sites for biopsy, although less valuable, include mediastinum, bone marrow, and spleen.

PATIENT EVALUATION

Once a diagnosis of sarcoidosis is made, the patient should be thoroughly evaluated for extent of disease. Careful examination of the lungs, the eyes, and the skin should be performed by specialists expert in these areas. Liver function tests, protein electrophoresis, and calcium levels should be obtained. An electrocardiogram is necessary. Chest x-ray and pulmonary function tests with diffusion studies should be ordered. Skin tests to detect anergy, using multiple antigens, should be performed. The Kveim test has been used for confirmation of a diagnosis of sarcoidosis, but because it is not standardized and because antigens may not be reliable or available, it is less important in evaluating the patient. The use of gallium scans and bronchial alveolar lavage is not necessary for routine evaluation of patients, but should be left to the physician's discretion. Appropriate biopsies, as mentioned previously, are helpful in confirming the diagnosis. Careful evaluation is necessary in order to define the organ systems involved and to best determine the prognosis and need for therapy.

PROGNOSIS

Mortality rates in sarcoidosis vary from 3 to 6%. Cardiac disease, progressive pulmonary disease, and neurosarcoidosis have been associated with the rare cases of death in these patients.

Morbidity in sarcoidosis can be severe. Blindness can result from untreated ocular disease, and pulmonary disease can cause fatigue and shortness of breath. Renal failure has been reported from granulomatous involvement of the kidney as well as from calcium deposits and from chronic urinary tract stones. Cosmetic deformities may occur in patients with cutaneous sarcoidosis, particularly in those with lupus pernio. Although many patients with pulmonary sarcoidosis may have resolution of their disease, the rates vary with the stage of pulmonary disease. Stage I sarcoidosis resolves in roughly 60% of patients, stage II resolves in 40% of patients, and stage III resolves in only 12% of patients.

Despite the aberrations noted in tests of cell-mediated immunity, untreated sarcoidosis is not associated with an increased number of infections. However, sarcoidosis has been linked to an increase in the frequency of malignancy. Several studies have reported an increased incidence of lung cancer and lymphoma. It is not clear, however, from the studies whether sarcoidosis is the primary disease, or whether a local sarcoidal reaction is the response to the malignancy.

TREATMENT

Acute sarcoidosis in which bilateral hilar adenopathy exists alone or in combination with erythema nodosum, uveitis, or arthritis is usually a self-limited disease and does not require specific therapy. Symptomatic therapy for the erythema nodosum or arthritis could include non-steroidal anti-inflammatory drugs such as aspirin or indomethacin. Acute uveitis can be treated with corticosteroid eye drops.

Chronic cutaneous lesions, particularly lupus pernio and indurated plaques, which can cause scarring, should be treated more aggressively. Topical corticosteroids have rarely been effective because of the lack of penetration into the dermis and because of the potential for epidermal atrophy. Intralesional corticosteroids are generally more effective but are still not dramatically so. Antimalarials, particularly hydroxychloroquine sulfate (Plaquenil) 200–400 mg per day, have been useful in treating patients with cutaneous sarcoidosis. Antimalarial therapy requires careful ophthalmologic monitoring. In addition, it has been noted that progressive systemic disease may occur despite antimalarial therapy. Cutaneous disease that has failed these measures and is significantly disfiguring may respond to systemic corticosteroids. Care must be taken not to induce flares of systemic disease when tapering the corticosteroids given for cutaneous manifestations. In addition, methotrexate, chlorambucil, and 13-cis-retinoic acid (isotretinoin) have been reported to be of value (in anecdotal reports) for treating cutaneous sarcoidosis.

Ocular sarcoidosis, which can lead to scarring and blindness, must be aggressively treated. Corticosteroid eye drops may be effective; however, patients who do not respond or who only respond partially may require intraocular corticosteroid injections or systemic corticosteroid therapy.

Progressive pulmonary disease is considered to be an indication for systemic corticosteroid therapy. Documented changes in pulmonary function tests as a result of therapy have been reported. In addition, changes in serum angiotensin converting enzyme (SACE) level and in abnormalities seen on bronchial alveolar lavage have been reported in patients treated with systemic corticosteroids. Alternative therapies that have been reported to be effective or that decrease corticosteroid dosage include antimalarials, oxyphenylbutazone, various antibiotics, and various immunosuppressive agents. However, too few studies are available to evaluate the effects of any agent reliably other than systemic corticosteroids.

In addition to chronic, scarring skin lesions, ocular lesions, and progressive pulmonary disease, the indications for systemic corticosteroid therapy include hypercalcemia, neurosarcoidosis, symptomatic cardiac sarcoidosis, and functional endocrinologic abnormalities.

Suggested Readings

Hanno R, Callen JP: Sarcoidosis: A disorder with prominent cutaneous features and their interrelationship with systemic disease. Med Clin North Am 64:847–866, 1980.

Izumi T: Sarcoidosis. Clin Dermatol 4:4, Oct–Dec 1986.

James DG: Dermatologic aspects of sarcoidosis. Quart J Med 28:109–124, 1959.

Olive KE, Kataria YP: Cutaneous manifestations of sarcoidosis: Relationship to other organ system involvement, abnormal laboratory measurements, and disease course. Arch Intern Med 145:1811–1814, 1985.

39

Cardiovascular Diseases and the Skin

JEFFREY P. CALLEN

Many of the multisystem disorders discussed in this text have associated cardiovascular abnormalities. Table 39–1 lists the cardiac abnormalities seen in these multisystem disorders. Table 39–2 lists cutaneous findings that may be observed in association with primary cardiovascular disorders. Table 39–3 lists those inherited disorders that are associated with both cutaneous and cardiac abnormalities. In this chapter, we discuss only those diseases not discussed elsewhere and only highlight some of the disorders.

CARCINOID SYNDROME (see Chapter 13)

Paroxysmal flushing of the face and anterior chest occurs in carcinoid tumors that have metastasized to the liver or that begin in the lung. The symptoms are due to release by the tumor of vasoactive substances, primarily serotonin. With continued disease, telangiectasias and sclerodermoid changes may occur on the affected areas. Asthmatic attacks may accompany the flushing episodes. Right-sided heart failure, tricuspid insufficiency, and/or pulmonic stenosis are the most common cardiac manifestations. In addition to the carcinoid syndrome, flushing may occur with pheochromocytoma or systemic mast cell disease.

DEGOS DISEASE (MALIGNANT ATROPHIC PAPULOSIS)

Degos disease is an arteriopathy in which small areas of cutaneous necrosis are pres-

ent, healing with an ivory, stellate scar. Similar lesions may be present in the gastrointestinal tract and may result in death from uncontrolled hemorrhage. Cardiac involvement is rare, but when it occurs it is manifested by pericarditis and/or pericardial effusions.

HEMOCHROMATOSIS (see Chapter 29)

Hemochromatosis is due to excessive iron deposition in the skin, heart, liver, and pancreas. The skin becomes darkened in a bronze tone; thus, the term "bronze diabetes" is used. Adult onset diabetes mellitus is common, as well as hepatic dysfunction with eventual cirrhosis. The heart is affected with supraventricular arrhythmias with or without congestive heart failure. The treatment of choice is to remove the excess iron stores by repeated phlebotomies.

RELAPSING POLYCHONDRITIS

Relapsing polychondritis is a rare disease characterized by recurrent episodes of inflammation affecting cartilaginous tissue. It is believed to be an "autoimmune" disease directed against type II collagen, which occurs only in cartilaginous tissue. The most common manifestation is the sudden onset of a tender, erythematous, warm, swollen external ear (Fig. 39–1; Plate VI *F*). The inflammation subsides spontaneously over a 1–2 week period, only to recur. Eventually

Table 39–1. CARDIOPULMONARY ABNORMALITIES IN MULTISYSTEM DISORDERS WITH PROMINENT CUTANEOUS FEATURES

Disease	Cardiopulmonary Manifestations	Cutaneous Features
Amyloidosis (see Chapter 17)	Congestive heart failure, conduction disturbances, cardiomegaly	Pinch purpura, waxy skin
Behçet's syndrome (see Chapter 6)	Pericarditis	Oral aphthosis, pathergy, pustular "vasculitis"
Carcinoid syndrome	Endocardial plaque–tricuspid insufficiency, pulmonic stenosis, right-sided heart failure, asthmatic attacks	Flushing, "sclerodermoid" changes
Dermatomyositis (see Chapter 2)	Non-specific EKG changes, conduction defects, pericarditis (rare), congestive heart failure (late)	Gottron's papules, heliotrope rash, poikiloderma
Degos disease	Pericarditis, pericardial effusions	Ivory scars, infarcts of skin
Diabetes mellitus (see Chapter 22)	Coronary artery disease	Necrobiosis lipoidica diabeticorum, etc.
Exfoliative erythroderma (see Chapter 11)	High output cardiac failure	Exfoliative dermatitis
Hemochromatosis (see Chapter 29)	Congestive heart failure, supraventricular arrhythmias	Generalized pigmentation
Kawasaki's syndrome	Coronary arteritis, coronary artery aneurysms, myocardial infarction	Glossitis, cheilitis, peeling of acral skin
Neonatal lupus erythematosus	Congenital heart block	Transient LE rash
Systemic lupus erythematosus	Verrucous endocarditis (mitral valve), pericarditis, coronary arteritis	"Butterfly" rash, photosensitivity, DLE, SCLE skin
Lipid disorders	Coronary artery disease	Xanthomas
Lymphomatoid granulomatosis	Angiocentric, angidestructive pulmonary vasculitis	Inflammatory plaque and nodules
Multicentric reticulohistiocytosis	Coronary artery disease	
Relapsing polychondritis	Tracheobronchial wall collapse, aortic insufficiency, dissecting aortic aneurysms	Beefy, red ears; floppy ears
Reiter's disease	Conduction defects, pericarditis (rare), aortitis–aortic insufficiency	Circinate balanitis, keratoderma, psoriasis-like dermatosis
Sarcoidosis	Conduction disturbances, congestive heart failure	Plaques, papules, nodules, etc.
Scleroderma	Conduction defects, cor pulmonale, pulmonary fibrosis, pericarditis, visceral Raynaud's phenomenon	Sclerosis, telangiectasis, calcinosis
Vasculitis	Coronary vasculitis	Palpable purpura

Table 39–2. CUTANEOUS FINDINGS THAT MAY BE OBSERVED IN ASSOCIATION WITH PRIMARY CARDIAC ABNORMALITIES

Cardiac Disorder	Cutaneous Changes
Coronary artery disease	Xanthomas, skin changes of diabetes, sclerosis (premature aging), earlobe crease(?)
Hypertension: pheochromocytoma	Café au lait spots, neurofibromatosis
Hypertension: renovascular	Scleroderma
Cholesterol emboli	Palpable purpura, necrosis
Bacterial endocarditis	Osler's nodes, Janeway's lesions, petechiae, purpuric pustules, splinter hemorrhages
Left atrial myxoma	Purpura (emboli)
Cardiovascular drugs	
Amiodarone	Photosensitivity
Beta-blockers	Flare of psoriasis
Minoxidil	Hypertrichosis
Quinidine	Petechiae, photosensitivity
Procainamide hydrochloride (Pronestyl)	Drug-induced lupus erythematosus
Thiazides	Photosensitivity

Table 39–3. INHERITED DISORDERS ASSOCIATED WITH CARDIOPULMONARY AND CUTANEOUS FINDINGS

Disease	Cardiopulmonary Manifestations	Cutaneous Changes
Cutis laxa	Aortic dilatation and rupture, pulmonary artery stenosis with cor pulmonale	Marked looseness of the skin
Ehlers-Danlos syndrome	Aortic, pulmonary artery dilatation; mitral, tricuspid valve prolapse; arterial rupture	Hyperelasticity, "cigarette paper" scars
Hereditary hemorrhagic telangiectasia	Pulmonary arteriovenous malformation	Telangiectatic mats
LEOPARD syndrome	EKG abnormalities	Multiple lentigines
Myxomas (Carney's syndrome, LAMB or NAME syndrome)	Atrial myxoma	Cutaneous myxoma, lentigines
Neurofibromatosis	Hypertension (pheochromocytoma)	Café au lait spots, neurofibromas
Pseudoxanthoma elasticum	Early onset atherosclerotic vascular disease, aortic aneurysm	Yellow macules on intertriginous surfaces
Tuberous sclerosis	Rhabdomyomas	Adenoma sebaceum, periungual fibromas, ash-leaf macule
Werner's syndrome	Premature atherosclerosis	Atrophy, sclerodermoid changes

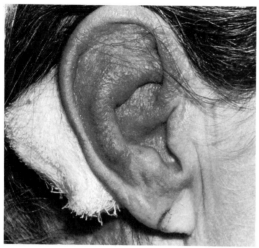

Figure 39–1. Erythematous eruption of the earlobe representative of relapsing polychondritis (see also Plate VIF).

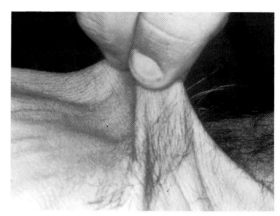

Figure 39–2. Hyperextensible skin seen in Ehlers-Danlos syndrome.

the cartilage may be damaged with a permanent deformity developing. Other tissues that contain cartilage are also affected, including the joints and trachea most commonly. The heart may be involved with aortic insufficiency or aortic aneurysms. The most dangerous development in this disorder is asphyxia and death as a result of tracheal collapse. Therapy is directed at blocking the neutrophilic inflammatory reaction in the cartilage. To this end, corticosteroids, immunosuppressives, and dapsone have been used.

EMBOLIC PHENOMENON

Emboli may occur from atrial myxomas, cholesterol deposits, or infections. The cutaneous lesions that result are due to a blockade of the small vessels in the skin. Thus, splinter hemorrhages, petechiae, purpura, and livedo reticularis are the most common findings. Cholesterol emboli or atheroembolism is not uncommon and usually is due to the dislodging of atheromatous plaques during angiography. Not only is the skin affected, but also central nervous system, ophthalmic, and renal disease may follow. The treatment is supportive.

EHLERS-DANLOS SYNDROME AND CUTIS LAXA

Ehlers-Danlos syndrome is a group of disorders that may include cutis laxa. These

patients have hyperelasticity of their skin and joints (Fig. 39–2) and with severe forms have multiple folds of skin (cutis laxa) (Fig. 39–3). In addition, "cigarette paper" scars form as a result of poor wound healing. Cardiac manifestations may include mitral valve prolapse, tricuspid valve prolapse, aortic dilatation with insufficiency, and arterial rupture.

LEOPARD SYNDROME

This is an autosomal dominant disorder that is manifested by *l*entigines, electrocardiographic (EKG) abnormalities, ocular hypertelorism, pulmonary stenosis, abnormalities of the genitalia, retardation of growth, and deafness (sensorineural). Multiple lentigines appear on the skin. The EKG abnormalities include axis deviation, prolonged P-R intervals, left anterior hemiblock, bundle branch block, and/or complete heart block. A hypertrophic cardiomyopathy (subaortic stenosis) is the most common anatomic alteration.

MYXOMAS

Multiple cutaneous lentigines, nevi, and myxomas have been reported in association with cardiac myxomas, testicular tumors, adrenal tumors, and pituitary adenomas. This association appears to be familial. These cases have been referred to by various acronyms (mnemonics) such as LAMB or NAME syndrome (*l*entigines, *a*trial myxoma, *m*ucocutaneous myxoma, and *b*lue nevi; or *n*evi, *a*trial myxoma, *m*yxoid neurofibromata, and *e*phelides).

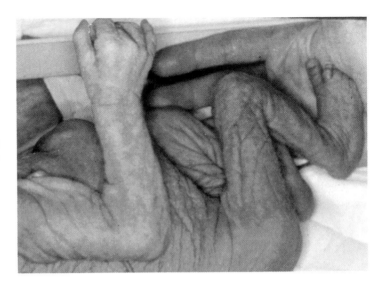

Figure 39–3. This male was born with loose skin representative of cutis laxa.

WERNER'S SYNDROME

Werner's syndrome results from premature aging. The skin becomes atrophic, weathered, and sclerotic. The nose may appear beak-like, and the voice takes on a high-pitched nasal quality. Coronary artery disease with myocardial infarction occurs at an early age, and is often the cause of death.

Suggested Readings

Carney JA, Gordon H, Carpenter PC, et al: The complex of myxomas, spotty pigmentation, and endocrine overactivity. Medicine *64*:270–283, 1985.
Franks AG Jr: Cutaneous aspects of cardiopulmonary disease. *In* Fitzpatrick TB, Freedberg IM, Eisen AZ, Wolff K, et al (eds): Dermatology in General Medicine, 3rd ed. New York, McGraw-Hill Book Co., 1987, pp. 1980–1997.

40

Cutaneous Nephrology

JEFFREY P. CALLEN

Patients with end stage renal disease frequently will manifest a variety of cutaneous disorders, including abnormal pigmentation, pruritus, a variety of infections, drug eruptions, and bullous dermatoses. In addition, there may also be certain disease states of the skin that are associated with an increased frequency of renal disease. In particular, many of the collagen vascular disorders may be associated with glomerulonephritis, the nail-patella syndrome has been associated with a nephrotic syndrome, neurofibromatosis may be associated with malignant hypertension and secondary renal failure, tuberous sclerosis may be associated with rhabdomyomas in the kidney, and Fabry's disease is associated with renal failure as a result of deposition of ceramide trihexoside in the kidney. Skin changes may occur because of the profound biochemical and metabolic changes associated with chronic renal failure. Finally, the skin may be predisposed to the development of many disorders because of the therapy for the renal failure with either chronic hemodialysis or renal transplantation. In this chapter, we discuss each of these issues.

CUTANEOUS CHANGES RELATED TO CHRONIC RENAL FAILURE

The patient with chronic renal failure is often anemic and will have a pale or sallow complexion. In addition, many of the patients develop a generalized hyperpigmentation. The skin often becomes xerotic and in some cases may even take on the appearance of ichthyosis. If the renal failure is allowed to progress, it becomes possible for the patient to develop uremic frost. Pruritus is a frequent finding in patients with chronic renal failure, especially in those on hemodialysis. The mechanism of the production of pruritus is not known, but it may be related to calcium-phosphorus balance and to the existence of secondary hyperparathyroidism. The pruritus may progress to the point at which the patient produces secondary skin lesions from the intense scratching and/or picking. Patients with secondary hyperparathyroidism may develop metastatic calcification in the skin, which is manifested as firm to hard nodules, often with a yellow or blue discoloration (Fig. 40–1; Plate VIIA). In some patients, the vessels can become calcified and cutaneous gangrene can result. The nails may also change in patients with chronic renal failure. The "half and half" nail may be distinctive to renal failure. It is manifested as a proximal white portion of the nail with a distal red or brown coloration.

SYSTEMIC DISORDERS WITH CUTANEOUS AND RENAL MANIFESTATIONS

The collagen vascular disorders have been discussed in depth elsewhere in this text; however, certain of these diseases have frequent renal involvement, which will be emphasized in this section. Lupus erythematosus (LE) is a multisystem disorder with

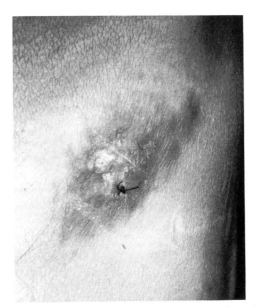

Figure 40–1. The nodular lesion shown represents metastatic calcification in a patient with chronic renal failure on hemodialysis (see also Plate VIIA).

prominent cutaneous disease. Fortunately, those patients with chronic cutaneous LE (discoid LE = DLE) and those with subacute cutaneous LE (SCLE) do not have high frequencies of renal involvement, and when renal disease is present it tends to be of a milder variety. Those patients with systemic lupus erythematosus (SLE) may have cutaneous findings such as photosensitivity, a malar rash, or a cutaneous vasculitis. These patients appear not to be protected from renal involvement, and in fact the appearance of the rash may herald a worsening of the renal disease. Renal disease in LE patients may be of many types, including a focal glomerulonephritis, a membranous glomerulonephritis, or a proliferative glomerulonephritis. Renal failure is among the poorest of prognostic findings in the LE patient, and even with aggressive therapy death can result from the renal disease. Patients with progressive systemic sclerosis (scleroderma) have a lower incidence of renal impairment than those with LE, but when it occurs it is often associated with rapidly progressive deterioration of renal function and death. The use of angiotensin converting enzyme inhibitors to treat the malignant hypertension has led to improved renal function. Patients with various vasculitic syndromes may have renal involvement induced by immune complexes. In particular, patients with polyar-

teritis nodosa, those with Wegener's granulomatosis, and those with Henoch-Schönlein purpura seem to have frequent renal involvement. Impairment of renal function is one of the major causes of mortality in the vasculitic syndromes; thus, its recognition and aggressive treatment are necessary.

Several inherited diseases have also been associated with cutaneous changes and potential renal disease. Neurofibromatosis has been associated with hypertension related to pheochromocytoma as well as to a renal artery stenosis. In some patients, recognition of the cutaneous signs has led to the discovery of the adrenal tumor. Patients with tuberous sclerosis can develop hamartomas that replace the normal kidney tissue and lead to impairment of renal function. Recognition of the cutaneous lesions, including ash-leaf macules, shagreen patches, periungual fibromas, and adenoma sebaceum, has led to the discovery of underlying renal hamartomas in some patients. Fabry's disease is a rare disorder that is inherited as an X-linked recessive trait. It is due to a defect of the enzyme alpha-galactosidase A (ceramide trihexosidase) and the accumulation of the lipid ceramide trihexoside in the tissues. In general, it is a disease of males, but female carriers can also show some evidence of mild disease. The cutaneous disease is characterized by angiokeratomas, small angiomatous lesions (Figs. 40–2 and 40–3; Plate VII A and B). Angiokeratomas can also occur in some other instances not associated

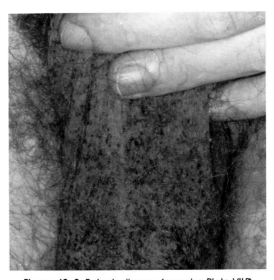

Figure 40–2. Fabry's disease (see also Plate VIIB).

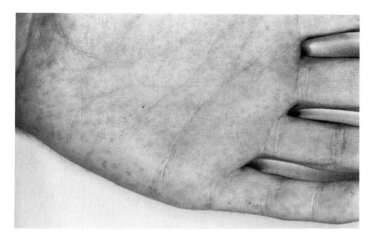

Figure 40–3. Fabry's disease (same patient as in Fig. 40–2) (see also Plate VIIC).

with systemic disease; in particular, their occurrence on the scrotal skin of older individuals is known as angiokeratoma of Fordyce and is a benign condition. The lesions of Fabry's disease are known as angiokeratoma corporis diffusum, since they occur on the trunk in a diffuse distribution. Renal disease develops in a majority of the patients and may first appear as lipiduria. Eventually the lipid deposition will lead to the development of uremia. Interestingly, renal transplantation can provide the missing enzyme in some cases and lead to clinical improvement. The nail-patella syndrome (Fong's syndrome) is a genetic disorder, inherited in an autosomal dominant fashion, that is characterized by hypoplasia of the nails (Fig. 40–4) and patella; skeletal abnormalities of the elbows, knees, and iliac crests; and frequently progressive renal failure. Proteinuria is an early sign of the renal involvement, and progressive deterioration of renal function occurs in about 30% of the patients.

Several other disorders may affect the skin and the kidneys, and have been discussed elsewhere in this text. Sarcoidosis frequently has cutaneous manifestations, but it infrequently involves the kidneys directly. However, the kidneys can become involved if hypercalcemia is left untreated. Diabetes mellitus may have profound effects on the kidneys, and it may also have cutaneous manifestations; however, it is rarely found that the cutaneous disease correlates with the kidney disease. Amyloidosis (AL type) frequently has cutaneous lesions and an associated nephrotic syndrome. The progressive impairment of renal function can lead to the patient's eventual demise.

CUTANEOUS CHANGES IN PATIENTS ON DIALYSIS

Patients undergoing hemodialysis frequently have or will develop cutaneous le-

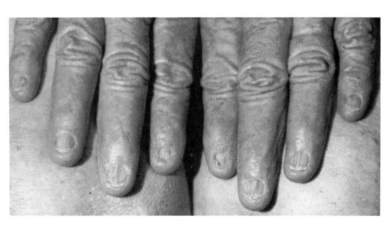

Figure 40–4. Nail-patella syndrome. Note the hypoplasia of the nails. Also, the patella are missing in this particular individual. (Courtesy of Dr. Neil A. Fenske, Tampa, FL.)

sions. The most common problem encountered is that of pruritus, but in addition these patients will also frequently have purpura secondary to the use of anticoagulants and to impaired platelet function. They may also have splinter hemorrhages. Infrequently, these patients may develop a bullous dermatosis or a perforating cutaneous disease.

Pruritus affects up to 80% of patients on hemodialysis at some time in the course of their treatment. The severity of the pruritus is divided about equally among mild, moderate, and severe forms. It is constant in roughly 25% of those affected. The relationship to the timing of the dialysis is very variable. The mechanism by which the pruritus occurs is not fully understood, but some theories propose mast cell proliferation and others relate pruritus to the presence of secondary hyperparathyroidism. Treatment with ultraviolet B light seems effective in many of the patients. Ultraviolet A light does not seem to be as beneficial. In addition, some authors have suggested that the ingestion of inactivated charcoal is helpful, but this may inactivate some oral medications.

There have been multiple reports of a cutaneous blistering eruption in patients on chronic hemodialysis that clinically and his-

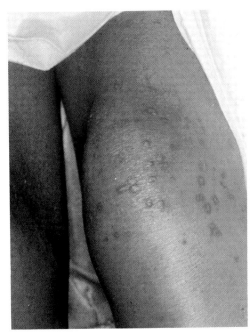

Figure 40–6. Multiple papular lesions are present in this patient with Kyrle's disease. The patient has diabetes and is on hemodialysis.

topathologically resembles porphyria cutanea tarda (PCT). Some of these patients have been shown to have biochemical changes of PCT, whereas others do not have these abnormalities. The eruption consists of small, fragile vesicles generally found on sun-exposed surfaces such as the dorsum of the hand (Fig. 40–5). Hyperpigmentation, scarring, and milia formation also occur. When circulating porphyrins are found, the treatment consists of an attempt to remove them, but in their absence the therapy involves photoprotection.

In unusual circumstances, patients may develop pruritic, hyperpigmented papular lesions that frequently contain a central keratinous plug (Fig. 40–6). This condition is known as Kyrle's disease, or "hyperkeratosis follicularis et parafollicularis in cutem penetrans." Originally, this disorder was thought to be associated with diabetes mellitus (most of the patients on dialysis who have this problem are also diabetics). In addition, this disorder seems to occur much more often in blacks, although white patients have also been affected. An effective treatment approach is the application of topical tretinoin (Retin-A), combined with therapy for the pruritus.

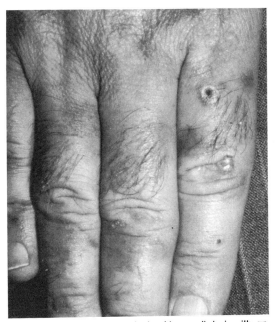

Figure 40–5. Bullous dermatosis of hemodialysis with an appearance similar to porphyria cutanea tarda.

CUTANEOUS MANIFESTATIONS IN RENAL TRANSPLANT PATIENTS

Some cutaneous problems that are unique to transplant patients relate to the use of immunosuppressive drugs to prevent transplant rejection. These same problems occur in patients with other organ transplants who are taking the same medications, but they do not seem to be as frequent in non-transplant patients on these medications. The changes that occur can be subdivided into (1) those that are caused directly by the medications used, (2) those that are due to infectious agents, and (3) those that are neoplastic. Almost all patients with renal transplantation will develop some cutaneous disease at some point in their course.

Most of these patients are taking systemic corticosteroids and will develop some changes of iatrogenic Cushing's syndrome. A common problem seen by dermatologists is the development of steroid-acne. This change occurs most often on the trunk, particularly on the back, and is manifested by small pustules, occasionally on an erythematous base. Other changes, such as cushingoid facies, striae, obesity, a redistribution of the normal body fat, and hirsutism, are also commonly seen.

Infections that complicate renal transplantation are those that are commonly found in the non-transplant population, but in addition there are a host of unusual infections that may present in an unusual fashion. Bacterial, viral, fungal, and protozoan infections may occur. Viral infections are particularly common in this population. Herpes simplex may have an unusual appearance, with chronic erosions or ulcerations occurring. The longer the patient has had a transplant, the greater the risk of developing multiple verrucae (warts) (Fig. 40–7). Warts in this group of patients are extremely difficult to treat; thus, if an individual skin lesion that could potentially be a wart is noticed, it should be removed. Warts have also been associated with the potential for development of cutaneous malignancy. Transplant patients who are exposed to scabies may develop an unusual infection in which the mite reproduces in an exuberant fashion. The lesions may become crusted and may become generalized. This type of infestation is known as Norwegian scabies. These patients are highly contagious, and the infection is often difficult to clear.

The development of cancer in this population is more common than in a similarly matched age group. Cancers that primarily account for this complication are squamous cell carcinomas of the skin. Sunlight is implicated as the inducer of these tumors; thus, sunscreens should be advocated for all transplant patients, with the exception of the most deeply pigmented individuals. Furthermore, the cancers that develop in these patients appear to behave in a much more aggressive fashion. The recognition of a potential skin cancer should be treated with the utmost urgency, and aggressive forms of therapy are indicated. Reduced immune surveillance may promote this change in tumor behavior. Another malignancy for which

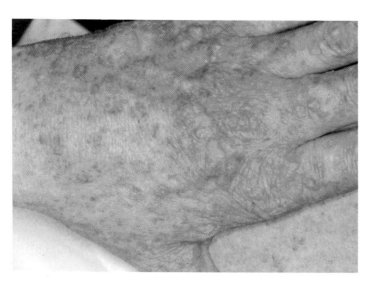

Figure 40–7. Multiple verrucous lesions are present on the hand in this individual with a renal transplant and on immunosuppressive therapy for 18 years.

these patients are at a greater risk is Kaposi's sarcoma. These patients are iatrogenically immunosuppressed, and the type of Kaposi's sarcoma that they develop is more akin to that seen in the AIDS population.

Suggested Readings

Dymock RB: Skin disease associated with renal transplantation. Aust J Dermatol 20:61–67, 1979.

Gilchrest BA, Rowe JW, Mihm MC Jr: Bullous dermatosis of hemodialysis. Ann Intern Med 83:480–483, 1975.

Gilchrest BA, Stern RS, Steinman TI, et al: Clinical features of pruritus among patients undergoing maintenance hemodialysis. Arch Dermatol 118:154–156, 1982.

Hood AF, Hardegen GL, Zarate AR, et al: Kyrle's disease in patients with chronic renal failure. Arch Dermatol 118:85–88, 1982.

Koranda FC, Dehmel EM, Kahn G, Penn I: Cutaneous complications in immunosuppressed renal homograft recipients. J Am Med Assn 229:419–424, 1974.

Poh-Fitzpatrick MB, Bellet N, DeLeo VA, et al: Porphyria cutanea tarda in two patients treated with hemodialysis for chronic renal failure. N Engl J Med 299:292–294, 1978.

41

Neurocutaneous Disease

JOHN J. ZONE

Discussions of neurocutaneous disease are frequently limited to descriptions of the 4 "phakomatoses." These conditions were grouped together because they shared central nervous system and retinal tumors (phakomas). The phakomatoses include the developmental disorders neurofibromatosis, tuberous sclerosis, Sturge-Weber syndrome, and von Hippel–Lindau syndrome, the first 3 of which have striking cutaneous manifestations. This discussion includes a variety of other developmental disorders as well as metabolic and infectious diseases in which cutaneous and nervous system findings are shared.

CLASSIFICATION

The relationship between the skin and the nervous system may be based on (1) a developmental abnormality, frequently a result of a shared embryogenesis; or (2) the systemic effect on both organ systems of a metabolic disorder, infection, or immune response. The developmental and metabolic disorders are primarily of genetic origin, whereas the infectious and immune abnormalities represent the response of the skin and nervous system to a common insult. The neural crest is a transient embryonic structure that gives rise to dorsal root ganglion cells, Schwann's cells, and autonomic ganglion cells, as well as melanocytes. Abnormalities of the neural crest cells lead to a myriad of clinical findings. Unfortunately, the resulting disease entities can seldom be

distilled to a pattern that can be totally explained by deductive reasoning. Disorders involving both the skin and the nervous system can be briefly categorized if one includes only the phakomatoses, but the list

Table 41–1. CLASSIFICATION OF NEUROCUTANEOUS DISEASE

A. Developmental disorders
  1. Dysplasia of neural crest cells
    a. Neurofibromatosis
    b. Tuberous sclerosis
  2. Vascular malformations
    a. Sturge-Weber disease
    b. Cobb's syndrome
    c. Ataxia-telangiectasia
    d. von Hippel–Lindau syndrome
  3. Pigmentary abnormalities
    a. LEOPARD syndrome
    b. Waardenburg's syndrome
    c. Incontinentia pigmenti
    d. Hypomelanosis of Ito
    e. Vogt-Koyanagi-Harada syndrome
  4. Epidermal nevus
  5. Ectodermal dysplasia
  6. Ichthyosis-associated syndromes
B. Metabolic disorders
  1. Angiokeratoma corporis diffusum
  2. Congenital hypothyroidism
  3. Amino acid abnormalities
C. Infectious disorders
  1. Viral
    a. Herpes simplex
    b. Herpes zoster
    c. Viral exanthem
  2. Bacterial: meningococcemia
  3. Rickettsial: Rocky Mountain spotted fever
  4. Spirochetes: syphilis
D. Immune disorders
  1. Henoch-Schönlein purpura
  2. Behçet's disease
  3. Lupus erythematosus

becomes very extensive if less common syndromes and systemic diseases involving both organ systems are included. The classifications in Table 41–1 include the classic neurocutaneous disorders, representative examples of various syndromes, and pertinent systemic disorders.

The term "phakomatosis" is derived from the Greek word "phakos" meaning "mother spot or mole." Although originally used to describe the retinal lesions of tuberous sclerosis, it has come to refer to a group of disorders including (1) tuberous sclerosis, (2) neurofibromatosis, (3) the Sturge-Weber disease, and (4) the von Hippel–Lindau syndrome. These disorders, as well as other vascular abnormalities, will be discussed in detail. The remainder of the developmental disorders represent disorders of epidermal cells and their appendages that share an ectodermal origin with the nervous system. The syndromes mentioned in Table 41–1 are rare but represent examples of probable neural crest abnormalities as well as poorly understood but well documented disorders involving both the skin and the nervous system. Metabolic, infectious, and immune disorders that involve both the nervous system and the skin are discussed in less detail because many of these conditions are reviewed in other chapters.

NEUROFIBROMATOSIS (VON RECKLINGHAUSEN'S DISEASE)

Neurofibromas may occur in several clinical settings: (1) sporadic solitary cutaneous tumors generally arising in adulthood and not associated with café au lait spots; (2) segmental neurofibromatosis, which is characterized by café au lait spots, cutaneous neurofibromas, and sometimes visceral neurofibromas limited to a sharply defined unilateral body segment; (3) acoustic neurofibromatosis, which is characterized by the constant finding of bilateral acoustic neuromas as well as café au lait spots and cutaneous neurofibromas; and (4) classic neurofibromatosis as described by von Recklinghausen, with multiple café au lait spots, multiple cutaneous neurofibromas, and a myriad of systemic involvement and marked variability of expression. This discussion is limited to classic neurofibromatosis, and the term "neurofibromatosis" is used to refer to only that disorder.

Pathogenesis

The incidence of neurofibromatosis is 40 per 100,000 live births. It has been shown to be inherited as an autosomal dominant trait when large kindreds are closely examined, although no specific gene abnormality or gene product has yet been identified. Fifty per cent of cases are estimated to be new mutations.

As stated previously, the neural crest is a transient embryonic structure that gives rise to dorsal root ganglion cells, Schwann's cells, autonomic ganglia, melanocytes, endocrine cells, and other tissues. The clinical findings of neurofibromatosis dictate a central importance of the neural crest in pathogenesis. There is a disturbance in melanin production with aberrant melanosomes demonstrated in café au lait spots. Hamartomatous proliferation of Schwann's cells and perineural fibroblasts produces tumorous growths around the cranial, spinal, and peripheral nerves. There is such patchy phenotypic expression of the gene that it is unlikely that an isolated morphologic defect is the cause of neurofibromatosis (as is seen in embryologic syndromes such as branchial cleft abnormalities). Riccardi has postulated that the primary defect in neurofibromatosis resides in the neural-crest-related secretory-membrane system of the Golgi complex and endoplasmic reticulum; that expression of the defect is determined by local cell-cell interactions involving neural crest and non–neural crest cells; and that the mast cell and its secretions participate in such interactions with the net effect of unmasking the otherwise latent presence of the neurofibromatous defect. This theory is far from proved but does have appeal in that it proposes a defect of cell-cell interactions that can be used to explain the wide variety of clinical findings.

Clinical Manifestations

Café au Lait Spots. These are present in virtually all patients with neurofibromatosis. Crowe first used the presence of 6 or more café au lait spots larger than 1.5 cm as a criterion for the disease (Fig. 41–1). Café au lait spots are usually present at birth but may take up to 1 year to develop. The lesions gradually enlarge with growth. Distribution of larger café au lait spots is random. They usually spare the face. Intertriginous areas are involved in 20% of cases, with freckle-like pathognomonic lesions (Crowe's sign) (Fig. 41–1). Hyperpigmentation may occur over plexiform neurofibromas. When such pigmentation extends to the midline, it often indicates that a tumor involves the spinal cord.

Neurofibromas. Neurofibromas begin to appear in late childhood and adolescence and gradually increase in size and number. Clinically, they are at first sessile, then become pedunculated, fleshy tumors that can be invaginated (buttonholing) (Fig. 41–2). They are composed of various combinations of neurons, Schwann's cells, fibroblasts, vascular elements, and mast cells. Subcutaneous neurofibromas occur either as discrete nodules on a peripheral nerve or as highly vascular diffuse plexiform neuromas (16% of cases) that involve a nerve trunk and may account for segmental hypertrophy and obstruction of neighboring vital structures. Both pregnancy and puberty are known to increase the number and size of neurofibromas. Malignant degeneration of neurofibromas into neurofibrosarcomas and malignant schwannomas unequivocally occurs in 2–3% of cases. Malignancy is most common

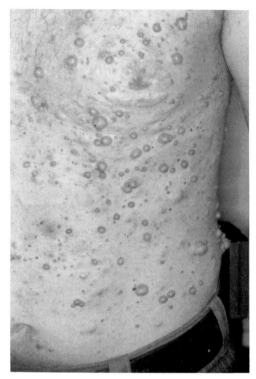

Figure 41–2. Multiple neurofibromas are present in this individual.

within a plexiform neuroma. Malignant degeneration is more common in patients greater than 50 years of age.

Lisch's Nodules. These pigmented iris hamartomas are present in 94% of patients age 6 years or older. They are asymptomatic and are not correlated with other manifestations or with severity of the disease.

Central Nervous System Involvement. Central nervous system (CNS) tumors develop in 3–10% of patients and include benign neoplasms such as optic nerve gliomas, acoustic neuromas, neurilemmomas, meningiomas, and neurofibromas. Such growths are presented clinically with symptoms and signs of CNS mass lesions. Optic nerve glioma is the most common of these tumors and may result in papilledema, retrobulbar neuritis, and eventually optic atrophy. Spinal tumors are presented with localizing peripheral signs. Malignant tumors, most commonly astrocytomas, may also occur.

Intellectual handicap involves about 40% of patients, although obvious retardation occurs in less than 5%. It does not worsen with time and does not correlate with the degree of skin involvement. Headaches oc-

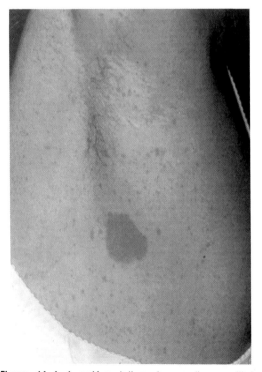

Figure 41–1. A café-au-lait spot as well as multiple freckles (Crowe's sign) in the axillary vault is seen in this patient with neurofibromatosis.

cur with increased frequency even in the absence of CNS tumors. Mild speech impediments are present in 30–40% of cases, and cerebrovascular compromise as a result of involvement of cerebral arteries with neurofibromas does occur. Major and minor motor seizures occur in less than 5% of cases in the absence of identifiable mass lesions or cerebral vascular involvement. An additional 26% of patients will have abnormal or borderline findings on electroencephalogram.

Macrocephaly is present in at least 27% of patients. This manifestation is more common after 6 years of age. There is no correlation between macrocephaly and impaired intellectual performance, seizures, or electroencephalographic abnormalities.

Musculoskeletal Disorders. Pseudarthrosis occurs in less than 1% of cases. This most frequently involves the tibia or the radius. It is characterized by congenital bowing of the involved bone with subsequent variable displacement of the joint (varying from a minimal radiologic abnormality to severe displacement with total loss of function). Radiographic bone abnormalities may also result from pressure by intraosseous or paraosseous neurofibromas.

Kyphoscoliosis occurs in at least 2% of patients. It is often associated with paravertebral neurofibromas; however, it is not certain if there is a cause-effect relationship between the two. Kyphoscoliosis usually has its onset in childhood and may rapidly progress to produce severe cardiorespiratory and neurologic compromise.

Gastrointestinal Disorders. Visceral tumors arise from intra-abdominal neural tissue and include neurofibromas, leiomyomas, and miscellaneous tumors. The most common complications are obstruction, intussusception, and hemorrhage caused by erosion or necrosis of pedunculated tumors. Persistent constipation occurs in 10% of cases and is due to disorganization of the tunica muscularis and Auerbach's plexus of the colon.

Endocrine Disorders. Aberrant endocrine function is not a regular finding in neurofibromatosis and although frequently mentioned is probably present in less than 1% of cases. Pheochromocytoma, often bilateral, is the most common endocrine abnormality. Medullary carcinoma of the thyroid and hyperparathyroidism are even less common.

Other reported endocrine associations probably occur only by coincidence.

Miscellaneous Disorders. Other findings that may be associated with neurofibromatosis are of significance because of their systemic implications. These include congenital pulmonary stenosis, idiopathic interstitial pulmonary fibrosis, and an extramural or intramural involvement of the renal arteries producing renal artery stenosis and hypertension.

Miscellaneous malignancies, including Wilms' tumor, rhabdomyosarcoma, and leukemia (especially xanthomatous leukemia), are much more common in patients with neurofibromatosis than in the population at large, for unknown reasons.

Differential Diagnosis

The diagnosis of neurofibromatosis can be made in 80% of the cases by identifying 6 or more café au lait spots greater than 1.5 cm. The remaining patients will frequently have multiple characteristic neurofibromas if they are post-pubertal. The diagnosis may be difficult to make in pre-pubertal children who do not have sufficient numbers of café au lait spots. In that situation, a positive family history, the presence of bone cysts, and evidence of spinal nerve involvement may help confirm the diagnosis. The CNS variant with bilateral acoustic neuromas is frequently associated with few cutaneous findings and therefore requires confirmation based on CNS findings.

Albright's syndrome consists of polyostotic fibrous dysplasia, endocrine dysfunction, melanotic macules, and precocious puberty in females. The melanotic macules of Albright's syndrome are also present at birth but tend to be unilateral, segmental, and frequently linear in arrangement. The border of the pigmented lesions in Albright's syndrome have been said to be serrated (likened to the coast of Maine), as opposed to the smooth borders of café au lait spots in neurofibromatosis. Further evaluation of this finding has found it to be of questionable diagnostic importance. Macromelanosomes are common in neurofibromatosis but are rare in Albright's syndrome. However, they have been found not to be specific for the café au lait spots of neurofibromatosis.

Patient Evaluation

Riccardi has published recommendations for extensive patient evaluation aimed at confirming the diagnosis, identifying complications, and monitoring progression. These recommendations include intelligence testing (IQ), psychologic evaluation, electroencephalography, audiography, slit-lamp examination, skeletal survey (with attention to the skull, optic foramina, and spine), cranial computed tomography (CT) scanning to include the orbits and optic chiasm, and measurement of 24-hour excretion levels of norepinephrine and epinephrine. This detailed evaluation is justified because 5–10% of patients will have significant findings and the remaining patients will benefit significantly from the reassurance of a negative evaluation.

Several important points concerning natural history should be kept in mind:

1. Progression in the number and size of all lesions is relentless throughout life.

2. The presence of one feature of the disease in no way correlates with the other features.

3. The severity of neurofibromatosis is not influenced by the severity of the maternal disease.

4. One cannot predict the course of neurofibromatosis based on the current severity of the disease.

Treatment

Malignant degeneration of neurofibromas is a constant threat. Surgical removal of rapidly enlarging lesions should be undertaken. In addition, removal of disfiguring or functionally compromising lesions is recommended. Anticonvulsants, analgesics, and H_1 antihistamines are useful for symptomatic therapy of appropriate manifestations.

Genetic counseling should make the patient aware of a 50% recurrence risk in both sexes with virtually 100% penetrance and variable expressivity. Pre-natal diagnosis is not possible.

The disease presents serious psychosocial problems. The various complications may involve sight, hearing, and learning as well as growth and development. Awareness of these problems and methods of coping with them are essential to decrease long-term morbidity.

TUBEROUS SCLEROSIS (BOURNEVILLE'S DISEASE)

Tuberous sclerosis is a disorder that classically consists of the triad of epilepsy, adenoma sebaceum, and mental retardation. However, a variety of other lesions may affect the skin, nervous system, heart, kidney, and other organs.

Pathogenesis

Tuberous sclerosis shows no racial, ethnic, or sexual predilection. The incidence is estimated at 5–7 per 100,000 live births. An autosomal dominant inheritance pattern may occur, but the majority of cases must be attributed to a gene mutation. The effective fertility is reduced by the frequently severe mental retardation. There is a high degree of penetrance when subtle clinical findings are included. The karyotype is normal, and a responsible gene or gene product has not yet been isolated.

The pathogenesis of this disorder no doubt involves an embryologic defect (possibly a deficiency of a controlling protein) that allows the hamartomatous proliferation of both mesodermal and ectodermal elements. These proliferations are usually focal and rarely undergo malignant transformation.

Clinical Manifestations

Facial Angiofibroma (Adenoma Sebaceum). The hamartomas called adenoma sebaceum are actually angiofibromas, and the sebaceous glands are actually generally atrophic. The lesions are erythematous, smooth papules involving the nasolabial folds, cheeks, and chin in a symmetrical distribution (Fig. 41–3). They are found in 70–90% of patients with tuberous sclerosis older than 5 years if the clinician closely examines the patient. When found, they are virtually pathognomonic of tuberous sclerosis. The main histologic findings are dermal fibrosis and dilatation of dermal capillaries.

Hypomelanotic Macules (Ash Leaf Macules). These consist of asymmetrically dis-

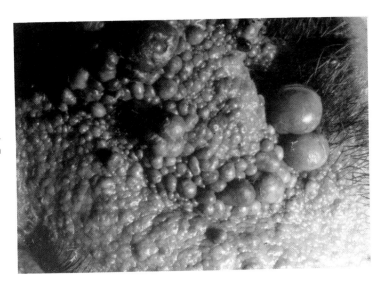

Figure 41–3. Multiple lesions of adenoma sebaceum in a patient with tuberous sclerosis.

tributed, hypopigmented macules that are most common over the trunk and buttocks and are rare over the face (Fig. 41–4; Plate VII D). They are usually greater than 1 cm in diameter and range in number from 3–4 to 100. Their configuration is usually leaf-like ("ash leaf macule"). They have been reported in 50–90% of cases of tuberous sclerosis. However, ash leaf macules are probably present at birth in the vast majority of patients with tuberous sclerosis (based on studies in which neonates were closely ex-

amined using a Wood's light). They persist throughout life and constitute the earliest cutaneous sign of tuberous sclerosis. Biopsy examinations reveal a normal number of melanocytes but a decreased intensity of melanization.

Ungual Fibromas (Koenen's Tumors). These are pink to flesh-colored papules ranging in size from 1 mm to 1 cm that arise from the toenail bed or less commonly from the fingernail bed (Fig. 41–5). They can be located in the lateral nail groove, under the nail plate, or along the proximal nail groove. They usually appear at puberty and are present in about 50% of cases. Histologically, they resemble facial angiofibromas, with fibrosis and capillary dilatation. Older lesions may contain large, stellate fibroblasts with a "glial appearance."

Shagreen Patch. These connective tissue hamartomas are plaques (Fig. 41–6) that are usually found on the trunk, particularly in the lumbosacral area. They vary in size from a few millimeters to 10 or more cm. They are yellowish-brown to pink in color and have a firm consistency. The lesions are rarely found in infancy and become more common after puberty, reaching a peak incidence of 70–80% of cases of tuberous sclerosis. The shagreen patch, however, differs neither clinically nor histopathologically in any way from other connective tissue nevi that may occur as isolated developmental defects in otherwise normal individuals.

Miscellaneous Nevoid Lesions. Café au

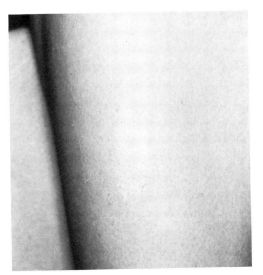

Figure 41–4. A hypopigmented spot on the thigh in the shape of an ash leaf is present in this patient with tuberous sclerosis (see also Plate VIID).

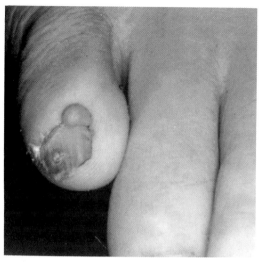

Figure 41–5. A periungual fibroma is present in this patient with tuberous sclerosis. (Courtesy of Dr. Neil A. Fenske, Tampa, FL.)

lait spots may occur as an isolated finding in 10–20% of tuberous sclerosis patients. Interestingly, Crowe found that 10% of the general population has one or more café au lait spots.

Fibromas of various sizes and shapes may occur in other locations. These include (1) large, asymmetrical fibromas of the face and scalp; (2) soft, pedunculated growths on the neck, trunk, or extremities (molluscum fibrosum pendulum); (3) grouped, firm papules of the neck, trunk, and extremities; and (4)

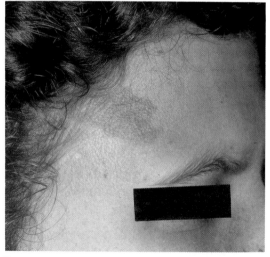

Figure 41–6. An erythematous plaque representative of a connective tissue nevus is present in this patient with tuberous sclerosis (shagreen patch).

pedunculated or sessile nodules of the buccal or gingival mucosa.

Central Nervous System Involvement. Focal or generalized seizures occur in over 80% of patients with tuberous sclerosis. These are largely related to "tuberous" tumors of the cerebral cortex. Cerebral tumors up to 3 cm in size represent hamartomas of glioblasts and neuroblasts. These tumors calcify in about 50% of patients and produce characteristic roentgenographic changes. Prior to known calcification (in infancy), the tumor may be recognized by CT. Neoplastic transformation to astrocytomas, glioblastomas, and meningiomas may be seen. Mental function gradually deteriorates with time, and 60–70% of patients demonstrate both seizures and mental retardation by 3 years of age.

Retinal and optic nerve involvement is the most frequent ophthalmic manifestation of tuberous sclerosis. It occurs in 50% of patients. Retinal gliomas may appear as peripheral, non-calcified lesions that are flat, white to salmon-colored, and circular (phakoma—"white spot"). They are frequently located superficial to a retinal vessel. The second type of retinal lesion is the classic nodular lesion resembling a mulberry, with clusters of small, glistening granules. Generally, the retinal lesions do not grow significantly and blindness is rare. Treatment is not necessary.

Renal Involvement. Two characteristic renal lesions occur in tuberous sclerosis: angiomyolipomas and renal cysts. The prevalence of angiomyolipomas increases with age (being present in greater than 90% of patients over the age of 10). They can be the sole manifestation of the tuberous sclerosis complex. Angiomyolipomas are usually multiple, bilateral, and innocuous. When they are symptomatic, the patient may manifest pain and/or hematuria. Renal failure is very rare. They range in size from a few millimeters to 20 cm, and the mass effect of the tumor is usually responsible for symptoms. There are multiple reports of malignant transformation of angiomyolipomas, but in none of these has metastasis occurred.

Renal cysts may be small and asymptomatic or large, producing renal impairment. Although the prevalence of such lesions is not known, the small cysts are felt to be common and large cysts are very rare.

Cardiac and Pulmonary Involvement. Cardiac involvement in tuberous sclerosis includes multiple, discrete rhabdomyomas, which occur in 30% of patients. The vast majority of patients with rhabdomyomas die during the first year of life, and the deaths are related to outflow obstruction or conduction defects.

Pulmonary involvement is rare and usually consists of diffuse leiomyomatosis. This produces a pattern on chest x-ray that may range from a fine reticular pattern to multiple cysts. Pneumothorax, progressive exertional dyspnea, and cor pulmonale may occur.

Miscellaneous Systemic Findings. A number of variable and non-specific findings have been reported. These include goiter, hypothyroidism, Cushing's syndrome, abnormal glucose tolerance tests, precocious puberty, adrenal hyperplasia, cystic radiographic lesions of the metacarpals and phalanges, pitted defects of dental enamel, and splenic hamartomas.

Differential Diagnosis

The characteristic skin ash leaf macules in children with seizures and/or mental retardation are sufficient to establish the diagnosis. However, the early stages of the disease and the forme fruste may give trouble in diagnosis. There is also a poor correlation of severity among the individual components of the disease. For example, young adults with normal intelligence may have angiofibromas and various systemic lesions. In such situations, the search for individual cutaneous or non-cutaneous components of the syndrome in a patient with an isolated finding confirms the diagnosis.

Patient Evaluation

A detailed family history with examination of family members is required. However, 85% of cases represent mutations and family history should not be used to rule out tuberous sclerosis. Studies that may support the diagnosis include skull roentgenograms for calcification and biopsy of appropriate skin lesions.

Patients with established cases should have a detailed ophthalmologic examination, looking for gliomas; CT scan of the brain to evaluate the severity of CNS involvement; chest roentgenogram to detect pulmonary involvement; echocardiogram to evaluate intracardiac tumors; and radiographic evaluation for renal masses. There is no set recommendation for periodic follow-up studies. However, symptoms in any organ system should prompt immediate evaluation for hamartomatous lesions.

Treatment

Genetic counseling is essential for adults with even minimal involvement from tuberous sclerosis, since their children may be severely affected. Symptomatic treatment with anticonvulsants is valuable. Surgical removal of extracutaneous hamartomas is indicated if symptoms become evident or if such lesions enlarge rapidly, indicating possible malignant degeneration. Removal of cutaneous lesions is for cosmetic reasons only.

STURGE-WEBER DISEASE

Sturge-Weber disease is characterized by a nevus flammeus, or port-wine stain, in the area of the ophthalmic branch of the trigeminal nerve (Fig. 41–7; Plate VII E). Cutaneous lesions are present at birth. In addition, there are ipsilateral leptomeningeal angiomas that lead to progressive calcification and degeneration of the underlying cerebral cortex. This degeneration may lead to seizure disorders, contralateral hemiparesis, and ipsilateral ocular involvement with angiomatosis of the choroid and glaucoma.

Pathogenesis

Sturge-Weber disease is believed to be genetically transmitted, although familial cases of the complete syndrome are rare. Dominant transmission with incomplete penetrance has been proposed on the basis of the finding that some family members may have mental retardation, angiomas in various locations, and seizures. Trisomy 22 has been reported in isolated patients, but no metabolic defect as the result of a gene abnormality has been identified.

The vascular abnormalities of Sturge-Weber disease probably represent a mesodermal defect that occurs in the fourth to eighth week of embryonic development. At this

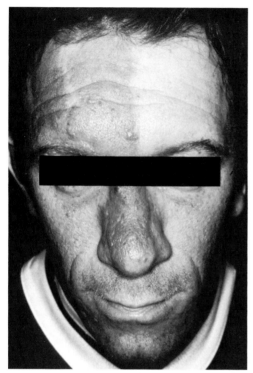

Figure 41–7. A unilateral port-wine stain is present in this man with Sturge-Weber syndrome (see also Plate VII*E*).

point, the ectoderm, which will form the skin, overlies the tissue that will eventually become the ipsilteral cerebrum. Subsequently, the leptomeningeal vessels develop into venous angiomas with a network and thin-walled ectatic venules filling the subarachnoid space. At birth, the port-wine stain is flat and grows in proportion to the growth of the child. The cerebral angiomas develop progressive loss of venous drainage with subsequent venous stasis and calcification. Calcification is believed to be the result of deposition of colloid fibers on a matrix of reticulin fibers with precipitation of calcium salts on reticulin fibers. This calcification increases throughout life. The combination of vascular ectasia and calcification then produces ischemia of underlying cerebral tissue with resultant diffuse cortical atrophy and the resultant nervous system abnormalities.

It has been proposed that the trigeminal distribution of the nevus flammeus represents a co-migration of skin vasculature and the underlying trigeminal nerve during embryogenesis. Occasional angiomas in the tri-

geminal nerve ganglion support this theory, but this hypothesis fails to explain the frequent findings of port-wine stains that intrude on neighboring cervical and contralateral dermatomes.

Clinical Manifestations

The port-wine stains are flat, vascular lesions ranging in color from pink to deep purple. The area of involvement may range from a single eyelid to bilateral extensive angiomas. Eight per cent of patients demonstrate unilateral involvement of the face, usually both above and below the palpebral fissure. When a nevus flammeus lies entirely below the ophthalmic branch of the trigeminal nerve (below the palpebral fissure and upper eyelid), cranial involvement is rare and the clinical skin abnormality is best termed nevus flammeus, or port-wine stain, rather than Sturge-Weber disease. As port-wine stains age, the vessel walls become progressively more ectatic, producing exophytic blueberry-like ectasias in mid-adult life.

The characteristic cerebral angiomas, calcification, and atrophy may occur in the absence of skin lesions in 5–14% of cases. Such cases are still termed Sturge-Weber disease but obviously do not fulfill the traditional criteria for the syndrome.

Cutaneous involvement of the upper eyelid is associated with intraocular abnormalities. Intraocular abnormalities occur in one half of the patients as angiomas of the conjunctiva, iris, or choroid. Angiomas of the choroid may produce glaucoma or retinal detachment that may be congenital or that may occur later in life. Angioid streaks of the retina and enlargement of the globe may occur. Oculocutaneous melanosis produced by ectopic dermal melanocytes presents as slate blue discoloration of the sclera and of the periorbital skin resembling nevus of Ota. This is not a common occurrence.

Oral mucous membranes and the tongue may show unilateral telangiectatic hypertrophy in addition to gingival hypertrophy. The latter may be greatly accentuated by pregnancy.

Seizures may begin shortly after birth but usually occur in late infancy or early childhood. Up to 20% of patients never develop seizures. Seizures frequently begin with febrile episodes that precipitate contralateral focal motor seizures. Generalized seizures develop later. Hemiparesis, hemiplegia, hemisensory defects, homonymous hemianopsia, and limb atrophy also occur.

Mental retardation may be minimal in early childhood but is progressive after the onset of seizures. Control of seizures by medical or surgical means may slow the progression of the mental defect.

Radiologic calcifications are seldom present at birth, but in early childhood the characteristic railroad track pattern of calcification develops. These fine double lines outline the convolutions of the underlying cerebral cortex. Electroencephalographic evidence of brain involvement usually occurs in early childhood.

Patient Evaluation and Treatment

Improvement of the appearance of cutaneous lesions is best accomplished with cosmetics (e.g., Covermark). Electrodesiccation usually produces unacceptable scarring. The argon laser offers theoretical benefit in that red-colored blood vessels should selectively absorb the laser energy that thereby selectively destroys the hemangioma. However, cosmetically unacceptable scarring frequently results and makes the treatment less acceptable than anticipated. Laser treatment is effective for shrinking oral lesions or for the papular ectatic lesions that develop later in life.

If the characteristic cutaneous lesion is present, the affected child should be aggressively evaluated and treated with the hope of averting brain damage. Computed tomography (CT) and cerebral angiography can evaluate CNS lesions early in life. Medical prophylactic treatment of seizure disorders as well as surgical removal of leptomeningeal angiomas may then be justified. When present, glaucoma should be controlled by medical or, if necessary, surgical means. Mental deterioration may not be severe in one half of patients, and such people may then lead relatively normal lives.

COBB'S SYNDROME

Cobb's syndrome is the association of a port-wine stain or cavernous hemangioma in a dermatomal distribution with an angioma of the spinal cord that corresponds to the cutaneous distribution. Neurologic deficits of spinal cord compression may then occur.

ATAXIA-TELANGIECTASIA (LOUIS-BAR SYNDROME)

Ataxia-telangiectasia is an autosomal recessive disorder consisting of progressive cerebellar ataxia, ocular and cutaneous telangiectasia, and variable immune deficiency. The immune deficiency predisposes the patient to recurrent sinopulmonary infections and to an increased incidence of neoplasia. Patients have a defect in cell growth and chromosomal integrity that is associated with an increased sensitivity to ionizing radiation.

Pathogenesis

The incidence is approximately 1 in 40,000 births, with the incidence of the asymptomatic heterozygote being as high as 1 in 100. Although this disorder is unequivocally genetic, the precise molecular defect is unknown. A mesodermal defect has been hypothesized, because mesodermal influence is necessary to regulate thymic development and blood vessel growth in the fetus.

There is significant hypersensitivity to clinical doses of x-ray. Fibroblasts and lymphoblasts are extremely sensitive to x-ray and to chemotherapeutic killing. In addition, cells from ataxia-telangiectasia patients have defective DNA repair following x-ray and fail to slow their rate of DNA synthesis. It appears that these defects in DNA synthesis and repair lead to degenerative CNS changes and to premature senescence, whereas abnormalities in tissue differentiation probably cause the failure of organ maturation and immunologic abnormalities.

Clinical Manifestations

Affected children have ataxia that becomes evident when they begin to walk. At the same time, problems with choreoathetosis, nystagmus, and difficulty in initiating voluntary eye movements develop. Telangiectasias develop between 2 and 8 years of age and occur first as wire-like vessels on the bulbar conjunctiva and later on the exposed areas of the auricle, the neck, and the flexor folds of the extremities. Other skin abnormalities may include premature graying of hair, loss of subcutaneous fat, vitiligo, and café au lait spots. Endocrine abnormalities frequently develop with time and include hyperinsulinism with insulin resistance, hypogonadism with delayed sexual development, and growth retardation. Recurrent sinopulmonary infections occur in most patients, with eventual bronchiectasis, respiratory failure, and death.

Defects in both cellular and humoral immunity are seen. Cellular defects are to be expected, in view of the consistent finding of an absent or hypoplastic thymus. Cellular defects include impaired skin test responses to recall antigens, reduced lymphocyte numbers, and decreased percentages of T cells. Two thirds of the patients have reduced *in vitro* proliferative response to mitogens and to specific antigens. Antigen challenge with foreign protein or with virus produces a poor antibody response related to abnormal antibody levels. Seventy per cent of patients are IgA-deficient, and 80% are IgE-deficient. These defects are caused primarily by defective antibody synthesis. There is persistent production of fetal proteins, as evidenced by the nearly constant finding of elevated serum alpha-fetoprotein levels.

Approximately 10% of patients develop malignancy, usually before the age of 15. Eighty per cent of these neoplasms are lymphoproliferative disorders, and 20% are carcinomas. This striking abnormality is no doubt related to compromised immune surveillance.

Treatment

Therapy is limited to treatment of infections, early detection of malignancy, and genetic counseling. Most patients die of infection or malignancy in childhood. The diagnosis may be suspected antenatally by the *in utero* elevation of alpha-fetoprotein concentration.

OTHER NEUROCUTANEOUS DISEASES

von Hippel–Lindau Syndrome. This condition is believed to be inherited as an autosomal dominant trait. It is characterized by single or multiple benign cerebellar tumors of capillaries. These tumors gradually increase in size, producing cerebellar signs. The retina may also be involved, with vascular proliferation. A port-wine stain may occur over the head and neck in some patients, but most patients have no cutaneous lesions.

LEOPARD Syndrome (Multiple Lentigines Syndrome). This is an autosomal dominant disorder characterized by the onset in early childhood of multiple lentigines involving the entire surface of the skin, including palms and soles but sparing mucous membranes. The components are L, lentigines; E, electrocardiographic abnormalities; O, ocular hypertelorism; P, pulmonary stenosis (subaortic stenosis also occurs frequently); A, abnormalities of genitalia (ovarian hypoplasia, undescended testes, or hypospadias); R, retardation of growth; and D, deafness (neural). Mental retardation may also occur. An embryonic abnormality of the neural crest could explain the auditory conduction defect, the lentigines, and the defective sympathetic cardiac innervation.

Waardenburg's Syndrome. A neural crest defect is also suggested in this autosomal dominant disorder, which combines piebaldism, depigmented macules on the skin, congenital deafness, and ocular hypertelorism. In this disorder, melanocytes are totally absent from the depigmented areas.

Incontinentia Pigmenti. Incontinentia pigmenti is an X-linked dominant disorder that is usually fatal *in utero* to affected males. It presents in the pre-natal period as scattered vesicular inflammatory lesions and progresses over a matter of months to verrucous lesions that are eventually replaced by hyperpigmentation (Fig. 41–8). In about 80% of the patients, other congenital abnormalities of the CNS, bones, eyes, and teeth may occur. CNS involvement occurs in 25% of the cases and may include epilepsy, microcephaly, mental retardation, and slow motor development. The genetic defect is unknown and represents an unusual combination of an inflammatory cutaneous disorder and congenital CNS abnormalities.

Hypomelanosis of Ito (Incontinentia Pigmenti Achromians). This disorder is believed to show autosomal dominant transmission. It is characterized by depigmented macules that are not preceded by the inflammatory patches noted in incontinentia pig-

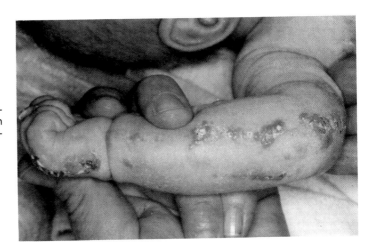

Figure 41–8. Multiple verrucous and vesiculated lesions in a linear distribution are present in this patient with incontinentia pigmenti.

menti. Pigmentary abnormalities may give a whorled or streaked appearance (Fig. 41–9; Plate VII F) and may be present at birth or may develop early in childhood. Nervous system abnormalities occur in about one half of the patients and may include seizures, electroencephalogram abnormalities, strabismus, and language retardation. Hypopigmentation tends to fade with age.

Vogt-Koyanagi-Harada Syndrome. This syndrome features depigmentation of the skin (especially of the eyebrows and eyelashes), headache, stiff neck, uveitis, and occasionally optic neuritis. Onset is associated with a febrile illness and is not known to be inherited or related to a pre-existent neural crest defect.

Epidermal Nevus (Nevus Unius Lateris, Systematized Nevus). This disorder is characterized by unilateral or occasionally bilateral verrucous papules or scaling plaques that are arranged in continuous or interrupted streaks (Fig. 41–10; Plate VII G). The lesions vary in color from yellow to brown and are usually asymptomatic. Histologically one sees benign hyperkeratosis, acanthosis, and papillomatosis of epidermal cells. There is no known hereditary predisposition. Epidermal nevi may be associated with skeletal deformities and CNS disease, including arteriovenous malformations, epilepsy, mental retardation, and peripheral nerve disorders. Although the lesions frequently appear to have a dermatomal distribution, there is no pathogenetic link between the skin lesion and a peripheral nerve, as is seen in herpes zoster. Rather, this association represents the coexistence of unexplained abnormalities in structures that share an ectodermal origin. Sebaceous nevi

have also been reported to be associated with similar CNS defects.

Ectodermal Dysplasia. Hidrotic ectodermal dysplasia is an autosomal dominant disorder characterized by dystrophic nails, hypotrichosis, palmoplantar keratosis, and dental abnormalities. Sweat glands are normal. Neural deafness, epilepsy, and mental retardation may occur.

Ichthyosis-Associated Syndromes. There have been multiple cases of congenital ab-

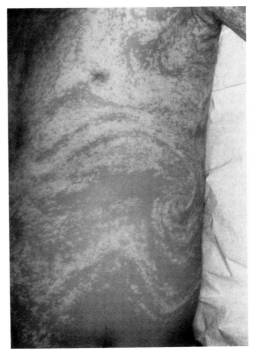

Figure 41–9. Hypopigmented swirls of skin in a patient with incontinentia pigmenti achromians (see also Plate VII F).

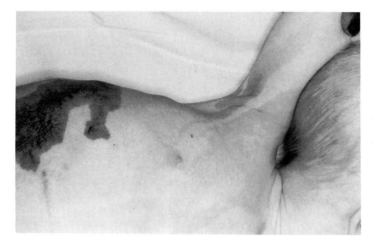

Figure 41–10. The patient shown has epidermal nevus syndrome with multiple anomalies, hemangiomas, and epidermal nevi, as represented by the fine, slightly pigmented skin (see also Plate VIIG).

normalities of the nervous system associated with ichthyosis, usually lamellar ichthyosis. These include the following:

1. Sjögren-Larsson syndrome, which is an autosomal recessive disorder characterized by lamellar ichthyosis, thickened palms and soles, mental retardation, epilepsy, and spastic diplegia or quadriplegia.

2. Rud's syndrome, which is believed to be a sex-linked disorder characterized by generalized ichthyosis of uncertain type in association with epilepsy and mental retardation.

3. Cases described by Tay that were characterized by lamellar ichthyosis, thickening of the palms and soles, pili torti, mental retardation, dwarfism, and progeria-like facies.

4. Jorizzo and coworkers described two patients in whom lamellar ichthyosis was found in association with involvement of the palms, soles, nails, and trichothiodystrophy. Subsequent patients have been reported as having IBIDS* syndrome or trichothiodystrophy. Associated defects included dwarfism, mental retardation, and defective teeth.

The remaining disorders listed in Table 41–1 include a variety of metabolic, infectious, and immune disorders in which both the skin and the nervous system are affected. For the most part, this occurs on the basis of circulating factors or pathogens that affect both organ systems. Many of these disorders

*Ichthyosis, brittle hair, intellectual impairment, decreased fertility, and short stature.

are discussed in other parts of the text. The clinical findings of these disorders will be briefly described.

Metabolic Disorders. Angiokeratoma corporis diffusum (Fabry's disease) is caused by defective galactosidase A (ceramide trihexosidase) (see Chapter 40). The characteristic cutaneous finding is that of clusters of dark red to blue-black angiectases, especially in the scrotum or umbilical areas. Neurologic findings frequently include extremity pain and paresthesias, which may be indicative of lipid infiltration of the vasa nervorum. Cerebral findings are multiple and result from multifocal small vessel involvement of cerebral arteries.

Congenital as well as acquired hypothyroidism may produce dryness and laxity of the skin with coarseness of the hair. If left uncorrected, congenital hypothyroidism may be associated with profound psychomotor maldevelopment.

Disorders of amino acid metabolism frequently cause abnormalities of hair and skin in combination with neurologic disease. The best known example is phenylketonuria, in which decreased pigmentation of hair and skin and frequently atopic dermatitis are associated with mental deficiency and epilepsy. A myriad of other cutaneous findings may be found in various aminoacidurias, which will not be detailed here.

Infectious Disorders. Both herpes simplex and herpes zoster represent an intimate pathogenic association between skin and peripheral nerves. Migration of latent virus along sensory nerves causes the characteristic lesions of cutaneous herpes infections.

Clinically, pain and tingling precedes the cutaneous eruption by hours to days. Viral exanthems may be of great help when searching for causes of encephalitis.

The remaining infectious disorders are self-explanatory. Bacterial sepsis may produce both meningitis and skin lesions of septic vasculitis, as typified by meningococcemia. Rocky Mountain spotted fever is characterized by a progression of erythematous papules of the extremities that subsequently become hemorrhagic. CNS findings include headache, occasionally meningeal symptoms, and even coma.

Immune Disorders. Immune disorders frequently affect both skin and nervous system, usually via inflammation of blood vessels. In such cases, neurologic symptoms may range from headaches to cerebral vascular accidents. Cutaneous findings include palpable purpuric papules (Henoch-Schönlein purpura). Behçet's syndrome may additionally show scattered, sterile pustules that progress to pyoderma gangrenosum–like le-sions. Lupus erythematosus is discussed elsewhere in the text.

Suggested Readings

Alexander GL, Norman RM: The Sturge-Weber Syndrome. Bristol, England, John Wright and Sons, Ltd., 1960.

Crowe FW, Schull WJ, Neel NV: A Clinical, Pathological, and Genetic Study of Multiple Neurofibromatosis. Springfield, IL, Charles C Thomas, 1956.

Gomez MR: Tuberous Sclerosis. New York, Raven Press, 1979.

Jorizzo JL, Crounse RG, Wheeler CE: Lamellar ichthyosis, dwarfism, mental retardation and hair shaft abnormalities. J Am Acad Dermatol 2:309–317, 1980.

Person JR, Perry HO: Recent advances in the phakomatoses. Int J Dermatol 17:1–13, 1978.

Riccardi VM: von Recklinghausen neurofibromatosis. N Engl J Med 305:1617–1626, 1981.

Solomon LM, Fretzin DF, Dewald RL: The epidermal nevus syndrome. Arch Dermatol 97:273–285, 1968.

Waldman TA, Misiti J, Nelson DL, Kraemer KH: Ataxia telangiectasia: A multisystem hereditary disease with immunodeficiency, impaired organ maturation, X-ray hypersensitivity and high incidence of neoplasia. Ann Intern Med 99:367–379, 1983.

42

Psychocutaneous Disease

JEFFREY P. CALLEN

The interplay between the skin and the psyche is important to physicians who treat patients who have disorders of either type. Abnormalities of the appearance often lead the patient to the physician's office. Skin disease can have a profound effect on the growth and development of the individual. For example, John Updike, a psoriasis sufferer, claims to have become a writer because of his skin problem. Conversely, severe psychologic disturbance can lead patients to manipulate their integument, with resultant cutaneous disease. It has been suggested that psychocutaneous disorders be divided into three subgroups: (1) primary psychologic disturbance with secondary cutaneous lesions that are produced or perceived by the patient, (2) organic skin disease with secondary psychologic effects, and (3) diseases in which there is an interplay between these factors. In this chapter, we deal primarily with the first group of disorders.

FACTITIAL DERMATITIS

Patients with factitial dermatitis have self-inflicted lesions. The patients deny or hide the mechanism by which they have produced the lesions. The patients may often delight in their ability to manipulate those in their environment, including family, friends, and physicians. A review of various published series of patients with this problem has suggested a female predominance. The patients rarely give a lucid history; often there is an illogical explanation given as to

the meaning of the skin lesions, or their natural history. The lesions, which are known to heal spontaneously, may persist for months or years. Lesions with angulated edges (Fig. 42–1), suggesting an exogenous cause, are present, yet the patient denies cutaneous manipulation. Cutaneous lesions may be produced by burns, which are ther-

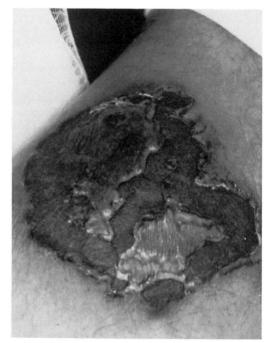

Figure 42–1. Factitial ulceration in a patient using lye to induce injury of the skin. Note the square corners and irregular margin. (Courtesy of Dr. Joseph J. Chanda, Melbourne, FL.)

mally or chemically induced; rubber bands may be used to produce ischemia and edema or trauma-inducing hemorrhage; or lesions may be produced by injection of foreign material. The lesions occur in a distribution consistent with sites that can be reached by the patient. There is rarely a symmetrical distribution. Lesions are seen in a similar stage and heal together. There is rarely an eruptive phase. Diagnosis of this type of problem is difficult, and treatment is even more difficult.

TRICHOTILLOMANIA

Trichotillomania is a psychocutaneous disorder that usually occurs in children and adolescents. It is manifested by patches of hair loss. The patches tend to be irregular, without total loss of hair, and they may contain multiple broken hairs within the patch. The injury is caused by a mechanical manipulation, often twisting, of the hair. Patients are often unconscious of their actions. Occasionally this type of hair pulling behavior is an attempt by the child to get the attention of the parent through the need for medical care.

DELUSIONS OF PARASITOSIS

Delusions of parasitosis are believed to be a monosymptomatic hypochondriacal psychosis. It is manifested by the patient's perception that insects are infesting and biting his or her skin. Such patients may present with multiple excoriations, and they may complain of severe pruritus. Frequently, patients present to the physician with a container filled with what they believe is biting them. On close examination of the contents, one usually finds a mixture of lint, dried scales, and various other inanimate particles. The care of these patients requires a compassionate approach combined with psychiatric evaluation when possible, and the use of anti-psychotic drugs such as pimozide.

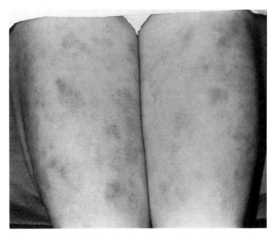

Figure 42–2. Multiple bruises in a patient with Gardner-Diamond syndrome (see also Plate VII*H*). (Courtesy of Dr. Neil A. Fenske, Tampa, FL.)

THE AUTO-ERYTHROCYTE SYNDROME (GARDNER-DIAMOND SYNDROME)

This syndrome has not unequivocably been proved to be psychogenic in its pathogenesis. The disorder occurs primarily in young women, often attractive but with significant emotional pathology. The disorder is manifested by the rapid development of unexplained non-inflammatory purpura (Fig. 42–2; Plate VII*H*). Laboratory studies of immune function and coagulation are within normal limits. It is said that the injection of autologous erythrocytes will reproduce the lesions. Manipulation of injection sites by the patient has been demonstrated in some individuals with this diagnosis. These patients, similiar to those previously discussed, are extremely difficult to treat.

Suggested Readings

Cotterill JA: Clinical features of patients with dermatologic nondisease. *Sem Dermatol* 2:203–206, 1983.

Lyell A: Delusions of parasitosis. *Sem Dermatol* 2:189–195, 1983.

Masters R: The psyche and the skin. *Neurol Clin* 5:483–498, 1987.

Ratnoff OD: The psychogenic purpuras: A review of autoerythrocyte sensitization to DNA, "hysterical" and factitial bleeding, and the religious stigmata. *Sem Hematol* 17:192–213, 1980.

Sneddon IB: Simulated disease and hypochondriasis in the dermatology clinic. *Sem Dermatol* 2:177–181, 1983.

43

Pregnancy and the Skin

JEFFREY P. CALLEN

Pregnancy is associated with alterations of endocrine and metabolic systems as well as with changes in the physiologic state of the body. These alterations can lead to normal changes in the skin, hair, and nails as well as to the pathologic conditions that are related to the pregnant state. Five broad areas will be discussed as follows: (1) physiologic changes related to hormonal changes; (2) changes in tumors that are influenced by pregnancy; (3) diseases specifically associated with pregnancy, in particular, the pruritic dermatoses; (4) genital infections that are of perinatal importance; and (5) the influence of pregnancy on dermatological as well as systemic disorders associated with cutaneous manifestations.

PHYSIOLOGIC CHANGES

Ninety per cent of pregnant patients develop some change in pigmentation involving the genitalia, areolae, scars, moles, or even generalized hyperpigmentation. A specific change in pigmentation known as melasma, or the "mask of pregnancy," has been reported in roughly 15–60% of pregnant women. Melasma consists of a hyperpigmentation that is usually on the cheeks, forehead, mustache area, and occasionally the neck. The pigmentation is irregular macular hyperpigmentation with occasional hypopigmented areas occurring within the hyperpigmented area. The disease is exacerbated by sun exposure and may be effectively prevented by sun avoidance as well as by using sunscreens. Melasma may also be present in non-pregnant individuals who are using oral contraceptives. The mask of pregnancy may be treated with topical hydroquinone, a depigmenting agent. Topical corticosteroids and topical retinoic acid may enhance the depigmenting effects of the hydroquinone.

During pregnancy, the rate of hair and nail growth increases and the nails may develop linear ridges occurring horizontally that are known as Beau's lines. Some degree of hirsutism may develop in certain individuals. In addition, during the pregnant state and surrounding the time of delivery the hair may convert from a normal anagen (growing) phase to a telogen (resting) phase. Usually 2–4 months following delivery, a telogen effluvium type of hair loss may occur. Eventually, however, the hair that is lost is replaced and therapy is not required for this process.

Eccrine activity increases during pregnancy, which may account for the hyperhidrosis reported by some patients. Decrease in apocrine (sweat gland) activity has been noted. An increase in sebaceous gland activity occurs during pregnancy; however, acne, a disease related to increased sebaceous gland activity, does not uniformly worsen during pregnancy. Enlargement of Montgomery's glands on the areola is a common clinical correlation of increased sebaceous gland activity and occurs in approximately 30–50% of pregnant women.

Vascular changes occur during pregnancy and are related to dilatation, fragility, and proliferation of the small cutaneous blood vessels. Manifestations of dilatation of these blood vessels include vaginal edema and erythema, diffuse palmar erythema, and hypothenar erythema. Patients with pre-existing Raynaud's phenomena may improve during pregnancy because of vascular dilatation. Varicosities affecting the leg veins as well as hemorrhoidal veins are common in patients during pregnancy; however, venous thromboembolic phenomena occur uncommonly. Proliferation of blood vessels may be manifested by development of pyogenic granulomas during pregnancy. Spider angiomas also occur.

CUTANEOUS TUMORS

Often the pregnant state has a profound influence upon tumors. Pyogenic granulomas are more frequent in patients who are pregnant. In addition, a tumor known as molluscum gravidarum (basically an enlarging skin tag) may occur on the neck, chest, or inframammary areas in the latter stages of pregnancy. Occasionally these tumors will regress following pregnancy; however, if they are large and bothersome they may be removed. Keloids may grow rapidly during pregnancy. Nevi may arise, grow, or change color during pregnancy. Neurofibromas present prior to pregnancy may increase in size, or new tumors may form during pregnancy. Neurofibromas do not regress post-partum.

The effect of pregnancy on dysplastic nevi and malignant melanoma has been debated. There are certain melanomas that contain estrogen receptors; thus, pregnancy may indeed have an effect on these patients. It has been stated that patients with stage I melanoma are not affected by pregnancy, but those who have stage II or III melanoma may develop spread of their disease during pregnancy. Controversy still exists regarding whether or not a patient who has had a melanoma should become pregnant.

PRURITIC DERMATOSES OF PREGNANCY

Pruritus in pregnancy can be a difficult problem to treat. It may be associated with both maternal and fetal complications. The presence of pruritus is not only alarming to the patient but also should alert the physician to potential serious complications and does warrant an appropriate evaluation.

Pruritus Gravidarum

This condition is characterized by an intense, generalized pruritus without primary skin lesions. It tends to occur in late pregnancy and abates quickly after delivery. It is the most common cause of pruritus seen in pregnancy, possibly occurring in up to 20% of all pregnancies. Pruritus gravidarum may be related to cholestasis, and minimal abnormalities are often noted on liver function tests, including an increase in bilirubin. Frank jaundice is rarely seen in these patients. In addition to the pruritus, the patients may have anorexia or nausea and occasionally diarrhea. Similar changes may be noted in patients who take oral contraceptives after the time of delivery. Patients with pruritus gravidarum may be at an increased risk for the development of cholelithiasis and possibly cholecystitis after pregnancy.

If the pruritus is mild, treatment may not be necessary. If treatment is necessary, the first line includes emollients and antihistamines as well as reassurance of the patient as to the transient nature of the disease. In patients who do not respond to these measures, cholestyramine given with supplemental fat soluble vitamins may be effective.

Herpes Gestationis

This pruritic dermatosis is a vesicular, bullous disease that is closely related to bullous pemphigoid. It is a condition that also occurs in non-pregnant individuals. The name refers to the grouping of the lesions (herpetiform) in a pregnant (gestational) individual rather than to an etiologic association. Thus, the name does not refer in any way to a herpesvirus infection. The exact incidence of herpes gestationis is not known, but it has been estimated to occur in 1 of 4000 pregnancies.

In a first pregnancy, clinical manifestations of herpes gestationis appear in the second and/or third trimesters. In subsequent pregnancies, an earlier onset is possible. In addition, lesions may occur in patients taking oral contraceptives. In the initial stages of the lesions, an intense pruritus occurs and urticarial papules or plaques may develop on the abdomen and trunk. Within several days, these lesions become vesicular and large blisters may also develop. Subsequently, the lesions can spread to involve the entire cutaneous surface. The healing process involves the formation of crusts, and residual hyper- or hypopigmentation may occur. Little or no scarring occurs unless lesions become infected or are significantly excoriated.

Histopathologic study of an early stage lesion reveals the non-specific finding of a perivascular lymphohistiocytic infiltrate. As the condition progresses, subepidermal bullae containing neutrophils and eosinophils can be observed. Herpes gestationis has a characteristic immunofluorescence microscopic pattern, which is the deposition of IgG and C3 in the basement membrane zone. On immunoelectronmicroscopy, the immunoglobulin is found within the lamina lucida. In addition, a circulating immunoglobulin that has been termed the HG factor (which appears to be an IgG) deposits in a similar area of the basement membrane zone.

Herpes gestationis rarely causes serious maternal complications, with the exception of secondary bacterial infections. Fetal complications have been reported, but there is some controversy over the exact risk to the fetus. The incidence of premature delivery may be as high as 23%, compared with less than 10% in the normal population. In addition, because the factor related to the disease appears to be a circulating immunoglobulin of the IgG class, it may cross the placenta and lead to a transient blistering disease in the neonate that is similar to that seen in the mother.

Herpes gestationis usually persists until the time of delivery, and it abates within a period of approximately 1 month following delivery. It frequently recurs with subsequent pregnancies, as a consequence of the use of oral contraceptives, and as a consequence of the development of hydatidiform mole or of choriocarcinoma.

Treatment of herpes gestationis depends on its severity and on the severity of the accompanying pruritus. It is not clear whether systemic corticosteroid therapy alters fetal prognosis. If prednisone is used, oral doses of 40–80 mg per day should be given and should be tapered as soon as possible.

Pruritic Urticarial Papules and Plaques of Pregnancy (PUPPP)

This dermatosis was first described in the late 1970s. It is probably the most common pruritic dermatosis of pregnancy and it appears to be harmless to the mother as well as to the fetus. It must be differentiated from early stages of herpes gestationis and from a condition known as papular dermatitis of pregnancy, which will be discussed later.

Although PUPPP seems to be an appropriate name, there is some debate about whether or not other terms might be used, such as polymorphic eruption of pregnancy. There are various other rashes described previously in the literature, such as Bourne's toxemic rash, Besnier's prurigo, and the late onset type of Nurse's prurigo gestationis. It seems that these disorders described in the medical literature under various names are variations of PUPPP.

PUPPP is characterized by urticarial papules and plaques that usually appear first on the trunk and on the proximal extremities (Fig. 43–1). It may spread to involve the entire cutaneous surface. These lesions are intensely pruritic. The lesions can be clinically indistinguishable from those that occur in the early stages of herpes gestationis. They often resemble erythema multiforme. The onset is usually in a primigravid patient late in the third trimester.

The histopathologic findings in PUPPP are non-specific, usually revealing a perivascular lymphocytic infiltrate. Eosinophils, epidermal changes, leukocytoclasis, and edema have been observed in individual patients. Abnormal laboratory findings are not a feature of PUPPP; thus immunologic tests are normal, as are tests for human chorionic gonadotropin and estrogen levels.

The lesions and the pruritus clear rapidly (within a day or two) after delivery. Some patients have had pruritus abate just prior to delivery. Maternal and fetal complications do not occur, although one neonate has been described with urticarial lesions similar to those seen in the mother. Recurrence of PUPPP in subsequent pregnancies is exceedingly rare.

Treatment of PUPPP depends on the se-

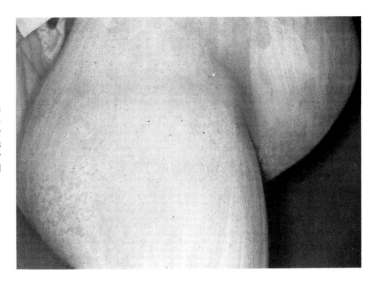

Figure 43–1. Multiple urticarial plaques in a patient with pruritic urticarial papules and plaques of pregnancy (PUPPP). Also, note that the patient has used calamine lotion topically to alter the appearance of these lesions and relieve the itching.

verity of symptoms and should include reassurance about the benign and transient nature of the disease, the use of emollients, and aggressive use of antihistamines. Corticosteroids should be avoided in these patients if at all possible. The use of diphenhydramine HCl has been acceptable to most obstetricians. Doses of these agents are increased to patient tolerance or to disappearance of pruritus.

Spangler's Papular Dermatitis of Pregnancy

In 1962, Spangler and associates described a very rare dermatosis in a group of pregnant patients. Since the initial description, it is not clear whether any other patients with this entity have been described. Spangler reported that 24-hour urinary levels of human chorionic gonadotropin were elevated beyond the limits that were considered normal for that stage of pregnancy. In addition, estriol and cortisol levels were depressed. The histologic and immunologic findings have been non-specific. Spangler believed this to be an allergic disorder and demonstrated a positive intradermal test to material obtained from placental extracts subsequent to delivery. It was believed that fetal mortality was associated with this condition and that corticosteroids were useful in preventing the fetal mortality. It is not known whether or not this condition is an actual entity.

Impetigo Herpetiformis

This rare skin eruption of pregnancy is identical to pustular psoriasis. Impetigo herpetiformis is characterized by sheets of small pustules on an erythematous base, the presence of fever, malaise, and often hypoalbuminemia and hypocalcemia. The pustules in this condition are sterile, although secondary infection can complicate the process. Severe systemic toxicity occurs and can result in death of the mother or fetus. The skin eruption occurs in late pregnancy and may also recur in subsequent pregnancies. Supportive therapy is indicated, as well as the use of systemic corticosteroid therapy.

EFFECTS OF PREGNANCY ON PRE-EXISTING SKIN DISEASES

Pregnancy has variable effects on pre-existing cutaneous disease. Skin diseases that are generally improved by pregnancy include psoriasis, atopic dermatitis, hidradenitis suppurativa, and Fox-Fordyce disease. Those that are generally worsened by pregnancy include pityriasis rosea, condyloma acuminatum, neurofibromatosis, tuberous sclerosis, and most of the collagen-vascular diseases. The effects of pregnancy on acne seem to be variable—some patients report worsening of acne during pregnancy, and others report improvement.

Erythema nodosum deserves special mention because it can be caused by pregnancy.

It also has been related to the use of oral contraceptives. When the disease does occur in a pregnant individual, it often occurs during the second trimester and persists until the time of delivery. The approach to therapy should be conservative, with avoidance of systemic therapy if at all possible.

Candidiasis develops more in pregnant women than in non-pregnant women, possibly because of greater intertriginous surface area, combined with hyperhidrosis, increased estrogen concentrations, and an altered immune response. Adequate hygiene plus topical therapy is usually effective in controlling candidiasis in pregnant women.

Condyloma acuminatum and neonatal herpes simplex infection assume special importance when noticed at the time of delivery. Active herpes simplex infection in the mother may result in the development of neonatal herpes simplex, including neonatal herpetic encephalopathy. It may be necessary for patients with active herpetic infections to have cesarean sections in order to prevent this problem. Mothers who have herpes simplex infection during pregnancy may be at increased risk of developing a disseminated infection, and the fetus may also be at risk. In addition, condyloma acuminatum not only may grow during pregnancy but also can be present in the birth canal. Children delivered to mothers who have had condyloma acuminatum may develop laryngeal papillomas as a manifestation of human papillomavirus infection. In addition, these laryngeal papillomas can be extremely difficult to treat. Thus, a cesarean section should be considered in a mother with condyloma acuminatum present at the time of delivery.

Lupus erythematosus may worsen or improve during pregnancy. In addition, fetal complications in mothers who have anti-Ro (SS-A) antibodies and possibly anti-nRNP (U_1RNP) antibodies may result in infants with neonatal lupus erythematosus (NLE). This syndrome not only may involve cutaneous disease but also may predispose neonates to congenital heart block. The risk of a fetus in a subsequent pregnancy for the development of NLE seems to be approximately 25%. Mothers of neonates with lupus erythematosus syndromes tend to be antibody positive for the Ro (SS-A) antibody. Although 50% of the mothers are asymptomatic, many of these women will eventually develop a connective tissue disease syndrome. Dermatomyositis will usually worsen during pregnancy, and in many patients the disease has occurred for the first time during pregnancy.

DRUG THERAPY FOR CUTANEOUS DISEASE IN PREGNANCY

In general, pregnant women should not be given systemic medications unless other therapy proves inadequate. In addition, it should be realized that topical medications are partially absorbed and should be delivered only when indicated. Certain medications appear to be "safe" during the pregnant state and include diphenhydramine HCl and topical corticosteroids. Use of any medication during pregnancy should be discussed with the patient's obstetrician and pediatrician whenever possible.

Suggested Readings

Callen JP: Pregnancy effects on the skin, common and uncommon changes. Postgrad Med 75:138–145, 1984.

Callen JP, Hanno R: Pruritic urticarial papules and plaques of pregnancy: A clinicopathologic study. J Amer Acad Dermatol 5:401–405, 1981.

Wade TR, Wade SL, Jones HE: Skin changes and diseases associated with pregnancy. Obstet Gynecol 52:233–242, 1978.

Winton GB: Dermatoses of pregnancy. J Assn Milit Dermatol 7:20–27, 1981.

44

Mast Cell Disease

JOHN J. ZONE

Mast cell disease includes a wide spectrum of clinical entities characterized by mast cell infiltration of tissue. The most frequent site of involvement is the skin. Systemic mast cell disease accounts for 10% of mastocytosis, but it usually occurs in conjunction with skin lesions. The hallmarks of cutaneous mast cell lesions are pruritus, swelling, and erythema on stroking of a lesion (Darier's sign). Confirmation of the clinical diagnosis in both cutaneous and systemic disease is made by demonstration in tissue of increased numbers of mast cells with characteristic metachromatic cytoplasmic granules on Giemsa's stain. Extensive disease in the skin or internal organs may produce headache, abdominal pain, diarrhea, flushing, tachycardia, and syncope. These symptoms are believed to be the result of mast cell degranulation with the release of histamine, prostaglandins, and other mediators.

The term "urticaria pigmentosa" refers to mast cell disease of the skin. However, many authors reserve this term for the maculopapular form of cutaneous disease and refer to other forms with specific terms (e.g., solitary mastocytoma).

PATHOGENESIS

Although there is a rapidly enlarging body of knowledge on the physiology of the mast cell, no well-accepted theory on the pathogenesis of mastocytosis syndromes exists. Familial aggregates of urticaria pigmentosa have been reported, but most cases are sporadic with both sexes being affected equally. Specific chemical stimulators of mast cell proliferation have been identified in culture systems of rodent mast cells, where mucosal mast cell growth is T cell dependent and requires interleukin 3. Nerve growth factor may also stimulate mast cell proliferation. However, the role of such growth factors in local tissue proliferation is speculative at this time.

The stimuli for mast cell degranulation in mastocytosis are physical and pharmacologic rather than immunologic in origin. Pressure, heat, and cold stimulate degranulation, as do pharmacologic agents, including aspirin, alcohol, morphine, codeine, quinine, radiographic dyes, and scopolamine.

Systemic and local release of mast cell mediators following activation is believed responsible for most signs and symptoms. The dramatic clinical findings in patients with mastocytosis are believed to be secondary to the production of large quantities of mast cell products rather than to a unique mediator produced by mastocytosis cells. Histamine release is accepted as the cause of local increased vascular permeability and pruritus. However, gastrointestinal symptoms and hypotension are poorly controlled by both H_1 and H_2 blocking agents and are likely related to prostaglandin release (PGD_2) or to the release of other biologically active metabolites of arachidonic acid. These other mediators may well be responsible for symptoms such as tachycardia, flushing, hypotension, nausea, vomiting, and diarrhea. Heparin release is the probable cause of prolonged bleeding at biopsy sites as well as of rare problems with hemorrhage in systemic mastocytosis. Determination of mediators causing specific symptoms is obviously critical to planning rational therapy.

Table 44–1. THE SPECTRUM OF MAST
CELL DISEASE

A. Cutaneous disease (urticaria pigmentosa)
   1. Localized mastocytoma
   2. Generalized
      a. Maculopapular
      b. Telangiectasia macularis eruptiva perstans
      c. Diffuse or erythrodermic
      d. Without clinically obvious skin lesions
B. Systemic disease
   1. Liver, spleen, or bones with or without cutaneous
      lesions
   2. Mast cell leukemia

CLASSIFICATION

A classification of the spectrum of mast cell disease is summarized in Table 44–1. The classification of the conditions demands close examination and biopsy of the skin, as well as a search for potential extracutaneous disease.

Cutaneous Disease

Localized mastocytomas are estimated to represent 10% of all cases of mast cell disease. Lesions are usually solitary, but up to 3 or 4 lesions may be seen. They are indurated plaques that are usually present at birth or that occur in early infancy. They affect both the extremities and the trunk, may occasionally be annular or linear, and range in size from a few millimeters to several centimeters. The color may vary from reddish-brown to yellow, and the surface may be smooth or have an orange peel appearance. Lesions frequently swell or urticate spontaneously, and bullae may develop, especially if the lesions are traumatized. Intense pruritus, flushing, and colic may be associated with urtication. A few mastocytomas in children have progressed to generalized urticaria pigmentosa, but this is rare. Mastocytomas usually resolve spontaneously over the first several years of life.

The maculopapular type of generalized cutaneous mastocytosis consists of multiple, scattered, red-brown, oval macules, papules, and plaques distributed predominantly over the trunk and proximal extremities (Fig. 44–1). Lesions are occasionally present at birth, but they usually develop within the first year of life. The borders are poorly demarcated, and hundreds of lesions may be pres-

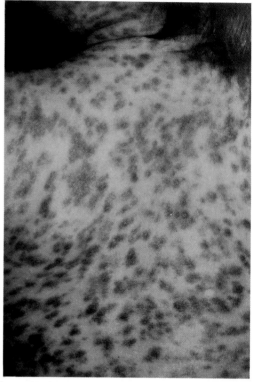

Figure 44–1. Multiple, slightly pigmented lesions of urticaria pigmentosa (mast cell disease).

ent in severe cases. Vesication of individual lesions is common before age 2. There is a rare generalized bullous variant that may be associated with a poorer prognosis. Maculopapular childhood mastocytosis frequently clears by adulthood, or it may persist as asymptomatic, lightly pigmented lesions. The maculopapular type may occur for the first time during adulthood and in such cases is likely to persist indefinitely. The adult form also carries an increased likelihood of attendant systemic symptoms of mastocytosis.

Telangiectasia macularis eruptiva perstans (TMEP) is a rare form of generalized cutaneous mastocytosis that occurs predominantly in adults. The chest and back are involved with numerous hyperpigmented macules that may be nearly confluent. Prominent telangiectasias are associated with the macular lesions. At times, only minimal urtication is elicited on stroking the affected skin.

The diffuse erythrodermic variant of mastocytosis is also very rare. It usually starts in infancy and is characterized by a yellowish pigmentation and a doughy consistency of the skin. Pruritus is intense, and large blisters may develop spontaneously or may follow trauma. Histologically, there is a dense band-like infiltrate of mast cells with a uniform appearance in the dermis. Systemic involvement is the rule in such patients.

Cutaneous mastocytosis has been reported in the absence of clinically apparent skin lesions. This may be a fairly common, previously unrecognized clinical syndrome. More than 90% of these patients present with systemic symptoms that include syncope or severe lightheadedness, flushing, pruritus, palpitations, and tachycardia. Additional symptoms may include abdominal cramps, diarrhea, vomiting, nausea, and severe headaches. Symptoms are accentuated by heat, exercise, and anxiety. A weal and flare response is evoked when normal skin of the chest is stroked. Evanescent erythematous papules are seen in some patients. Biopsy of clinically normal appearing chest skin reveals greater than 10 mast cells per high-powered field (normal is less than 6). When such biopsies are performed, it is best to anesthetize around, but not in, the area to be biopsied to avoid mast cell degranulation in the specimen. The increase in the number of mast cells in the skin is frequently not great, and review by a dermatopathologist skilled in such interpretation is essential. Over two thirds of patients reported to date have had elevated levels of urinary prostaglandin D_2 metabolites between attacks. Dramatic increases were noted when patients were evaluated during attacks. Recognition of this symptom complex warrants skin biopsy and screening for increased urinary prostaglandin metabolites, where such testing is available.

Systemic Disease

Systemic mastocytosis is characterized by infiltration of the bone marrow, liver, spleen, lymph nodes, or gastrointestinal tract with aggregates of mast cells. The central nervous system does not contain mast cells and is not affected in systemic mastocytosis. Systemic symptoms and signs such as flushing, headache, and diarrhea frequently occur in the absence of internal organ involvement and may simply reflect the systemic effects of release of mediators from cutaneous mast cells, rather than being a sign of systemic involvement.

Systemic mastocytosis has been reported in association with all of the cutaneous types of mastocytosis. However, systemic involvement is exceedingly rare in association with solitary mastocytomas, common in TMEP, and the rule in patients with the diffuse erythrodermic form of the disease. Systemic infiltration in the maculopapular variant of urticaria pigmentosa is common (greater than 70%) with adult onset, but it occurs in less than 15% of cases of childhood onset. Most of these patients have limited, asymptomatic systemic involvement. The incidence of detecting systemic involvement is largely related to the intensity of the effort made to detect it. A small percentage of patients with systemic involvement develop widespread and progressive disease.

Webb and colleagues reviewed their experience with 26 patients with systemic mast cell disease. The presenting symptoms ranged from pruritus and flushing to fatigue, weakness, and bone pain. Common physical findings included lymph node enlargement (40%), splenomegaly (50%), hepatomegaly (45%), and skin lesions (56%). Extra-abdominal lymph nodes frequently show mixed cellular involvement, making a definite diagnosis difficult, but splenic involvement is characterized by definite mast cell infiltration. Liver involvement is characterized histopathologically by a portal infiltrate of mononuclear cells that on special staining prove to be mast cells.

Bone involvement is present in 75% of patients with systemic mast cell disease, as evaluated by skeletal survey with conventional roentgenograms. Generalized bone lesions are the rule, although localized involvement may occur. Osteoporosis and osteosclerosis may occur together or separately and are presumably due to focal resorption of bone, with sclerotic areas being caused by reactive new bone formation. Bone infiltration may be responsible for localized musculoskeletal complaints. Bone marrow aspiration typically shows aggregates of mast cells associated with granulocytic hyperplasia and eosinophilia. Examination of the peripheral blood reveals anemia (40%), leukocytosis (30%), thrombocytopenia (20%), eosinophilia (15%), or monocytosis (15%). However, circulating mast cells (4–16%) and basophilia (0–2%) are rare.

Gastrointestinal involvement includes a response to circulating mediators, abdominal pain, malabsorption, and peptic ulcer disease. Actual infiltration of bowel tissue is unusual.

Death from complications of systemic mast cell disease occurs in less than 10% of patients with systemic disease, assuming that malignant transformation does not take place. Most severe complications are related to hematologic problems, including myelofibrosis and pancytopenia.

Mast cell leukemia is a rare manifestation of systemic mast cell disease, and typically it has a rapidly progressive course with a mean survival of 6 months. The diagnosis is suspected when there is a substantial increase in circulating mast cells as seen in the peripheral smear. There is a strong association of mast cell leukemia with peptic ulcer disease, presumably owing to mast cell mediator release. Extensive infiltration of lymph nodes, liver, spleen, and bone marrow with the malignant infiltrate is the rule.

DIFFERENTIAL DIAGNOSIS

The diagnosis of cutaneous mast cell disease hinges upon urtication of skin lesions after stroking (Darier's sign) with subsequent biopsy confirmation. Urticaria pigmentosa lesions may resemble xanthomas, multiple melanocytic nevi, or a drug eruption in color and texture. The other lesions should have a negative Darier's sign. Patients with urticaria and some "normals" may demonstrate weal formation on stroking the skin (dermatographism). The lack of a primary macular or papular lesion in dermatographism is usually evident. Insect bites may also appear as weals or even as bullae and are differentiated on the basis of time course. The diffuse erythrodermic type of mastocytosis can clinically be confused with infiltrative conditions such as histiocytosis X.

Biopsy confirmation is extremely helpful for skin lesions, and it usually resolves any diagnostic questions. The pathologist needs to be instructed to perform specific mast cell staining for granules. Without special stains, mast cells can be confused with fibroblasts, pericytes, and histiocytes.

Histologic confirmation of TMEP and cutaneous mastocytosis without skin lesions may be difficult. Numbers of mast cells are only slightly increased in these disorders. Care should be taken in the biopsy procedure to avoid degranulating mast cells. Specimens need to be interpreted by a dermatopathologist with expertise in this area. It should also be remembered that some inflammatory dermatoses such as lichen simplex chronicus and atopic dermatitis may demonstrate minimal increases in numbers of cutaneous mast cells.

The symptoms of the mastocytosis syndrome are most easily confused with those of carcinoid syndrome. The best way to differentiate the two is obviously by biopsy. If no cutaneous lesions are present, bone marrow aspiration or biopsy of a bone lesion can reveal mast cells. In general, one expects characteristic 24-hour urine findings (e.g., high 5-HIAA) in carcinoid syndrome and elevated histamine levels in mastocytosis. However, on occasion carcinoid syndrome may show elevated urinary histamine concentrations.

PATIENT EVALUATION

A histologically confirmed diagnosis of cutaneous mastocytosis dictates a variable response, depending on the clinical syndrome. Detailed history to detect symptoms of mastocytosis syndrome should be undertaken. Physical examination specifically looking for adenopathy or hepatosplenomegaly should be performed. Disease arising in childhood requires little further evaluation if there are no systemic symptoms or physical findings. A complete blood count provides reassurance as to the benign nature of the disorder. Detailed study would suggest that up to 15% of children with urticaria pigmentosa may have asymptomatic extracutaneous disease. There seems to be little need to search for bone lesions, since it would not change therapy in the absence of symptoms. The majority of patients show gradual resolution through childhood. However, if specific symptoms develop (e.g., bone pain), detailed evaluation of that finding should be undertaken.

Biochemical abnormalities resulting from poorly regulated mast cells are surprisingly difficult to quantify. Elevated excretion of both histamine and PGD_2 has been described. Determination of histamine metabolites in the urine is considerably more specific and sensitive than is the determination of histamine itself. Measurement of PGD_2 and its metabolites may also show marked elevations, especially during attacks. The reliability of such testing is very dependent on the expertise of the specific clinical laboratory. If values are minimally elevated, repeat evaluation should be undertaken.

There is an eight-fold greater incidence of systemic mast cell disease developing in an adult with urticaria pigmentosa than in a child. Detailed history, physical examination, complete blood count, and chemistry profile are appropriate in adults. The presence of hepatosplenomegaly or adenopathy should prompt detailed evaluation for systemic mast cell disease. The finding of anemia, leukopenia, or thrombocytopenia should prompt bone marrow biopsy with concern that mast cell infiltration may be the cause. Radiologic skeletal survey is likely to aid in the diagnosis of systemic mast cell disease. The results of this evaluation are of importance because they rule out other, more severe causes of clinical findings, particularly reticuloendothelial malignancy.

Malignant mastocytosis is known to develop in some cases of urticaria pigmentosa. Unfortunately, we cannot predict which patients will be affected. Patients and families can be reassured that development of malignant mastocytosis is rare, especially with the childhood variety.

TREATMENT

There is no consistently effective therapy to eradicate the benign proliferation of mast cells. Symptoms can be minimized by avoidance of known precipitating factors, such as heat, rubbing, and heavy exercise, and by mast cell releasing drugs, including nonsteroidal anti-inflammatory drugs, salicylates, and narcotics. Although the symptoms of mastocytosis have traditionally been attributed to the release of histamine, antihistamine therapy has generally not been found to ameliorate the systemic symptoms, especially not the hypotension and flushing. The combination of H_1 and H_2 blockers may improve symptoms further, but it seems likely that many of the systemic symptoms are related to overproduction of the potent vasodilator PGD_2.

Oral disodium cromoglycate has been given to patients with systemic mastocytosis with good response of wealing, flushing, diarrhea, and abdominal pain. Cromolyn prevents release of mediator from mast cells and represents a low risk basic therapy for symptoms. Unfortunately, the drug is poorly absorbed and is quite expensive. TMEP has been reported to be quite resistant to treatment, although no detailed studies have been performed.

There is little information on the symptomatic relief of generalized mastocytosis without clinically obvious skin lesions. High dose salicylate (3.9–5.2 gm per day) has been tried and has been successful in some patients.

Local treatment may improve symptoms in lesions limited to the skin. Psoralen and ultraviolet A light (PUVA) therapy has been somewhat successful in the treatment of generalized cutaneous disease. Injection of lesions with 0.25 ml of triamcinolone acetonide 40 mg per ml produces involution of individual lesions. Similar results have been obtained using 0.05% betamethasone dipropionate under occlusion. If an individual cutaneous lesion is of of excessive concern, it can be excised.

Suggested Readings

Barton J, Lavker RM, Schechter NM, Lazarus GS: Treatment of urticaria pigmentosa with corticosteroids. Arch Dermatol 121:1516–1523, 1985.
Caplan MR: The natural course of urticaria pigmentosa. Arch Dermatol 87:146–157, 1963.
DiBacco RS, DeLeo VA: Mastocytosis and the mast cell. J Am Acad Dermatol 7:709–722, 1982.
Kendall ME, Fields JP, King LE: Cutaneous mastocytosis without clinically obvious skin lesions. J Am Acad Dermatol 10:903–904, 1984.
Klaus SN, Winkelmann RK: The clinical spectrum of urticaria pigmentosa. Mayo Clinic Proc 40:923–931, 1965.
Olafsson JH: Cutaneous and systemic mastocytosis in adults. Acta Derm Venereol Suppl 115:1–43, 1985.
Roberts LJ, Fields JP, Oates JA: Mastocytosis without urticaria pigmentosa: A frequently unrecognized cause of recurrent syncope. Trans Assoc Am Physicians 95:36–45, 1982.
Travis WD, Li CY, Hoagland HC, Travis LB, Banks PM: Mast cell leukemia: Report of a case and review of the literature. Mayo Clinic Proc 61:957–966, 1986.
Webb TA, Li CY, Yam LT: Systemic mast cell disease: A clinical and hematopathologic study of 26 cases. Cancer 49:927–938, 1982.

45

Bullous Diseases

JOHN J. ZONE

Bullous diseases of the skin represent a systemic problem because of their potential severity with extensive mucocutaneous involvement and the potential for secondary infection and/or fluid loss. In addition, these diseases are associated with a variety of systemic disorders both directly and indirectly. They demand immediate diagnosis and therapy.

PEMPHIGUS

Pemphigus is characterized by intraepidermal acantholytic vesicles and bullae involving stratified squamous epithelium of both cutaneous and mucosal surfaces. Affected skin in pemphigus vulgaris reveals flaccid blisters that generally develop on non-inflamed skin; are readily broken; and progress to large, weeping, denuded areas (Fig. 45–1). Oropharyngeal erosions are common and may be the presenting sign. Superficial pemphigus (pemphigus foliaceus) may be idiopathic or may be endemic to certain areas of Brazil (fogo selvagem). Both forms of the disease are characterized by deposition of IgG antibody, which reacts with epidermal cell surface antigen and stimulates acantholysis.

Pathogenesis

The pathogenetic process in pemphigus is that of an organ-specific autoimmune disease. Perilesional skin and frequently serum demonstrate the presence of an IgG class autoantibody directed against a cell surface antigen of squamous epithelium. Why pemphigus patients become intolerant of this antigen is uncertain.

Several lines of evidence support the hypothesis that the pemphigus antibody is responsible for the acantholysis. Pemphigus antibody produces acantholysis when added to normal human skin in organ culture and results in detachment when added to epidermal cell cultures. Further convincing evidence of the pathogenetic role of pemphigus antibody has been provided by the demonstration that IgG fractions purified from the serum of patients with pemphigus can induce a disease in neonatal mice that reproduces the clinical, histologic, and immunologic features of human pemphigus.

It is believed that the pemphigus antibody subsequently stimulates the release of plasminogen activator. It has been proposed that the activation of plasminogen to plasmin by plasminogen activator may then actually be responsible for the loss of epidermal cell attachment. Although this in vitro phenomenon can occur in the absence of complement, the presence of complement accentuates the pemphigus antibody–mediated cell detachment and provides a mechanism for loss of epidermal cell cohesion in addition to the plasminogen-plasmin system.

Although the stimulus for pemphigus antibody formation is unknown, the endemic nature of pemphigus foliaceus in Brazil suggests the involvement of an infectious agent. Most of the cases in Brazil occur in the population residing near rivers, and an insect vector for a microorganism has been proposed. Whether pemphigus in other geographic areas is precipitated by similar events is unknown. D-Penicillamine may produce pemphigus (predominantly pem-

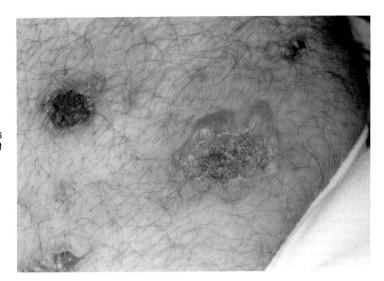

Figure 45–1. Vesicular and bullous lesions with slight erosions in a patient with pemphigus vulgaris.

phigus foliaceus) in patients being treated for rheumatoid arthritis, Wilson's disease, scleroderma, or other penicillamine responsive disorders. Consequently, it is likely that a variety of stimuli may give rise to epidermal antigen intolerance.

The disease has been described in all races and ethnic groups but is more common in persons of Jewish descent and in those people having the HLA-A10 genotype. The biologic role of this genetic predisposition is unknown.

Classification

There are 2 histopathologically distinct forms of pemphigus. Pemphigus vulgaris is characterized histopathologically by a suprabasilar cleft formation, and pemphigus foliaceus is distinguished by blister formation within or just beneath the granular layer. Both types show reduced cohesion and detachment of epidermal cells (acantholysis). In pemphigus vulgaris and, to a lesser extent, pemphigus foliaceus the blister may extend into surrounding non-blistered skin by applying shearing pressure to perilesional tissue (Nikolsky's sign).

Pemphigus vulgaris is the most common form of pemphigus and is generally seen in the fourth or fifth decade of life. It has, however, been described both in children and in the elderly. Prior to the use of corticosteroids, 50% of patients with the disease

died within the first 12 months, most frequently from cachexia, sepsis, and/or electrolyte imbalance, which were secondary phenomena.

Pemphigus vegetans is a rare variant of pemphigus vulgaris. Proliferative and verrucous lesions with surrounding pustules gradually develop from denuded bullae on intertriginous cutaneous surfaces. Such lesions were more common in the era before the development and use of corticosteroids and may represent a partial response of the host to the blistering process. Histopathologically one sees epidermal proliferation with hyperkeratosis, papillomatosis, and frequently intraepidermal abscess formation containing eosinophils.

Pemphigus foliaceus is generally less severe than pemphigus vulgaris. The superficial blisters rupture easily, producing shallow erosions and crusting. Lesions occur on the chest, back, and scalp and may produce a seborrhea-like scaling. Clinical blistering may be totally absent. The disease remains localized for long periods of time but occasionally may disseminate.

Fogo selvagem is endemic to Brazil. It occurs in children and young adults and is characterized by desquamation, erythroderma, and an intense burning. Histopathologically and immunopathologically, it is indistinguishable from pemphigus foliaceus.

Pemphigus erythematosus (Senear-Usher syndrome) represents a localized variant of pemphigus foliaceus characterized by erythematous lupus-like malar dermatitis. Patients frequently manifest an abnormal antinuclear antibody test as well as the presence of pemphigus antibody. Direct immunofluorescence microscopy may show immunoglobulin and complement components along the basement membrane as well as characteristic pemphigus antibody deposition. This disorder is believed to represent the coexistence of lupus erythematosus and pemphigus foliaceus.

Penicillamine therapy has been associated with a variety of autoimmune disorders, including pemphigus vulgaris and pemphigus foliaceus. Pemphigus foliaceus accounts for 70% of the penicillamine-induced cases, and pemphigus vulgaris composes the remainder. The development of pemphigus may occur with a wide range of dosage and is often a late complication of therapy. After discontinuation of penicillamine therapy, approximately half of the patients have their disease resolve in 4 months, whereas the other half require suppressive corticosteroid therapy over a longer period of time.

Pemphigus has occurred in association with thymoma and myasthenia gravis. The types of pemphigus include pemphigus vulgaris, pemphigus foliaceus, and pemphigus erythematosus. There is little, if any, association between the clinical activities of the coexistent disorders. The concurrence is believed to involve an underlying failure of thymic-dependent lymphocytes in suppressing autoimmune disease.

Patients with pemphigus have had associated solid tumors as well as reticuloendothelial malignancy. The tumor types as well as the types of associated pemphigus are variable. In only 1 case has a parallel course been noted with resolution of the pemphigus when the tumor was removed. Consequently, although weak association with malignancy has been described with pemphigus, it is not worthwhile to search for malignancy in the absence of other clinical signs.

Other sporadic and poorly understood associations with pemphigus include those with pernicious anemia, red blood cell aplasia, rheumatoid arthritis, and lymphomatoid granulomatosis.

Differential Diagnosis

The differential diagnosis of blistering disorders of the skin ranges from a wide variety

Table 45–1. BLISTERING DERMATOSES

1. Subcorneal vesicles
   a. Bullous impetigo
   b. Staphylococcal scalded skin syndrome
   c. Miliaria
   d. Subcorneal pustular dermatosis
2. Spongiotic blisters
   a. Eczematous disorders, including allergic contact dermatitis, stasis dermatitis, irritant dermatitis, fungal dermatitis, etc.
   b. Incontinentia pigmenti
3. Ballooning degeneration of epidermal cells
   a. Herpes simplex
   b. Herpes zoster and varicella zoster

of banal dermatoses to more serious and progressive disorders such as pemphigus, bullous pemphigoid, and epidermolysis bullosa acquisita. These disorders require clinical, histopathologic, and immunopathologic evaluation for definite diagnosis. When the etiology of blistering disorders cannot be recognized, biopsy is warranted. Subsequent decisions are made on the basis of these findings. Histopathologic characteristics of potential blistering disorders that will not be discussed here in detail are listed in Table 45–1.

Acantholysis is the hallmark of immunologically mediated pemphigus, but it may also be seen in transient acantholytic dermatosis, Darier's disease, and familial benign pemphigus. In transient acantholytic dermatosis, there is involvement of the trunk with pruritic papulovesicles. It is frequently precipitated by sun exposure or heat and lasts for weeks to months, although some chronic cases have been described.

Darier's disease (keratosis follicularis) is an autosomal dominant disorder characterized by yellowish-brown, crusted papules on the scalp, intertriginous areas, and seborrheic areas of the face and trunk. The disease is slowly progressive and seldom is overtly bullous. Lesions are frequently perifollicular. Although acantholysis is suprabasilar, as in pemphigus vulgaris, characteristic dyskeratotic changes (corps ronds and grains) occur within the epidermis.

Familial benign pemphigus (Hailey-Hailey disease) is an autosomal dominant disorder characterized by multiple grouped erythematous vesicles in intertriginous areas. Mucosal surfaces are usually spared. There is extensive loss of intercellular bridges with partial coherence of cells.

The clinical pattern of these acantholytic disorders is usually distinctive from that of pemphigus. If confusion exists, direct immunofluorescence of perilesional skin is negative for IgG deposition in these disorders, whereas pemphigus patients demonstrate characteristic IgG deposition.

Patient Evaluation

Close examination of all mucous membranes is indicated. Oral involvement is the rule. Esophageal involvement as well as vulvar involvement may occur. Significant esophageal symptoms may occur, and stricture may develop. Consequently, esophageal symptoms mandate endoscopy and possible biopsy. Patients presenting with blistering skin disorders that cannot be easily explained (e.g., friction blisters and contact dermatoses) require biopsy. If there is histopathologic acantholysis, biopsy of perilesional skin for direct immunofluorescence should be performed. Deposition of intercellular IgG confirms the diagnosis of pemphigus. Indirect immunofluorescence microscopy demonstrating pemphigus antibodies in the serum further confirms the diagnosis and may be valuable in therapy because changes in antibody titer in a patient usually correlate with disease activity. Disappearance of antibody from the serum frequently precedes remission.

Chest x-ray to rule out an associated thymoma and a search for clinical symptoms of myasthenia gravis are part of good clinical care, but low yield of positive findings is to be expected. Culture of potentially infected lesions and close attention to protein loss and malnutrition are necessary in severe cases. Chest x-ray, tuberculosis skin test, CBC, and blood glucose determination should be undertaken prior to initiating corticosteroid or immunosuppressive therapy.

Treatment

Initial therapy of pemphigus involves complete suppression of blistering with oral prednisone (usually 60–80 mg daily). Corticosteroids are then continued in sufficient doses to suppress blistering until serum antibody titers become negative, at which time tapering of therapy should be attempted. Because therapy may need to be continued for years, corticosteroid side-effects become a major clinical problem. Corticosteroid

sparing may be accomplished by the addition of an immunosuppressive agent. Systemic methotrexate (oral, intravenous, or intramuscular) can be used in dosages of 30–50 mg per week, but may aggravate oral ulcers. Cyclophosphamide is effective in oral dosages of 75–150 mg/kg/day, and oral azathioprine may be used in dosages of 1–3 mg/kg/day. Close attention should be paid to a variety of potential side-effects, including leukopenia, liver damage, teratogenesis, sterility, oral ulcers, and cystitis, depending on the specific agent used. Gold therapy has been shown to be effective in the treatment of pemphigus vulgaris, probably on the basis of an immunosuppressive effect. Weekly doses of intramuscular gold (25–50 mg) are given, and total dosages greater than 1000 mg are frequently necessary before there is a significant therapeutic effect. After initial control, the weekly doses can be gradually decreased and eventually stopped, depending on disease activity. Major side-effects include dermatitis, glomerulonephritis, and bone marrow suppression.

Plasmapheresis may be useful in patients poorly controlled on conventional therapy. Six-liter exchanges on 3 separate occasions over a 3-week period are necessary to lower the antibody titer significantly. Corticosteroids and/or immunosuppressives are then necessary to maintain the improvement.

BULLOUS PEMPHIGOID

Bullous pemphigoid (BP) is a cutaneous disorder characterized by subepidermal vesicles and bullae. The blisters are tense and, unlike the lesions of pemphigus vulgaris, do not rupture easily and rarely produce large areas of denuded skin (Fig. 45–2). Oropharyngeal lesions occur commonly, and the disorder may frequently be limited to mucosal surfaces (mucous membrane pemphigoid). Cutaneous blisters generally arise from erythematous or urticarial plaques. BP is generally a self-limited disease, and in contrast to pemphigus vulgaris the mortality is low even in the absence of corticosteroid therapy. However, BP is a potentially serious disease because it occurs in older individuals whose compromised status predisposes them to infection and complications of corticosteroid therapy. BP is characterized by the deposition of IgG antibody that reacts with basement membrane antigen in the

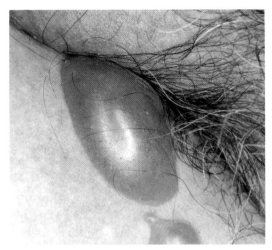

Figure 45–2. Tense blister formation on a slightly erythematous base in an intertriginous location, representative of bullous pemphigoid.

lamina lucida. This antibody then presumably stimulates loss of dermal-epidermal adherence.

Pathogenesis

Although the specific mechanism responsible for blister formation is unknown, there is good evidence that IgG anti–basement membrane antibody and complement are pivotal. Perilesional skin and frequently serum demonstrate the presence of IgG autoantibody directed against an antigen present in the lamina lucida. BP antigen is a 220,000 dalton glycoprotein that is secreted by basal cells into the area of the basement membrane, where it then becomes available for reaction with autoantibody. The BP antigen is a normal component of the basement membrane zone, but, as is the case in pemphigus, patients become intolerant to this antigen for unknown reasons.

It is believed that BP antibody is the primary cause of inflammation and eventual blister formation. The antibody is deposited at the site of separation in the lamina lucida. Intracorneal injection of BP antibody in rabbits has produced histologic separation of the epithelium. Immunofluorescent studies show that the BP antibody binds to the basement membrane zone in such cases. Superficial injection of BP serum in guinea pigs has produced dermal inflammation and blistering in some instances. However, multiple other attempts at demonstrating the

pathogenicity of the BP antibody by passive transfer experiments have been unsuccessful. In general, it is believed that BP antibody is responsible for the initiation of inflammation, although the supporting evidence is much weaker than is the case in pemphigus.

Current wisdom suggests a role for complement in the pathogenesis of BP lesions. Complement deposits have been detected in the lamina lucida, and BP antibody has been shown to activate complement in vitro. Gammon and coworkers have shown that formation of antigen-antibody complexes in the basement membrane zone leads to the adherence of leukocytes to the basement membrane zone in vitro. The stimulus for leukocyte attachment is activated complement components released by immune complex activation. Subsequent release of inflammatory mediators, including proteases and reactive oxygen intermediates, is then believed to be responsible for the separation.

Isolated reports have indicated that patients with BP may develop further blistering on exposure to ultraviolet light. The mechanism for this enhancement of blistering is unknown.

Classification

The term BP is generally reserved for patients demonstrating a chronic, vesiculobullous eruption involving at least to some extent non-mucosal surfaces. Some patients' biopsy specimens demonstrate a heavy inflammatory infiltrate around dermal blood vessels with an admixture of neutrophils, eosinophils, and mononuclear cells. The prominence of the eosinophil infiltration serves to differentiate this disorder from dermatitis herpetiformis histopathologically. The second histopathologic type is characterized by a sparse inflammatory infiltrate of mononuclear cells around superficial dermal blood vessels in the presence of prominent vesiculation in the basement membrane zone. BP has been described in pre-pubertal children, but it is most common in the sixth and seventh decades of life. In the precorticosteroid era, many cases resolved without treatment, although occasional patients developed aggressive and severe disease.

Many clinical variants of BP exist that fulfill the histopathologic and immunopathologic criteria for bullous pemphigoid. The most common is the generalized form with tense vesicles and bullae present in flexural areas. Localized variants include the Brunsting-Perry type of pemphigoid, benign mucous membrane pemphigoid (cicatricial pemphigoid), and a localized pre-tibial type of pemphigoid. The pathogenesis of these conditions is believed to be similar to that of BP, although the reason for localized disease and scarring is poorly understood.

In the Brunsting-Perry variant, scarring and blister formation occur on the head and neck with concomitant oral involvement. Benign mucous membrane pemphigoid is characterized by oral and eye lesions, although other mucous membranes may also be involved. Prominent secondary scarring occurs in a high percentage of cases. Eye involvement may result in conjunctival synechiae with obliteration of the conjunctival sulcus. Subsequent scarring of the cornea may produce blindness, making the disorder far from benign. Direct immunofluorescence microscopy of perilesional tissue reveals anti–basement membrane zone antibody in approximately 80% of the cases. However, indirect immunofluorescence studies reveal circulating anti–basement membrane zone antibodies in only about 10% of cicatricial pemphigoid patients.

An occasional patient demonstrates tense bullae limited to the pre-tibial area. Such cases are immunopathologically and histologically identical to BP, and no definite reason for the localized nature has been established. It has been suggested that a BP antigen may be distributed regionally, accounting for specific distributions.

There have been numerous case reports suggesting an association between BP and internal malignancy. However, rarely has concurrent onset or parallel course been documented. Ahmed and coworkers, as well as Stone and Schroeter, were able to find no increased rate of malignancy in their BP patients. Thus, BP is best considered not to be a cutaneous marker of internal malignancy.

BP has been reported in association with a wide variety of other autoimmune disorders, including lupus erythematosus, pernicious anemia, thyroiditis, polymyositis, and rheumatoid arthritis. Of these associations, the association with rheumatoid arthritis is especially strong, and it has been suggested that both exist because of a similar pathogenetic mechanism.

Differential Diagnosis

The initial diagnostic approach to blistering disorders is reviewed under the differential diagnosis of pemphigus. If biopsy confirms that the blister is subepidermal, direct immunofluorescence microscopy of perilesional tissue is indicated. BP characteristically demonstrates linear deposition of IgG along the basement membrane. Some cases of mucous membrane pemphigoid have also been described as having IgA along the basement membrane.

Dermatitis herpetiformis is differentiated by its clinical appearance (see later discussion), as well as by the characteristic deposition of granular IgA in perilesional tissue. Linear IgA disease (IgA bullous pemphigoid) shows characteristic deposition of IgA along the basement membrane as the predominant and usually the only immunoglobulin. This is an important differentiation, because linear IgA disease is sensitive to sulfone therapy.

Erythema multiforme may also show a subepidermal blister. Characteristic involvement of the palms and soles with target lesions (minor type) or involvement of mucous membranes and skin (major type) in an acute fashion is characteristic of erythema multiforme. Biopsy of erythema multiforme reveals individually necrotic keratinocytes, and direct immunofluorescence fails to reveal anti–basement membrane zone antibody. Occasional patients with erythema multiforme may have immunoglobulins in superficial dermal blood vessels.

Bullous lupus erythematosus usually occurs in patients who fulfill the American Rheumatism Association (ARA) criteria for systemic lupus erythematosus. In addition, the disorder shows granular deposition of immunoglobulin along the basement membrane zone. Such deposition may be sufficiently intense to give a band-like pattern that can be confused with BP. However, patients with bullous lupus erythematosus histopathologically demonstrate a neutrophilic infiltrate similar to that of dermatitis herpetiformis.

Bullous forms of lichen planus exist that are distinguished by an intense mononuclear infiltrate adjacent to the basement membrane zone, absence of anti–basement membrane zone antibodies, and characteristic epidermal changes of lichen planus, which allow differentiation.

Epidermolysis bullosa of the junctional and dystrophic types may show a blister at the dermal-epidermal junction. Such cases are characterized by onset of blistering early in childhood, absence of the inflammatory infiltrate, and negative direct immunofluorescence. The scarring, progressive nature of these disorders is easily distinguishable clinically.

Porphyria cutanea tarda also shows subepidermal blistering, which occurs in sun-exposed areas. Histologically, the dermal papillae irregularly extend into the floor of the bulla cavity, and direct immunofluorescence microscopy is negative. Epidermolysis bullosa acquisita is discussed in detail in a following discussion.

The mucous membrane lesions of benign mucous membrane pemphigoid must be differentiated from those of oral lichen planus, erythema multiforme, aphthous stomatitis, Behçet's syndrome, and pemphigus. The differentiation from oral lichen planus and erythema multiforme can usually be made histopathologically. Aphthous stomatitis lesions tend to be small and punched-out. Bechçet's syndrome need only be considered if other components of the syndrome, including genital ulceration, pustular dermatosis, and iritis, are present. None of these disorders demonstrate anti-–basement membrane zone antibodies.

Patient Evaluation

Close examination of all mucosal and cutaneous surfaces is necessary. Esophageal involvement may produce stricture, and patients with esophageal complaints should be considered for endoscopy and possible biopsy. In the presence of symptoms and/or signs found by the general physical examination that suggest the possibility of internal malignancy, evaluation of those findings should be undertaken. However, no detailed evaluation to rule out the possibility of malignancy is otherwise necessary. Bacterial culture of potentially infected lesions is necessary. Evaluation of the patient's general status, including CBC, chemistry profile, and urinalysis, is advisable because many of the patients will have associated complicating clinical problems attendant with their age. Chest x-ray and tuberculosis skin testing should be undertaken prior to starting corticosteroid and/or immunosuppressive therapy.

Several studies have attempted to correlate the titers of BP antibody with disease activity. The data suggest that a close correlation does not exist in most patients. However, the disappearance of antibody from the serum usually heralds the onset of spontaneous remission; consequently, periodic evaluation of BP antibody titer (every 3–6 months) is of value. Rarely, in some patients the antibody titer may correlate very well with disease activity.

Treatment

The majority of patients with BP have a complete clinical remission following effective therapy. The mainstay of therapy for BP is parenteral corticosteroids. Oral prednisone, 40–60 mg daily, is generally adequate for initial treatment and may be the only treatment necessary. With this agent, individual blisters resolve generally within a 2–3 week period and new blister formation ceases. A major complication of treatment is related to corticosteroid side-effects, including increased susceptibility to infection, potential gastrointestinal bleeding, onset of diabetes mellitus, and possible development of psychiatric abnormalities. These problems may well be severe, in view of the elderly age group afflicted. Consequently, close attention to complications is necessary.

Azathioprine, 1–3 mg/kg/day, is an especially effective agent when used to spare corticosteroid dosage in patients with BP. The onset of effect is slow; thus, after 4–6 weeks of treatment with azathioprine, corticosteroid doses can be gradually tapered. Cyclophosphamide is effective and may be used in severe cases in the manner described for pemphigus.

Mucous membrane pemphigoid, if localized, may be treated with topical corticosteroid preparations, but it usually requires systemic corticosteroid therapy. Dapsone may be helpful in controlling the oral lesions, but it is often ineffective in preventing progressive ocular disease. Therapy with dapsone should be given in doses similar to those described for dermatitis herpetiformis. Eye involvement in cicatricial pemphigoid is particularly serious and warrants aggressive therapy. If initial response to oral corticosteroid therapy is not forthcoming, aggressive treatment with cyclophosphamide is indicated. However, ophthalmic involvement may be resistant to all therapies.

Localized BP of the extremities as well as some mucosal disease may be successfully treated with intradermal injection of small amounts of triamcinolone acetonide (2.5 mg per ml) used in combination with potent topical corticosteroids.

EPIDERMOLYSIS BULLOSA ACQUISITA

Epidermolysis bullosa acquisita (EBA) is an acquired bullous disease distinguished by involvement of extensor surfaces with blisters that characteristically heal with scarring by formation of milia, and by the history of traumatic induction of the blisters (Fig. 45–3). The blisters are formed by separations below the basement membrane. Immunoglobulin and complement deposition is present in a linear pattern along the basement membrane zone as seen on direct immunofluorescence microscopy, and circulating IgG anti–basement membrane zone antibody is frequently present. However, serologic studies demonstrate that this anti–basement membrane zone antibody reacts with antigens distinct from the bullous pemphigoid (BP) antigen.

Pathogenesis

Because immunoglobulin and complement deposits are found at the basement membrane zone and some patients have circulating basement membrane zone antibodies, it is likely that this disorder has an immunopathogenesis similar to that of BP. However, the immune deposits of EBA are localized to the sub–lamina densa area. Woodley and colleagues have identified a basement membrane zone protein that serves as an antigen for the autoantibodies in this disorder. This antigen consists of 290,000 and 145,000 dalton components. Studies of basement membrane zone extracts reveal this antigen to be distinct from the BP antigen. What kind of effect this unique antigen has on subsequent immunopathogenesis is unknown.

Classification

EBA is a sharply defined entity on the basis of its immunopathologic findings. However, there appear to be a spectrum of clinical and histopathologic manifestations of EBA. The classic clinical and histopathologic presentation of EBA closely resembles that of porphyria cutanea tarda, but the patients have normal uroporphyrins. Specifically, blisters arise on a non-inflammatory base over the extensor surfaces and heal with the formation of milia. However, an inflammatory variant that closely mimics BP or drug-induced bullous erythema multiforme also occurs. The histopathology of this inflammatory variant consists of a marked inflammatory infiltrate of the upper dermis with neutrophils. This inflammatory variant is frequently associated with nail dystrophy.

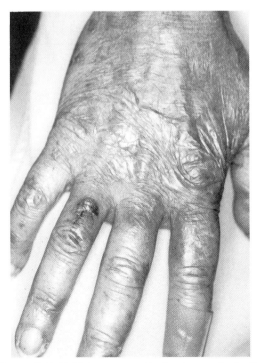

Figure 45–3. Multiple scars and bullae in a patient with epidermolysis bullosa acquisita. Note the similarity to porphyria cutanea tarda.

Differential Diagnosis

The differential diagnosis of subepidermal blistering disease is described under BP. Differentiation of EBA from other forms of epidermolysis bullosa includes the adult onset, as well as a negative family history of EBA. Differentiation from BP on the basis of direct immunofluorescence alone may be impossible; however, immunoelectron microscopy will reveal the deposition of immunoglobulin below the lamina densa.

Separation of epidermis from dermis using heat and saline produces a separation in the lamina lucida. Indirect immunofluorescence of EBA sera with this substrate will reveal antibody that adheres to the roof of the induced separation in cases of BP. The circulating antibody of EBA will adhere to the base of such induced separations.

Patient Evaluation

The evaluation of patients with EBA is essentially the same as that for patients with BP. Correlation of antibody titer with disease activity has not been well evaluated.

Treatment

Therapy of EBA is essentially that of BP. However, this disorder is more resistant to treatment with systemic corticosteroids and may well require aggressive therapy with immunosuppressives. The efficacy of plasmapheresis or gold therapy in this disorder has not been established.

DERMATITIS HERPETIFORMIS

Dermatitis herpetiformis (DH) is characterized by involvement of extensor surfaces with grouped, erythematous papulovesicles (Fig. 45–4). Biopsy demonstrates a blister at the basement membrane with accumulation of neutrophils in the dermal papillary tips. Perilesional skin demonstrates the pathognomonic deposition of granular IgA in dermal papillary tips.

Greater than 90% of patients with DH have the HLA-B8DR3 genotype, compared with 20% of controls. This offers a unique background on which gluten sensitivity and the subsequent IgA immune response develop. The circulating antibody responsible for the deposition of IgA in skin has not yet been identified, and indirect immunofluorescence studies are predominantly negative. The skin disease as well as the associated gluten sensitive enteropathy improves with dietary restriction of gluten.

Pathogenesis

The details of the associated gluten sensitive enteropathy of DH are discussed in Chapter 28. Two main hypotheses on the immunopathogenesis of DH exist. The first involves an immune response to gluten; the second involves gluten sensitive enteropathy as a "sieve."

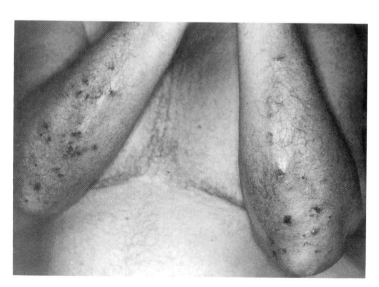

Figure 45–4. Multiple excoriated lesions and vesicles in a symmetrical distribution with some suggestion of grouping in a patient with dermatitis herpetiformis.

It has been proposed that gluten sensitive enteropathy represents a localized immune response to gluten. The gluten antigen could then induce antibodies to gluten, which travel to skin either dissociated or in the immune complex form. In the skin, the IgA antibody presumably would bind to an as yet unidentified antigen and then activate the inflammation via complement activation. Subsequent influx of neutrophils and release of elastase and other proteases could then produce blisters. Supporting this hypothesis is the fact that anti-gluten antibodies of IgA class have been identified in 20–50% of patients. Likewise, IgA containing circulating immune complexes have been identified in the circulation of 20–40% of patients. However, they are not present at all in some cases. Studies of IgA immune complex levels following ingestion of gluten have given inconsistent results, making this mechanism questionable. Further characterization of the IgA antibody in the skin awaits isolation of the IgA antibody in sufficient quantities to allow evaluation of its antigenicity. There have been no successful studies of inducing DH lesions in animals by passive transfer.

The "sieve" theory of immunopathogenesis would suggest that the role of gluten is to produce a defective mucosal barrier. Foreign proteins not necessarily related to gluten could then enter the circulation and produce an IgA immune response that then travels to the skin and produces inflammation. This theory has not been investigated in detail to date, but it is supported somewhat by studies conducted by Zeedijk and colleagues, who have produced total clearing of DH with an elemental diet.

Clinical Features

The term DH has come to be reserved for patients with characteristic granular IgA deposition in perilesional skin. The main clinical differentiation is with "linear IgA disease."

Linear IgA disease has 2 distinct clinical morphologies. The first that occurs in approximately one half of patients is involvement of the elbows, knees, and buttocks with characteristic grouped papulovesicles that are indistinguishable from those of granular IgA disease. The histopathologic appearance is nearly identical, but immunopathology shows linear deposition of IgA along the basement membrane in a pattern similar to that of bullous pemphigoid (BP). This disorder has been separated from DH because of studies that indicate that the HLA-B8DR3 genotype is present in a smaller percentage of cases (greater than 90% of granular IgA patients, 30–40% of linear IgA patients, and 20% of normal controls). In addition, gluten sensitive enteropathy has been noted on small bowel biopsy in only about 20% of patients, compared with greater than 85% of patients with granular IgA disease. Response of linear IgA disease to gluten free diet therapy has not been studied. The second clinical presentation is that of multiple, scattered vesicles and bullae in a morphology similar to that of BP. This morphology has given rise to the term "IgA bullous pemphigoid," but most authorities now refer to this disorder as linear IgA disease. The differentiation is important, because the treatment of choice in linear IgA disease is dapsone rather than systemic corticosteroids and immunosuppression, as is used in BP.

Thyroid disorders have been reported in multiple cases of DH. These disorders include hyperthyroidism, hypothyroidism, thyroid nodules, and asymptomatic goiter. Thyroid microsomal antibodies are seen in 40% of patients with DH. The abnormal findings are especially prominent in females, and some thyroid abnormality may occur in as many as 50% of female DH patients. It appears that this abnormality is associated with the HLA-B8DR3 genotype rather than with a specific mechanism in which DH stimulates thyroid disease or vice versa.

Lymphoma is known to occur with increased prevalence in patients with gluten sensitive enteropathy. There are multiple case reports of abdominal lymphoma in patients with DH. The only controlled study of this phenomenon was performed by Leonard and suggested a slight increase in the incidence of lymphoma (4%) in patients with DH. It was suggested that this incidence may be decreased by a gluten free diet, although there are insufficient data to support this conclusion at the present time. An extremely large study would be necessary to evaluate the statistical validity of the association between DH and lymphoma. Consequently, it is best to assume at this time that the incidence is approximately that of celiac disease, and appropriate evaluation should be performed if signs of lymphoma develop.

Differential Diagnosis

The differential diagnoses are that of subepidermal blistering disease, reviewed under the heading of bullous pemphigoid. Direct immunofluorescence is essential to differentiate between linear IgA disease and granular IgA disease.

Patient Evaluation

Close clinical examination for thyroid nodules and thyromegaly is indicated as a baseline and at return visits. Detailed history of bowel symptoms, including bloating after eating, recurrent abdominal pain, diarrhea, and steatorrhea, is frequently revealing. Patients who do not have obvious signs of gluten sensitive enteropathy may frequently note improvement in these minimal symptoms when gluten free diet therapy is instituted.

A CBC, chemistry profile, and urinalysis are indicated as baseline studies in all patients with DH. This approach not only screens for the malabsorption problems discussed previously, but also represents a baseline for subsequent abnormalities that may be induced by dapsone therapy. We routinely determine serum thyroxine levels as a baseline in view of the high incidence of thyroid abnormalities. Glucose-6-phosphate dehydrogenase levels should be checked as a baseline in patients who are black or of Southern Mediterranean origin, since catastrophic hemolysis may result in deficiency states.

Treatment

Dapsone is the drug of choice in the therapy of DH. Treatment with dapsone will adequately suppress (but not cure) the disease. Dapsone treatment will require continued monitoring and may be associated with significant side-effects. Dapsone is available in 25 mg and 100 mg tablets. Initial treatment with 50 mg of dapsone by mouth daily usually improves symptoms within 24–48 hours in adults. Correspondingly smaller doses should be used in children. When it is taken daily, dapsone levels reach a steady state within 7 days. Maintenance therapy is then adjusted on a weekly basis to maintain adequate suppression of symptoms; the average maintenance dose is 100 mg daily. Occasional new lesions (2 or 3 per week) are to be expected and are not an indication for altering daily dosage. Minor fluctuations in disease severity do occur and are probably related to oral gluten intake. Application of potent topical corticosteroid gel may be helpful in relieving symptoms of individual lesions. Hemolysis is the most common side-effect of treatment. Dapsone is a strong oxidizer and produces a dose-related oxidant stress on normal aging red blood cells. Initial reduction of hemoglobin by 2–3 gm is common, but subsequent partial compensation by reticulocytosis is the rule. Methemoglobinemia is seldom a severe problem, but it may be tolerated poorly in patients with cardiopulmonary decompensation. Other dose-related side-effects are rare in doses of less than 200 mg daily. These include toxic hepatitis, cholestatic jaundice, psychosis, and both motor and sensory neuropathy. Hypoalbuminemia may occur after chronic use. Carcinogenicity of dapsone has been reported in mice and rats, but has not been documented in humans. Rarely, infectious mononucleosis syndrome with fever and lymphadenopathy occurs.

Treatment with a gluten free diet is successful in greater than 70% of the cases if the diet is adhered to for a minimum of 6–12 months. In such cases, initial suppression of symptoms with dapsone is usually necessary. When gluten restriction allows a decrease in dapsone requirement, the patient can gradually taper the dosage. Complete control of skin disease on a gluten free diet obviates the need for hematologic follow-up. It also serves to treat the cause rather than the symptoms of the disease. Disadvantages of gluten free diet therapy include inconvenience in the diet, which some patients may find unappetizing. It must be stressed that the patient should actively participate in the decision regarding starting a gluten free diet. Individual patients vary in their willingness to take medications or adhere to diets over a prolonged period of time.

After initial baseline information is collected, a CBC should be checked weekly for 6 months and semiannually thereafter.

Chemistry profile should be checked at 6 months and then annually to monitor for possible hepatotoxicity, changes in renal function, and hypoalbuminemia.

Suggested Readings

Ahmed AR, Maize J, Provost TT: Bullous pemphigoid: Clinical and immunologic followup after successful therapy. Arch Dermatol 113:1043, 1977.

Alexander JO: Dermatitis Herpetiformis. London, WB Saunders Co., Ltd., 1975, pp. 1–346.

Anhalt GJ, Labib RS, Voorhees JJ, et al: Induction of pemphigus in neonatal mice by passive transfer of IgG from patients with the disease. N Engl J Med 306:1189–1196, 1982.

Briggaman RA, Gammon WR, Woodley DT: Epidermolysis bullosa acquisita of the immunopathological type (dermolytic pemphigoid). J Invest Dermatol 85:79s–84s, 1985.

Callen JP: Internal disorders associated with bullous diseases of the skin. J Am Acad Dermatol 3:107–119, 1980.

Cunningham MJ, Zone JJ: Thyroid abnormalities in dermatitis herpetiformis. Ann Intern Med 102:194–196, 1985.

Gammon WR, Merritt CC, Lewis DM, et al: Functional evidence for complement-activating immune complexes in the skin of patients with bullous pemphigoid. J Invest Dermatol 78:52, 1982.

Jordon RE, Kawana S, Fritz KA: Immunopathologic mechanisms in pemphigus and bullous pemphigoid. J Invest Dermatol 85:72s–78s, 1985.

Katz SI: The epidermal basement membrane zone—structure, ontogeny, and role in disease. J Am Acad Dermatol 11:1025–1037, 1984.

Leonard JN, Tucker WFG, Fry JS, et al: Increased incidence of malignancy in dermatitis herpetiformis. Br J Med 286:16–18, 1983.

Lever WF: Pemphigus and pemphigoid: A review of the advances made since 1964. J Am Acad Dermatol 1:2, 1979.

Roenigk HH, Ryan JG, Bergfeld WF: Epidermolysis bullosa acquisita. Arch Dermatol 103:1–10, 1971.

Zone JJ, Petersen MJ: Dermatitis herpetiformis. In Thiers BH, Dobson R (eds): Pathogenesis of Skin Disease. New York, Churchill Livingstone, Inc., 1985, pp. 159–183.

Zone JJ, Ward J, Boyce E, et al: Penicillamine-induced pemphigus. J Am Med Assoc 247:2705–2707, 1982.

46

The Hair, Nails, and Mucous Membranes

JOHN J. ZONE

HAIR DISORDERS

In utero, embryonic hair follicles produce fine, soft hair referred to as lanugo hair. This hair is normally shed 2–3 months before birth and is replaced by vellus hair, which is soft, less than 2 cm in length, and unpigmented. Longer, coarse, medullated, pigmented hair that begins growth on the scalp in infancy is termed "terminal hair." At puberty, vellus body hair, under the influence of androgens, converts to terminal hair in certain body sites. This change starts in the pubic region and progresses to involve various parts of the abdomen and eventually involves the axilla. Subsequently, terminal hair may develop on various parts of the trunk and extremities.

Hypertrichosis is defined as growth of hair that is not androgen dependent and is excessive for the site and age of the patient. In contrast, hirsutism is characterized by an excessive growth of terminal hair in women on androgen dependent areas of the body. Hirsutism is discussed in Chapter 25.

Hair loss is termed alopecia and may be divided into 2 groups: non-scarring alopecia and scarring alopecia. Exhaustive discussions of hair loss are the subject of entire textbooks. Discussion here will be limited to the more common abnormalities associated with systemic disease.

Pathogenesis

The activity of the hair follicle is cyclical. Individual hair follicles sequentially demonstrate a growing phase termed "anagen," which lasts from 2 to 6 years; and a resting, or "telogen," phase, which lasts 3–6 months. These are separated by a brief transitional phase termed "catagen." Thus 85% of hairs are in the anagen phase at any given time, 1–2% are in catagen, and the remainder are in the telogen phase. The duration of each phase in a given individual is controlled by a number of factors, including heredity, age, and body location.

The hair shaft is produced by the expanded lower part of the follicle, the hair bulb, which is an epidermal structure with a rich capillary blood supply. Rapidly dividing cells of the matrix surround the hair bulb and produce the column of compact keratin recognized as the hair. Melanocytes in the matrix provide pigment to the hair. At the end of the anagen phase, mitosis slows, the middle region of the hair bulb becomes constricted, and the base of the hair becomes keratinized to form a club. A thin epithelial column beneath the club connects to the dermal papilla. The cells of the dermal papilla eventually come to rest as a cluster of undifferentiated cells immediately beneath the epithelial sac containing the club hair. This hair characterizes telogen and demonstrates the characteristic club morphology of telogen noted in 15% of hairs when hairs are plucked from the scalp. After a varying period of rest, the germinative cells of the epithelial sac increase their metabolic activity; they grow downward, engulfing the dermal papilla, and a new anagen phase begins. Scalp hair has a much longer anagen phase than body hair, accounting for its longer maximum growth length. Chemotherapeutic drugs inhibit mitosis of the rapidly dividing cells of the hair bulb in the anagen phase. As a result, the hair abruptly narrows and eventually falls out.

Normally, hair follicles in humans are asynchronous, resulting in 100 hairs of a total of 100,000 scalp hairs being lost daily, and such normal shedding is barely perceptible. However, in telogen effluvium a disproportionate number of hair follicles enter the telogen phase simultaneously and large numbers of hairs fall out in a short period of time. Hair follicles are presumably "shocked" into telogen phase by a stressful life event such as childbirth, severe disease, or emotional trauma. Two to four months later, the telogen hair is shed as the next anagen phase begins and a dramatic, delayed hair loss takes place. Hair regrowth is evident within 6–12 months.

The rate of hair growth is normally about 0.37 mm per day. Steroid hormones, especially estrogens, increase the duration of telogen, and thyroxine decreases its duration. The rate of growth of body hair (not scalp hair) is decreased by anti-androgens and increased by androgens.

Non-scarring alopecia is usually diffuse and is frequently related to systemic effects on the hair cycle, as in telogen effluvium; or to metabolic effects on the matrix, such as hypothyroidism, nutritional deficiencies, or antimitotic effects of chemotherapeutic drugs. The exact biochemical pathogenesis of diffuse hair loss in conditions such as telogen effluvium and hypothyroidism is unclear.

Scarring alopecia is usually related to localized inflammatory or infiltrative processes of the scalp that actually destroy individual hair follicles. In such disorders, the scalp changes represent cutaneous lesions of systemic diseases rather than generalized metabolic effects. Cutaneous lesions include disorders such as lupus erythematosus, sarcoidosis, metastatic carcinoma, and syphilis.

Table 46–1. NON-SCARRING ALOPECIA IN SYSTEMIC DISEASE

Telogen effluvium
Hypothyroidism and hyperthyroidism
Cushing's syndrome
Cirrhosis
Nutritional deficiency
Rheumatologic inflammatory disorders
Drug-induced

However, it should be remembered that any locally infiltrative disorder may produce scarring alopecia and that the scarring alopecia is not necessarily an indication of systemic disease.

Alopecia

Diffuse Non-scarring Alopecia

Diffuse hair loss that occurs in the absence of inflammation in association with systemic diseases is for the most part non-specific. The patient usually complains of hair "thinning," or falling out, after washing. Extensive loss must occur before it is clinically apparent to the physician. In even extensive cases, a decrease in the number of hairs is still subjective and inflammation is absent. Table 46–1 provides a differential diagnosis of possible causes. Telogen effluvium and hair loss secondary to chemotherapy have been discussed. Diffuse alopecia as well as loss of lateral eyebrows (Queen Anne's sign) is frequent with hypothyroidism whether the thyroid dysfunction is primary or secondary to hypopituitarism. Up to 50% of thyrotoxic patients may also show diffuse, non-specific hair loss. This finding is related to atrophy of the epidermis and its appendages, and histologically only keratin plugs may remain in hair follicles.

Cirrhosis from any cause decreases body hair growth in parallel to the severity of the liver disease. Men with cirrhosis tend to have loss of axillary and pubic hair. This has been assumed to be secondary to hyperestrogenism.

Protein-calorie malnutrition is rare in the United States, although severe diarrhea that occurs after gastrectomy or that is due to ulcerative colitis may produce similar clinical findings. In such situations, the hair becomes dystrophic, the growth rate falls, the hairs become reddish brown, and the percentage of telogen follicles increases. Similarly, malabsorption associated with gluten sensitive enteropathy and pancreatic insufficiency may produce diffuse hair loss. Essential fatty acid deficiency and zinc deficiency produce dryness and redness of the scalp with sparse, brittle hair. The cutaneous effects of these deficiency states are readily reversed with appropriate supplementation.

Diffuse hair loss is present in greater than 50% of the patients with systemic lupus erythematosus and is a reliable enough finding that it was included in the original American Rheumatologic Association criteria for the classification of systemic lupus erythematosus. In acute lupus erythematosus, there is diffuse shedding of dry, fragile hairs that break easily. Short, broken hairs are frequently seen at scalp margins. Dermatomyositis may produce similar hair loss in 15–20% of cases. In Sjögren's syndrome, the hair may be dry, sparse, and brittle, and diffuse alopecia may involve the pubic and axillary hair as well as the scalp.

A wide range of drugs may produce diffuse hair loss. Chemotherapeutic agents inhibit mitoses in the matrix and subsequently lead to narrowing and fracturing of the hair shaft. Common offenders include cyclophosphamide, azathioprine, methotrexate, colchicine, doxorubicin, and prednisone. Both heparin and coumarin cause diffuse alopecia in up to 50% of patients, for uncertain reasons. Other commonly used drugs that cause diffuse alopecia include levodopa, propranolol, cholesterol binding resins, and antimalarial drugs. As a rule, such alopecia lags weeks to months behind the institution of drug therapy.

Scarring Alopecia

Table 46–2 lists systemic disorders in which scarring alopecia may be a prominent finding. The clinical findings in these disorders are described in depth in appropriate chapters of this text. Scarring alopecia is usually sharply demarcated and may be associated with induration and inflammation. Scalp nodules fixed to the dermis with overlying alopecia are especially characteristic of metastatic carcinoma. When such clinical findings are noted, biopsy is essential and will usually readily differentiate these conditions. When chronic scarring supplants

Table 46–2. SCARRING ALOPECIA IN SYSTEMIC DISEASE

Discoid lupus erythematosus
Scleroderma
Cicatricial pemphigoid
Sarcoidosis
Benign and malignant lymphoreticular disorders
Metastatic carcinoma
Infections
    Lupus vulgaris
    Leprosy
    Tertiary syphilis
    Leishmaniasis

inflammation, definitive diagnosis may become impossible.

Patient Evaluation

The initial approach to alopecia is differentiation between diffuse and localized disease. With diffuse hair loss, the loss is distributed evenly over the scalp. This is to be differentiated from androgenetic alopecia, in which there is frequently bitemporal and vertex involvement, and is also to be differentiated from the patchy hair loss seen in secondary syphilis and alopecia areata.

Evaluation of diffuse hair loss should include a "hair pull" if telogen effluvium is suspected. In this maneuver, 5–10 hairs are grasped firmly and pulled from the scalp. This should be repeated in neighboring areas so that 30–40 hairs can be examined. This must necessarily include both hairs that are firmly anchored to the scalp and those that can be easily removed. Normally, one sees 15–20% club hairs, indicating that they are in the telogen phase. Telogen hair roots show a club shape, smooth contours, and a loose sheath. In contrast, anagen hairs will show an intact root sheath that is firm and the root will appear angulated or fractured. It should be remembered that an increased number of telogen hairs may also be seen in early androgenetic alopecia, thyroid disorders, and some nutritional deficiencies.

Hair counts may be helpful in confirming the diagnosis of hair loss and in quantifying its severity. If the patient saves all of the hairs lost while washing or brushing the hair, less than 100 hairs should be lost daily.

The differentiation between scarring and non-scarring alopecia is then made by examination of the scalp. The clinical diagnosis of scarring may be difficult and frequently requires a hand lens and a close search. In scarring alopecia, the scalp is usually thin and atrophic and visible hair follicles are decreased in number or are absent. Virtually all cases of scarring alopecia demand a biopsy. Biopsies should be performed in areas of active inflammation and nodularity if possible. Biopsies from atrophic areas are frequently non-specific.

Treatment

Treatment of diffuse alopecia secondary to the etiologies listed in Table 46–1 is primarily treatment of the underlying disorder. Reassurance for the patient that hair will regrow is important in telogen effluvium. Hair loss associated with thyroid disorders, Cushing's syndrome, and nutritional disorders resolve after several months' correction of the underlying problem.

Scarring alopecia secondary to the causes listed in Table 46–2 frequently results in permanent and sometimes progressive hair loss. Discoid lupus erythematosus, cicatricial pemphigoid, and sarcoidosis usually respond to topical or intralesional corticosteroid therapy with slowing of the scarring process. Antimalarial drugs are effective in halting the progression of lupus erythematosus. Management of alopecia from the neoplastic and infectious etiologies listed in Table 46–2 depends on aggressive treatment of those causes.

Tertiary syphilis may produce scarring scalp nodules. There are also classic findings of secondary syphilis that are characterized by a patchy, non-scarring alopecia with a "moth-eaten" appearance.

Hypertrichosis

Hypertrichosis is defined as excessive growth of hair for the site and age of the patient. This may be localized or generalized, congenital or acquired. (Differential diagnosis is listed in Table 46–3.) Congenital hypertrichosis is seldom associated with internal disease, except in the instance of hypertrichosis over a congenital melanocytic nevus, in which case the lesion may be a precursor for malignant melanoma. In contrast to the usually benign nature of congenital hypertrichosis, acquired hypertrichosis lanuginosa may be a dramatic presentation of an internal malignancy (see Chapter 13). In this disorder, there is rapid growth of fine, poorly pigmented long hair, especially on the face, forehead, nose, and ears. Such hair may be present for weeks to months before

Table 46–3. DIFFERENTIAL DIAGNOSIS OF
HYPERTRICHOSIS

Congenital hypertrichosis
Acquired hypertrichosis lanuginosa
Head injury and encephalitis
Lipoatrophic diabetes
Cornelia de Lange's syndrome
Drug-induced
Porphyria

the underlying carcinoma is diagnosed. The mechanism of hypertrichosis in this and in the following disorders is unknown.

Hypertrichosis has been reported 1–4 months after head injury and rarely after encephalitis. Lipoatrophic diabetes (Lawrence-Seip syndrome) is associated with a progressive increase of non-scalp hair. Clinically, patients have hepatosplenomegaly and insulin resistant diabetes, and they lack subcutaneous adipose tissue. Cornelia de Lange's syndrome includes generalized hypertrichosis, physical and mental retardation, and variable somatic and ocular problems. Systemic therapy with minoxidil or cyclosporin A is regularly associated with impressive generalized hypertrichosis, although the mechanism is poorly understood. Phenytoin, corticosteroids, and streptomycin cause similar findings, less frequently.

Hypertrichosis is a feature of porphyria cutanea tarda, erythropoietic protoporphyria (EPP), erythropoietic porphyria (EP), and variegate porphyria. It occurs predominantly on sun-exposed skin, being most prominent in the area lateral to the eyebrow. It also appears on the forehead, cheeks, and chin and may involve other exposed areas. There have been a number of case reports in which hypertrichosis has occurred irregularly in association with generalized disease. These disorders include anorexia nervosa, dermatomyositis, hypothyroidism, and hyperthyroidism.

Patient Evaluation

In the evaluation of hypertrichosis, it should first be determined whether the disorder is localized or generalized and whether it is congenital or acquired. In localized hypertrichosis, an underlying nevus or a nearby site of inflammation is usually found. Long-term inflammation or rubbing of the skin may result in long, coarse hair. Congenital hypertrichosis is usually not associated with systemic findings and demands no further evaluation. The diagnosis of Cornelia de Lange's syndrome, including physical and mental retardation, is obvious if one is aware of the syndrome. A good history is often sufficient to diagnose head injury, encephalitis, or drug-induced hypertrichosis. Lipoatrophic diabetes is easily diagnosed by the findings of lipoatrophy and glucose intolerance. Patients with porphyria often show subtle hypertrichosis limited to sun-exposed areas, and they may have a history of photosensitivity. Patients with porphyria cutanea tarda and variegate porphyria show elevations of 24-hour urinary porphyrins, whereas individuals with EP and EPP show elevations of red blood cell and stool porphyrins.

Treatment

Treatment of hypertrichosis is for cosmetic rather than medical reasons. Contrary to popular belief, cutting or shaving hair influences neither the rate of growth nor the caliber of the hair shaft. Consequently, localized shaving and depilatories are always a reasonable option. Epilation provides permanent correction in localized areas but is painful and may result in scarring.

NAIL DISORDERS

Nail abnormalities reflect disorders of keratinization and are historical markers of metabolic and vascular events that affect the keratinization process. The visible topography of the nail units used as the basis for clinical descriptions consists of the lateral nail fold, the nail plate, the lunula, the cuticle, and the proximal nail fold (Fig. 46–1). The sagittal section of the nail unit reveals the matrix beneath the proximal nail fold and lunula; the nail bed beneath the nail plate; and the hyponychium, which is

immediately proximal to the distal nail groove (Fig. 46–2). The vast majority of nail abnormalities are due to local factors, including trauma, infection, and chemicals. However, this discussion will focus on the less common systemic associations with specific nail disorders.

Pathogenesis

Cell kinetics and the mechanics of nail growth are central to the understanding and treatment of diseased nails. Disorders that affect those processes will be discussed briefly here.

The nail matrix is the area of mitotically active epithelium that eventually forms the non-desquamating compact keratin of the nail plate. It may be seen clinically as the lunula (Fig. 46–1) or may not be visible. The proximal portions of the matrix contribute keratin to the surface of the nail plate, the mid-portion of the matrix provides keratin to the central nail plate, and the distal portion of the matrix contributes keratin to the ventral nail plate. The nail bed and periungual tissues do not contribute to the formation of the nail plate, although the hyponychium adheres to the nail plate via desquamating epithelium. Consequently, the source of nail plate defects can be localized to specific areas of the matrix. Pitting of the nails, which is common in psoriasis, is believed to be related to psoriatic matrix involvement with resultant parakeratotic columns of nail keratin. Subsequent desquamation of these columns results in clinical pitting. Such pitting, as well as other forms of psoriatic nail dystrophy, are seen in about one third of patients with uncomplicated psoriasis but in up to 80% of psoriatic arthritis patients. However, pitting is not specific for either psoriasis or psoriatic arthritis because numerous dermatitides in the vicinity of the proximal nail fold may cause parakeratotic foci in the matrix and therefore pitting.

The keratinization process produces nail plate at a rate varying between 1.9 and 4.4 mm per month in fingernails. Toenails grow at one third to one half the speed of fingernails. Temporary ineffectual keratinization results in transverse grooves of the nail plate, termed "Beau's lines." Such grooving occurs at the time of general body trauma or meta-

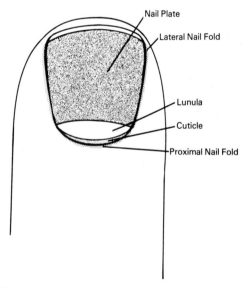

Nail Plate

Lateral Nail Fold

Lunula

Cuticle

Proximal Nail Fold

Figure 46–1. The visible typography of the nail unit.

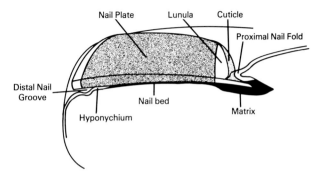

Figure 46–2. Sagittal section of the nail unit.

bolic stress. However, it can also occur from local trauma and from chemotherapeutic agents that interrupt cell division. Measuring the distance from the proximal nail fold to the leading edge of Beau's lines and dividing by an average growth rate of 3 mm per month allow a rough estimate of the time elapsed since the precipitating event.

The hardness of the nail plate is related to its high sulfur content, in the form of cysteine; poor ability to hold water, because of low lipid content of the nail plate; and highly developed junctional structures. It is not a result of calcium content, as is commonly believed. Brittle fingernails result from failure of the adhesive factors. Humid environment enhances softness, and dryness enhances brittleness. Brittleness is frequently caused by a variety of traumatic and chemical exogenous insults, but it may also be related to systemic problems. Inadequate blood supply from arterial insufficiency as well as from Raynaud's phenomenon may produce brittle or longitudinally ridged nails. Iron deficiency leads to relative hypoxia, producing brittle nails. Iron deficiency may also lower the cysteine content of the nails and therefore may make the fibrous proteins of the nail plate less stable. Uncommon systemic causes of brittle fingernails via uncertain mechanisms include tuberculosis, bronchiectasis, hypopituitarism, hyper- and hypothyroidism, diabetes, gout, osteoporosis, sarcoidosis, and amyloidosis. Koilonychia, or "spooning" of the nails, may be an expression of the brittle nature of the nails produced by iron deficiency. However, koilonychia is more frequently familial or idiopathic.

The nail plate is loosely attached to the underlying nail bed by virtue of the keratin-izing cells of the nail bed epidermis. Separation of the nail plate from the nail bed is termed onycholysis.

Onycholysis occurs distally and sometimes laterally and involves the formation of a cleft separating the nail plate from the hyponychium. The accumulation of debris in this cleft then gives the nail an opaque color in this area. Onycholysis is a finding in many systemic diseases, but no common mechanism has been established. Onycholysis frequently occurs in thyroid disease, especially in thyrotoxicosis. However, nonsystemic causes of onycholysis predominate and include fungus, bacteria, trauma, maceration, cosmetics, paronychial cutaneous diseases, and malignancy. The combination of ultraviolet light plus various medications is also known to produce photo-induced onycholysis. Implicated medications include the systemic administration of tetracycline, chloramphenicol, and psoralen.

A variety of insults can affect the color of the nail plate during its formation or during its subsequent journey over the nail bed to the free edge of the nail plate. If pigmentation of the nail plate is due to internal causes, the transverse discoloration of the nail plate follows the shape of the lunula. In contrast, the transverse pigmentation of the nail plate that is due to external factors will usually follow the configuration of the proximal nail fold. Nail pigmentation is commonly induced by many medications. These are well reviewed by Daniel and Scher. Longitudinal pigmented bands may be produced by doxorubicin hydrochloride (Adriamycin), bleomycin, cyclophosphamide, melphalan, fluoride, and antimalarials, but are also common in darkly pigmented people with no evidence of systemic disease. Transverse dark bands may be produced by doxorubicin hydrochloride, cyclophosphamide, daunorubicin, and quinacrine. Other chemotherapeutic agents, including methotrexate and nitrogen mustard, produce diffuse hyperpigmentation of the nail plate on the basis of matrix toxicity. A blue lunula and bluish nail bed is considered a classic finding of argyria, but drug toxicity, including that of doxorubicin hydrochloride and antimalarials, may impart a similar appearance to the nails.

Abnormalities in the nail bed such as pigmented nevi and melanoma will not affect the nail plate itself, unless they involve the matrix. However, such pigmented lesions may produce linear pigmented subungual debris. Increased levels of ACTH or melanocyte-stimulating hormone (MSH) may be responsible for horizontal pigmented bands. Transverse white bands of the nail (leukonychia) are most commonly due to trauma and can usually be differentiated from abnormalities from systemic causes. Systemic causes tend to (1) involve multiple nails; (2) spread across the entire width of the nail; (3) have the contour of the lunula; and (4) correlate with the time of the systemic insult. "Mee's lines" are transverse white striations that appear in the nails after acute arsenic poisoning. They are usually single, broad bands, but they may be multiple. It is now known that many systemic insults may initiate Mee's lines. Mee's lines represent a defect in the nail plate itself.

In contrast, Muehrcke's lines are double lines that represent an abnormality of the vascular bed of the nail. Squeezing of the distal digit will cause the lines to disappear temporarily. They do not indent the nail plates, and the exact pathogenesis has not been explained. They are frequently associated with hypoalbuminemia from a variety of causes, and they disappear when the plasma albumin concentration is above 2.2 gm per dl.

Splinter hemorrhages are formed by the extravasation of blood from the longitudinally oriented vessels of the nail bed. The blood then attaches to the nail plate and moves distally with nail growth. Trauma is the most common cause of splinter hemorrhages. However, septicemia and immune-mediated vasculitis may also be responsible. Findings that make a systemic etiology more likely include proximal location and simultaneous appearance in multiple nails.

Clubbing is characterized by an increase of the angle formed by the proximal end of the nail plate and the proximal nail fold. The normal angle of approximately 160 degrees is increased to 180 degrees or greater. Unilateral clubbing is usually related to vascular lesions such as Pancoast's tumors, erythromelalgia, or lymphadenitis. When a single nail is involved, clubbing is usually traumatic. Bilateral clubbing is due to respiratory abnormalities in approximately 80% of patients. Bronchiectasis and bronchitis make up the majority of the cases, although chronic infections and neoplasms may also be responsible. Congenital heart defects, cirrhosis, chronic diarrhea, and subacute bacterial endocarditis may also be responsible. Seemingly idiopathic cases are frequently hereditary or congenital.

Hypertrophic osteoarthropathy in its complete form includes (1) clubbing; (2) hypertrophy of the extremities with soft tissue proliferation; (3) peripheral neurovascular disease, such as cyanosis, erythema, and hyperhidrosis; (4) bone pain as a result of proliferative periostitis; (5) joint pain and swelling; and (6) muscle weakness. It is associated with malignant tumors of the chest in more than 90% of the cases.

Pachydermoperiostosis is an idiopathic condition that is frequently familial and consists of clubbing in combination with thickening of the legs and forearms that involves both the bones and soft tissue.

Classification

Nail findings are associated with many systemic diseases. The more significant findings not discussed previously are outlined in Table 46–4 and are largely self-explanatory.

Nail abnormalities may be associated with gastrointestinal disease. Terry's nails have an abnormal white appearance, except for a distal pink band that is just proximal to the free end of the nail plate. These nail changes are commonly seen in cirrhosis. Cronkhite-Canada syndrome includes non-familial gastrointestinal polyposis with alopecia, skin pigmentation, and nail abnormalities. The nails are thick, white, and brittle and may take on a triangular shape.

Hyperthyroidism is frequently associated with onycholysis. The nail may show a free edge that is undulated and curves upward.

Table 46–4. NAIL CHANGES ASSOCIATED WITH SPECIFIC ORGAN SYSTEMS

A. Cardiovascular diseases
  1. Aortic insufficiency: Quincke's pulse
  2. Heart failure: reddish lunulae
  3. Vasculitis: splinter hemorrhages and periungual infarcts
  4. Ischemia: non-specific dystrophy
B. Gastrointestinal diseases
  1. Cirrhosis: flat nails, Terry's nails, Muehrcke's lines, Beau's lines
  2. Chronic active hepatitis: clubbing, white nails, splinter hemorrhage
  3. Hemochromatosis: koilonychia, leukonychia, longitudinal striations
  4. Cronkhite-Canada syndrome: thick, white, brittle nails that may take on a triangular shape
  5. Plummer-Vinson syndrome (esophageal web): koilonychia
C. Endocrine disorders
  1. Acromegaly: thick, short, wide, flat nails
  2. Diabetes mellitus: yellowish nails and proximal nail bed telangiectasia
  3. Hypothyroidism: slow growth, longitudinal sulci, brittle nails, onycholysis
  4. Hyperthyroidism: Plummer's nail
D. Pulmonary disease
  1. Clubbing
  2. Yellow nail syndrome
E. Renal disease
  1. Chronic renal failure: half and half nails, Mee's lines, Muehrcke's lines, splinter hemorrhage
  2. Nail-patella syndrome: triangular lunula, ulnar-sided nail dystrophy, discoloration, absent or dystrophic nails
F. Rheumatologic disorders
  1. Reiter's syndrome: similar to psoriasis
  2. Systemic lupus erythematosus and dermatomyositis: periungual telangiectasia and hyperkeratotic cuticles
  3. Scleroderma and Raynaud's phenomenon: periungual telangiectasia, tightening of the skin, distal digital infarcts

The most notable nail finding in pulmonary disease other than clubbing, which was discussed previously, is the yellow nail syndrome (Fig. 46–3). In this disorder, the nails show a greatly slowed rate of growth and swelling of the periungual tissue. The nail plate has a yellowish discoloration, is thickened, and excessively curves from side to side. It has been found in association with tuberculosis, bronchiectasis, bronchitis, and chronic obstructive pulmonary disease. A multitude of other associations have also been described, including lymphoma, melanoma, adenocarcinoma of the endometrium, carcinoma of the larynx, rheumatoid arthritis, and treatment with penicillamine.

Chronic renal failure is strongly associated with the "half and half nail" (Lindsay's nails). In this disorder, the proximal nail has a whitish, ground glass appearance, whereas the distal nail has a brownish discoloration caused by increased melanin. The pathogenesis of this abnormality is poorly understood.

The nail-patella syndrome is an autosomal dominant disorder characterized by absent

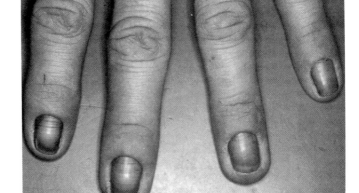

Figure 46–3. Yellow nail syndrome.

or markedly decreased patella, renal abnormalities, and nail findings that include triangular lunula and ulnar-sided nail dystrophy.

Patient Evaluation

Nail findings require close clinical examination. All 20 nails should be examined. In general, fingernails provide better information than toenails because trauma and slow growth more commonly affect toenails. The combination of a good chronologic history of events and knowledge of nail growth may frequently allow for the reaching of significant conclusions. Examination for fungus is essential if onycholysis or subungual debris is present.

Biopsy of the nail bed or matrix is unlikely to be of assistance in the differential diagnosis of the systemic disorders discussed here. However, in the presence of tumor or pigmented lesions, biopsy is essential. Biopsy can be performed either through the nail plate with a sharp, disposable punch or by routine surgical excision following avulsion of the nail. Avulsion is performed after digital block anesthesia using blunt dissection.

Treatment

In most cases, the acquired nail deformities discussed will reverse themselves when the underlying condition is treated. However, slow nail growth produces a 1- to 2-month delay before evidence of change is detectable. The vast majority of nail findings associated with systemic disease provide only minor cosmetic problems and need no treatment. Nail abnormalities secondary to disorders of keratinization, such as psoriasis, may be treated with topical or intralesional corticosteroid therapy to the posterior nail fold. Improvement in the deformity gradually occurs with new nail growth. Excessively keratotic nails may be chemically removed using a preparation of 40% urea, 20% anhydrous lanolin, 5% white wax, and 35% white petrolatum under occlusion.

MUCOUS MEMBRANE DISORDERS

Mucous membrane changes associated with systemic disease are for the most part components of syndromes described elsewhere in the text, and only salient features of the mucosal findings will be discussed here. Oral ulcerations and infiltrative lesions may be unique findings, allowing definite diagnosis, and will be discussed in more detail.

Pathogenesis

Oral ulcers are most commonly idiopathic in the form of aphthous stomatitis, but they may be clinically indistinguishable from ulcerations produced by a variety of systemic diseases. These lesions usually begin as erythematous macules that then become pustular and subsequently ulcerate. Many investigators believe that the pathogenesis of aphthous ulcers is immunologic in origin, but the details are poorly understood.

Classification and Differential Diagnosis of Oral Ulcerations

Mucosal ulceration usually is presented clinically as shallow, erythematous lesions and ulcers that may become purulent. Occasional localized lesions do not demand evaluation, but large, persistent erosions should prompt a search for a cause.

Leukemia may produce oral ulceration as well as cheilitis and is frequently associated with gingivitis and persistent bleeding. Leukopenia, whether secondary to drugs or as a part of a cyclic neutropenia, usually produces severe ulcerations and sloughing of mucous membranes. Up to 25% of patients with systemic lupus erythematosus may have shallow oral ulcers as part of their disease. Atrophic as well as discoid lesions may also occur in the mouth.

Both Crohn's disease and ulcerative colitis may be associated with oral ulcerations beginning as small pustules on the gingival or buccal mucosa. Rarely, such lesions may become proliferative and extensive, at which point they are referred to as "pyostomatitis vegetans." The severity of lesions usually parallels the severity of the underlying bowel disease.

Oral ulcers of Behçet's disease are indistinguishable from aphthous stomatitis and can only be separated when other components of the syndrome are identified, especially genital ulceration, iritis, and pustular skin lesions.

Pemphigus vulgaris and bullous pemphigoid may both be present with oral ulcerations, because vesicles and bullae are quite friable and are easily eroded in the mouth; however, the primary lesion is seldom pustular. Routine histopathology may be difficult to obtain, and direct immunofluorescence of perilesional tissue is frequently diagnostic. Oral pemphigoid is sometimes referred to as benign mucous membrane pemphigoid, but it is neither benign nor limited to the mucosa, since it may cause blindness and involve the skin. The term cicatricial pemphigoid is therefore preferred.

Erythema multiforme, or Stevens-Johnson syndrome, may be limited to the mouth. Definitive diagnosis is best made by demonstrating the classic histologic findings. Making such a diagnosis may allow for effective treatment by pointing to an etiologic medication or underlying herpetic infection.

Miscellaneous Disorders of the Oral Cavity

Miscellaneous conditions that affect the oral cavity and that are described elsewhere bear brief mention. The new onset of multiple pigmented macules on the lips, tongue, and buccal mucosa over weeks to months is a characteristic finding of Addison's disease and should prompt detailed evaluation for other laboratory and clinical findings of that disorder. Peutz-Jeghers syndrome is also characterized by hyperpigmented mucosal macules; however, such pigmentation usually arises over several years, is hereditary, and is associated with intestinal polyposis.

Gingival hypertrophy is frequently associated with phenytoin therapy for seizure disorders. However, sudden onset of this finding should prompt biopsy and search for blood dyscrasias.

Cirrhosis may be responsible for sublingual varicosities with the development of collateral circulation in the setting of portal hypertension.

Diabetes may be associated with severe gingivitis, periodontal abscesses, and cheilitis. Such findings are usually due to secondary bacterial or yeast infection and may improve significantly with improved oral hygiene.

Infiltrative Lesions. Firm infiltrative lesions of scleroderma may occur in mucosal stroma as elsewhere, but the disease is rarely limited to the mucosal surfaces. Macroglossia may occur in hypothyroidism, but it is a classic finding in primary amyloidosis. Gradual enlargement of the tongue with the development of waxy nodules and areas of hemorrhage is a classic finding in amyloidosis. Infiltrative tumors of local origin provide the main differential diagnosis for these systemic infiltrative disorders.

Glossodynia. A painful, burning sensation of the tongue may be associated with iron or vitamin B_{12} deficiency. In both instances, atrophy and loss of papillae are seen. Other causes of glossodynia include diabetes, zinc deficiency, and hypoestrogenism. Unfortunately, many cases defy an etiologic diagnosis.

Patient Evaluation

Examination of mucous membranes must be carried out in a systematic fashion with good lighting. Sequential examination should be performed of both the dry and mucous surfaces of the lips, the buccal mucosa, the hard and soft palate, and the mucosal buccal folds. Individual lesions as well as cervical and submandibular lymph nodes should then be palpated. If lesions are present on the oral mucosa, other mucosal surfaces, such as nasal, conjunctival, and genital mucosa, should be closely examined.

Persistent lesions warrant biopsy for routine histopathology. Nodules should be biopsied in their thickest and most indurated area. Ulcers and erosions should be biopsied at the edge of the lesion. Specimens for direct immunofluorescence microscopy should not be taken from lesional tissue, but from adjacent, clinically normal tissue, since immunoreactants are frequently destroyed by inflammatory infiltrates.

Treatment

The oral ulcerative disorders related to systemic disease are best treated by treatment of the underlying disorder. However, the oral ulcerations associated with inflammatory bowel disease may persist after definitive therapy of the bowel problem. Local corticosteroid therapy may be helpful in the form of potent topical corticosteroids, corticosteroid sprays usually used for pulmonary problems, or intralesional triamcinolone acetonide. Viscous lidocaine or diphenhydramine suspensions will produce local analgesia and/or anesthesia and will decrease discomfort.

Suggested Readings

Daniel CR III, Sams WM Jr, Scher RK: Nails in systemic disease. Derm Clin 3:465–483, 1985.

Daniel CR, Scher RK: Nail changes secondary to systemic drugs or ingestants. J Am Acad Dermatol 10:250–258, 1984.

Kechijian P: Onycholysis of the fingernails: Evaluations and management. J Am Acad Dermatol 12:552–560, 1985.

Norton LA: Nail disorders. J Am Acad Dermatol 2:451–467, 1980.

Rogers RS: Recent advances in erosive, ulcerative, and bullous diseases of the oral mucosa, Part I. Prog Dermatol 12:1–4, 1978.

Rogers RS: Recent advances in erosive, ulcerative, and bullous diseases of the oral mucosa, Part II. Prog Dermatol 12:5–10, 1978.

Rook A, Dawber R: Diseases of the Hair and Scalp. Oxford, England, Blackwell Scientific Publications, 1982.

Shklar G, McCarthy PL: The Oral Manifestations of Systemic Disease. Boston, Butterworth Publishers, Inc., 1976.

Drug Reactions

JEFFREY P. CALLEN

A drug reaction is defined as any and all unwanted effects related to the administration of a drug. In today's environment of "polypharmacy," drug reactions may take on a new meaning because physicians not only must treat single drug reactions but also must take into consideration drug-drug interactions that can result in untoward ef-

Table 1. PATTERNS OF CUTANEOUS ADVERSE DRUG REACTIONS AND
MOST COMMON ETIOLOGIC AGENTS

Acneiform Lesions Androgens Corticosteroids Halogenated compounds Lithium Tar containing preparations	**Lichenoid Eruptions** (Figs. 2 and 3) Gold salts Antimalarials Propranolol and related compounds Phenytoin Phenothiazines
Alopecia Cytotoxic drugs (cyclophosphamide, methotrexate, etc.) Anticoagulants Vitamin A derivatives	**Photosensitivity Reactions** Tetracyclines Thiazides Phenothiazines Sulfonamides Sulfonylureas NSAID Nalidixic acid Para-aminobenzoic acid
Eczematous Eruptions Antibiotics Diuretics Hypoglycemics	
Erythema Multiforme Antibiotics (sulfonamides and penicillins) Phenytoin Barbiturates	**Purpura** *Thrombocytopenic* Thiazides NSAID Phenothiazines Quinidine and related compounds
Erythema Nodosum Oral contraceptives Halogenated compounds Antibiotics Sulfonylureas Sulfonamides Thiazide derivatives	*Vasculitis* Antibiotics Thiazides and similar compounds Phenytoin Thiouracils
Exfoliative Dermatitis Pyrazolon derivatives Phenytoin Lithium Gold salts	**Toxic Epidermal Necrolysis** Allopurinol Barbiturates Phenytoin Hypoglycemics
Fixed Drug Eruptions (Fig. 1) Phenolphthalein Tetracycline Barbiturates Non-steroidal anti-inflammatory drugs (NSAID)	

Table 2. DRUGS UNLIKELY TO CAUSE AN ADVERSE GENERALIZED CUTANEOUS DRUG REACTION

Digitalis	Aminophylline
Antacids	Diazepam
Acetaminophen	Insulin
Spironolactone	Multivitamins
Nitroglycerin	

Table 3. DRUGS CAUSING MOST FREQUENT CUTANEOUS DRUG REACTIONS

Amoxicillin	Allopurinol
Trimethoprim-sulfamethoxazole	Cephalosporins
	Quinidine
Ampicillin	Blood or blood products
Other penicillins	Diuretics

Table 4. SYSTEMIC REACTIONS TO TOPICALLY APPLIED DRUGS

Drug	Reaction
Corticosteroids	Adrenocortical suppression Iatrogenic Cushing's syndrome
Phenol	Dizziness, vascular collapse
Podophyllin	Coma, fetal toxicity
Lindane	?Neurotoxicity
Nitrogen mustard	Pancytopenia

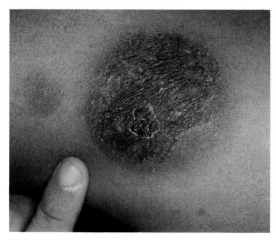

App. Fig. 1. Violaceous plaque of a fixed drug reaction as a result of therapy with thioridazine hydrochloride (Mellaril) (see also Plate VIIIA).

fects. It has been estimated that between 18 and 30% of hospitalized patients have a drug reaction, and of the patients hospitalized about 5% are hospitalized because of a drug reaction.

Certain measures can be used in an attempt to prevent drug reactions. The physician should attempt to limit the number of drugs given to a patient. Also, a therapeutic end-point should be defined, at which time the drug should be discontinued. The physician must be aware of the chemical and pharmacologic characteristics of a drug in order to predict and prevent drug interactions or predictable reactions. The physician must also consider the effects of the patient's disease on the potential for a drug interaction; for example, if the renal function is impaired, certain drugs cleared by the kidney, such as methotrexate, will be more toxic.

In Tables 1 to 3, *some* of the potential drug reactions are listed that are important because of their occurrence on the skin (App. Figs. 1, 2, and 3; Plate VIIIA). Included in Tables 4 and 5 are agents used to treat skin disease that have important systemic consequences. In each case the list is not exhaustive, but those agents that are the most common ones involved in the reaction are presented.

Table 5. REACTIONS TO DRUGS COMMONLY USED IN DERMATOLOGICAL PRACTICES

Drug	Adverse Reaction
Acne therapy	
Antibiotics	Candidosis
	Photosensitivity
	Colitis
Isotretinoin	Hypertriglyceridemia
	Pseudotumor cerebri
	Teratogenicity
	Hyperostosis
Corticosteroids	Iatrogenic Cushing's syndrome
Methotrexate	Cytopenias
	Hypersensitivity pneumonitis
	?Hepatotoxicity
Antimalarials	Ocular toxicity
	Myopathy, cardiomyopathy
Dapsone	Hepatotoxicity
	Methemoglobinemia
	Hemolytic anemia
Ketoconazole	Hepatotoxicity
	Adrenal suppression
Griseofulvin	?Hepatotoxicity
	Phototoxicity

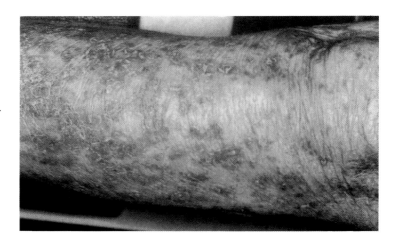

App. Fig. 2. Lichen planus–like eruption caused by captopril.

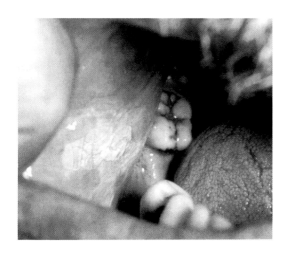

App. Fig. 3. Lichen planus on the buccal mucosa in a patient treated with gold.

Regional Approach to Diagnosis

JOSEPH L. JORIZZO

Certain dermatoses discussed in this book are listed in the following table by body region most typically affected. The lists of diseases that typically affect a given location cannot be used as a complete differential diagnosis for each region because dermatoses that are not associated with systemic signs and symptoms are not included.

Table 1. DERMATOSES WITH SYSTEMIC IMPLICATIONS: A REGIONAL APPROACH

Generalized	Scalp	Face	Oral Cavity	Intertriginous	Genital	Acral
Exfoliative erythroderma	Alopecia	Acne	Lichen planus	Candidiasis	Psoriasis	Reiter's syndrome
Urticaria	Scarring alopecia (e.g., discoid lupus erythematosus)	Photoallergic reactions	Reiter's syndrome	Acrochordons (Skin tags)	Lichen planus	Erythema multiforme
Erythema	Non-scarring alopecia	Phototoxic reactions	Behçet's disease	Acanthosis nigricans	Reiter's syndrome	Vasculitis
Drug	Patterned (e.g., alopecia areata, secondary syphilis, androgenic alopecia)	Lupus erythematosus	Angioedema	Glucagonoma syndrome	Behçet's disease	Pigmented purpuric eruption (i.e., capillaritis)
Viral		Dermatomyositis	Stevens-Johnson syndrome		Stevens-Johnson syndrome	
Erythema multiforme		Scleroderma (e.g., en coup de sabre)	Toxic epidermal necrolysis		Fixed drug eruption	Scleroderma (CREST syndrome)
Pemphigus vulgaris		Herpes simplex	Pemphigus vulgaris		Syphilis	
Bullous pemphigoid	Diffuse (e.g., telogen effluvium, thyroid disease)	Herpes zoster	Bullous pemphigoid		Gonorrhea	Secondary syphilis
Cutaneous T cell lymphoma		Impetigo	Lupus erythematosus		Chancroid	Porphyria cutanea tarda
Neurofibromatosis		Erysipelas	Syphilis		Granuloma inguinale	Kaposi's sarcoma
		Tuberculosis	Herpes simplex		Lymphogranuloma venereum	
	Psoriasis	Leprosy	Viral enanthem		Herpes simplex	
	Scleroderma (e.g., en coup de sabre)	Sarcoidosis	Candidiasis		Candidiasis	
	Herpes zoster	Amyloidosis	Amyloidosis		Extramammary Paget's disease	
	Folliculitis	Xanthelasma				
	Angiosarcoma					

Index

Page numbers in *italics* refer to illustrations;
page numbers followed by t indicate tables.